CANCER CURED

VICTORY OVER THE WAR ON CANCER

MARK SLOAN

ENDALLDISEASE
PUBLISHING

CANCER CURED
Copyright © 2019 by Mark D. Sloan

Library and Archives Canada Cataloguing in Publication

Sloan, Mark, 1985-, author
    Cancer cured : victory over the war on cancer / Mark Sloan.
Issued in print and electronic formats.
ISBN 978-0-9947418-3-7 (hardcover).--ISBN 978-0-9947418-0-6 (softcover)
ISBN 978-0-9947418-2-0 (Kindle).--ISBN 978-0-9947418-1-3 (PDF)
    1. Cancer. 2. Cancer--Treatment. I. Title.
RC261.S66 2017   616.99'4   C2017-901124-3
                                                        C2017-901125-1

Dedicated to my mother

Contents

BOOK I: THE CANCER INDUSTRY

1. SURGERY 1

2. CHEMOTHERAPY 21

3. RADIOTHERAPY 37

BOOK II: CANCER - THE METABOLIC DISEASE

6. TARGETING THE TUMOR MICROENVIRONMENT 105

7. ORANGES 121

8. COCONUT OIL 161

ACKNOWLEDGEMENTS

Although the research and writing that went into this book amounted to a few thousand hours of my time and many hardships, in no way would it have been possible without the life's work of Dr. Raymond Peat. For a life devoted to courageously exploring the unknown in search of empirical truth, and for preserving, consolidating and advancing the quintessential observations reported by a number of maverick scientists over the past 150 years and then freely sharing your interpretations with the world - it's time that your work be known and understood by all. Your guidance and generosity in responding to the many questions I had during the writing process of this book have been instrumental.

Last but not least, I'd like to thank my father for putting up with me all these years - and also for handing down the work ethic, discipline and fortitude that was needed to complete this work.

MY STORY

MY ENTRANCE INTO this world came on mother's day in the spring of 1985 – and it came in epic fashion. With my mother's umbilical cord wrapped tightly around my neck, nurses and doctors scrambled to free me from my umbilical neuse before it was too late. I can only imagine how my parents must have felt as they watched the doctor yank me from the womb and race to uncoil the cord from my neck. Fortunately, the efforts of the medical personnel paid off and my mother and father had a brand new son.

Growing up in Ontario, Canada with my parents and sister was not unlike that of your typical two-child family, but we were unique in some ways. One of the things that separated us from the herd was that my father ran his own business, which he started from scratch after finding out he and my mother had their first baby on the way. He knew the job he had couldn't provide the life he wanted for his family, so he risked everything and made it happen. While working day and night trying to build a successful business, my mother spent her time cooking, cleaning and taking care of my sister and I at home.

I had a great set of friends. I remember playing street hockey with them like it was yesterday. After putting down the sticks we would play tag, swim, light fires and most days you could find me riding my 3-wheel 'big wheelie' bike. In winter, we would carve tunnels into the mountain of snow piled high at the top of our street and *whiz* snowballs at each other. Aside from having to wake up early to attend school and the uncomfortable reality that success in school seemed to be about mindlessly repeating what we were told, things were going well. But as we all learn eventually, life is fragile, and things can change in an instant.

On a cold morning in grade 7, my father sat my sister and I down on the couch in the living room and told us he had an announcement to make. Although I was hoping to hear about an upcoming family vacation somewhere warm, I knew by his expression that the news was not going to be good.

He told us our mother had cancer.

The cancer was on her cervix and only about the size of a baby fingernail; and although I didn't know much about cancer at the time, hearing that doctors had detected it early and were going to rush her in for surgery and radiation made me feel hopeful.

Then our father told us it was too much for him to run a business and be a father and a mother to us at the same time, so he was flying in our aunt Kim from Alberta to help out for a number of months while mom recovered. My sister and I were both big fans of our aunt Kim and uncle Bob from out west, so we felt like we had just won the lottery.

Following surgery and radiation treatments, doctors assured us they 'got it all' and that my mother was cancer-free. My father wanted to make sure the cancer wasn't going to return so he took her to the best naturopathic doctor he knew, who put her on a number of dietary supplements. My father also did some research of his own and discovered Essiac - the famous 4-herb tea blend that nurse Renee Caisse of Bracebridge, Ontario had used to allegedly cure cancer patients for about 50 years until her death in 1978. He ordered the herbs and brewed them carefully following the instructions and administered it to my mother a number of times.

Unfortunately, after my mother's surgical and radiation therapy treatments, cutbacks at the hospital prevented us from having further testing done to assess her health. Eight months later, when we were finally able to have doctors run some follow-up tests, they encountered an aggressive cancer in her hip area: doctor's recommended chemotherapy and more radiation. Feeling afraid and out of options, we rushed her in for treatment once again.

The dramatic decline of her health following chemotherapy and radiotherapy treatments was obvious. I remember lying in bed late at night at the age of 11, hearing her pace back and forth in the living room below, struggling not to cry so we could sleep undisturbed. I don't think she knew it at the time but I could hear every sob, every whimper and every call out to God to put an end to her suffering.

Why was my mother in pain? I thought we had some of the best doctors in the country using the best treatments available to heal her, yet everything the doctors had done just seemed to make things worse. I felt angry and confused.

After a few long and difficult months, I woke up one morning to a scene in my living room that I will never forget: with tears rolling down his cheeks, my father sat my sister and I down on the couch next to aunt Kim and told us our mother was gone. I felt shocked and overwhelmed. I remember holding my breath to try and avoid feeling the intense emotions welling up inside me.

Dad spoke about the scene in the hospital earlier that morning right before our mother had died. Together with her mother and father, her five brothers and sisters and a priest from our local church, they formed a circle around her hospital bed and prayed. Aunt Kim told us the presence she felt in the room during those last moments was unlike anything she had experienced before. Dad agreed. The very last thing my mother did while laying on her hospital bed, he added, just seconds before exhaling her final breath and being received by God, was lift her arms straight up towards the heavens above.

Losing my mother was like losing my biggest fan; it was the ultimate setback in my development growing up, and it happened at the worst possible time - right before starting high school. What's worse, every time I was around people I felt like my emotions needed to be kept secret; like I needed to pretend that I was okay, and that if anybody ever truly understood how I felt, they wouldn't want to be around me because it would be too uncomfortable for them.

My family and I tried counseling, but I knew the therapist was only there because he was getting paid, so it ended up making me feel even angrier. I needed my mother - not some imposter pretending to care. My bottled up emotions had no place to go, so inside they remained. I accepted an award for *diligence and determination* at grade 8 graduation and moved on to highschool.

At highschool, I spent most of my time in the weight room; every lunch, every break, and sometimes I would even skip class to workout. I loved it in there! I felt like once again I had a group of friends I could trust; friends who shared a similar interest in fitness and were striving to become something better. Strength training provided me with the opportunity to continually challenge myself and break through my own limitations. It was in the gym where I first discovered that although there were plenty of guys who were bigger than me, none of them could outwork me. I remember in grade 11, weighing just 160lbs, my record shoulder press was 110lbs in each hand for 8 reps.

But far more than any muscle or strength I happened to gain, the weight room was the first place I had known where it was both safe and beneficial for me to express my anger. Finally I had found a way to channel the throbbing stockpile of emotions inside me into something useful; something that would benefit me and perhaps inspire others.

After graduating high school, I went on to college and earned a diploma in Fire Sciences. Along the way I learned a few things: First, very little of what was taught in the course was actually useful for preparing me to work as a firefighter. Somehow going into a 100% concrete structure with fire gear on and spraying water onto a steel crate of burning wood doesn't quite capture the reality of a fire scene. Secondly, even though I had the fastest time running up and down stairs with a hose on my back during tryouts for the *Firefighter Combat Challenge*, I learned that firefighting is a political man's game - and since I don't play games, someone slower got the spot on the team instead. Last but not least, the most valuable lessons in college are learned outside of class. In my final year, one of my roommates showed me a documentary that made me question my entire reality and the world around me. I wasn't sure if the information was true or not, but I knew I had to find out.

From an early age I had been drawn towards books on self-help and nutrition. I loved the fact that I could read about different theories and then test them myself to see what worked and what didn't. Constant and never-ending improvement was the path I was on from the beginning and I never had any doubt that I could change the world or accomplish whatever I wanted to in life.

With the age of the internet in full swing, suddenly I found myself on a quest for truth; broadening my horizons and obsessively exploring all avenues of research I could find - in books, articles and documentaries - for 8, 10, sometimes 12 hours or more per day. I also spent a lot of time integrating this newfound knowledge into my own articles and documentaries, then sharing my work with whoever was interested through my website and the power of social media. Almost 10 years after my search for truth began - it hit me.

I realized that my mother's death was not a tragedy, but an opportunity. She gave me a story to tell that could move people and a mind that could find the answers the world was literally dying to know; I realized that my mother died so my life could have purpose.

In return for this gift, I made a promise to her in my heart that I would find the cause and cure for cancer so that no child would have to go through what my sister and I did, ever again. I knew that once I found the answers and shared them with the world, the legacy of my mother would transform from a victim of cancer to a hero who inspired her son to save lives and change the world.

INTRODUCTION

IT'S BEEN NEARLY 50 years since the *War on Cancer* was declared, and yet more people are diagnosed with cancer and dying from the disease than ever before.[1]

I find it extraordinarily difficult to believe that after spending $500 billion dollars on cancer research since 1970,[2] the cancer establishment has come up with literally nothing useful for preventing or curing the disease. If it's true, then they are incompetent and their astonishing lack of advancement is undoubtedly the most spectacular failure in human history. But if cures or effective treatments have been systematically suppressed from the public, then their actions are criminal in nature and blood from over 530 million people[3] could be on their hands. Whatever the case may be, I intend to make it clear.

Up until this point on humankind's pursuit to end cancer, our primary mistake has been entrusting the same people who profit from treating cancer to provide us with a cure. I haven't spoken to anyone who didn't understand this concept - there is no money in a cure. Why would an industry that generates over $125 billion dollars a year[4] put itself out of business? It wouldn't.

So who then do we look to for answers?

In 1947, the young American physicist Ernest Sternglass wrote a letter to Albert Einstein telling him about the work he had been doing to reduce radiation doses during X-ray fluoroscopy. To his surprise, Einstein showed great interest in his work and invited the 23-year-old to meet with him at Princeton University, where they talked for 5 hours. "And that had an enormous effect on my life. Because among other things, he encouraged me to pursue my theory and I finally got it all published," recalls Sternglass.[5]

At the end of their conversation, Einstein issued a very important warning: "Don't go back into academia," he said. "They will kill every bit of originality out of you. In order to become a full professor, you have to get approved on every level and you cannot question the existing ideas too much or else you won't get promoted... have a shoemaker's job for the rest of your life, so that you can do something useful for humanity."

My purpose in writing this book is to explore the possibility that, hidden among the enormous amounts of information drifting through the vast reaches of cyberspace, a cure for cancer has already been found. And while a doctor might fear losing his medical license or job for completing such work, a layperson with no medical background like myself can fearlessly make a controversial conclusion when the evidence warrants one. This pure and unobstructed curiosity combined with discipline and an intention to simplify complex information will render a final product on the cutting edge of science that can be understood by those who need it.

FOR THE TIME IS AT HAND

The American Cancer Society estimates that almost half of everybody alive today will develop cancer at some point in their lives,[6] and the World Health Organization predicts a 50% rise in cancer diagnosis' by the year 2020.[7]

Unless we figure out what is fuelling this explosion of cancer rates and alter our course, a time will soon come when nobody escapes the ravages of this disease. The future of human civilization is at stake and only one thing is certain - if the answers are out there, they will be found.

REFERENCES

1. The American Cancer Society. (2017). All Cancer Facts & Figures. Available: https://www.cancer.org/research/cancer-facts-statistics/all-cancer-facts-figures.html. [January 31, 2017].

2. Lizzie Parry. (2014). 'The war on cancer may NEVER be won': Cure 'could be impossible' because the disease is so highly evolved. Mail Online. Available: http://www.dailymail.co.uk/health/article-2731765/The-war-cancer-NEVER-won-Cure-impossible-disease-highly-evolved.html. [January 31, 2017].

3. Kelsey Campbell-Dollaghan. (2013). Infographic: How People Died In The 20th Century. Available: https://www.fastcodesign.com/1672161/infographic-how-people-died-in-the-20th-century. [January 31, 2017].

4. Mariotto AB, Yabroff KR, Shao Y, Feuer EJ, Brown ML. Projections of the cost of cancer care in the United States: 2010-2020. J Natl Cancer Inst. 2011;103(2):117-28.

5. GLOBAL NUCLEAR COVER UP: Ernest Sternglass. Berkeley, 2006. r3VOLt23. YouTube. Available: https://www.youtube.com/watch?v=CLw2ISdx9eo. [January 31, 2017].

6. The American Cancer Society medical and editorial content team. (2016). Lifetime Risk of Developing or Dying from Cancer. Available: http://www.cancer.org/cancer/cancerbasics/lifetime-probability-of-developing-or-dying-from-cancer. [January 31, 2017].

7. World Health Organization. Global cancer rates could increase by 50% to 15 million by 2020. Available: http://www.who.int/mediacentre/news/releases/2003/pr27/en.[January 31, 2017].

BOOK 1

THE CANCER INDUSTRY

CHAPTER 1

SURGERY

A SURGEON'S FIRST instinct when he sees a patient with a tumor is to reach for his scalpel and carve it out of them. This makes it easy to assume patients are benefitting from the treatment, but removal of a tumor isn't simply a local phenomenon with no other biological consequences.

Although surgical removal of a tumor is widely accepted today as beneficial and necessary, it was not long ago that the prevailing public attitude towards tumor resection (and other cancer treatments used today) was so disapproving and hostile that it can be difficult for people to imagine. "It should be forbidden and severely punished to remove cancer by cutting, burning, cautery and other fiendish tortures," wrote 15th century renaissance physician Paracelsus.

Whether you've been cut by a criminal in the street because you refused to give him your wallet, or by a surgeon on an operating table because you gave him your wallet, the act of cutting into the body is traumatic and inflicts damage.

In this chapter we will investigate the impact of surgery on health and determine if tumor removal is beneficial for a person with cancer.

MILLIONS OF POINTLESS OPERATIONS EVERY YEAR

Common sense tells us that if a surgical procedure isn't needed then it shouldn't be performed. Nevertheless, some studies estimate that as many as 30% of certain surgeries are performed unnecessarily,[1] and some claim the numbers are actually much, much higher.

A 1995 report by Milliman & Robertson, Inc. concluded that nearly 60 percent of all surgeries performed are medically unnecessary,[2] but even that number is considered low by the late American pediatrician Dr. Robert Mendelsohn who wrote, "My feeling is that somewhere around ninety percent of surgery is a waste of time, energy, money, and life."[3]

Research on unnecessary surgery began in 1974, after a US congressional report estimated that 2.4 million unnecessary surgeries were performed every year, killing nearly 12,000 patients.[4] This report caught the eye of Harvard professor and former surgeon Lucian Leape, who has been following this line of research ever since.

Leape's take today? "Things haven't changed very much."[5]

A 2016 review of the latest research on unnecessary surgery states, "Worldwide every year millions of patients go under knife, but many of them are enduring great pain and shelling out thousands and dollars for surgeries they don't really need."[6]

Not only are many people put 'under the knife' needlessly, but Australia's top surgeon Dr. Ian Harris says that many commonly-performed operations of today "are no better than placebo."[7] In his new book *Surgery, The Ultimate Placebo*, Dr. Harris lists a number of "placebo surgeries," including spinal fusion for back pain, knee arthroscopy, coronary stenting, some shoulder surgery and appendix removal, laparoscopy for bowel adhesions and repairs of ruptured tendons and some fractures.

2

CORONARY ARTERY BYPASS SURGERY

One of the most common and expensive surgeries performed in America today is the coronary artery bypass - a procedure that grafts a new vein in place of a damaged one supplying the heart. According to Dr. Mark Hyman and Dr. Mark Liponis in their book *Ultraprevention*, "Bypasses are the single most commonly performed unnecessary surgery in the country." I reviewed the scientific literature to find out if there was any support for this claim, and the evidence seems to agree.[8-10]

A Closer Look...

- The first ever clinical trial on coronary artery bypass surgery was published in *The Lancet* in 1977 and compared heart disease patients who underwent bypass surgery with ones who received drug treatment only. Results showed that survival at four years was 3% lower in those who underwent surgery.[8]
- In the Coronary Artery Bypass Study of 1984, 780 heart disease patients were randomly assigned either surgical or drug treatments and evaluated 5-years later. "The five-year probability of remaining alive and free of infarction [heart attack] was 82 per cent in the patients assigned to medical therapy and 83 per cent in the patients assigned to surgery (not significant)."[9]
- A 1999 study from the journal *Circulation* compared the effectiveness of coronary angioplasty, coronary artery bypass surgery and drug treatment on heart disease patients. After a 5-year follow-up, researchers found that all three treatments "yielded a similar incidence of acute myocardial infarction and death."[10]

Despite clear evidence showing that cardiac bypass surgery provides no benefit to patients, more than 200,000 procedures are performed every year in the United States.[11] A 2016 study published in *The American Journal of Cardiology* asked 101 US hospitals what they charge for coronary artery bypass surgery, and of the 53 hospitals that responded, the average cost for the procedure was $151,271, ranging from $44,824 to $448,038. Buyer beware: the study found "no evidence to suggest that hospitals that charge higher prices provide better quality of care."[12]

As it turns out, cracking open people's chests and dicing up their arteries remains a treasured source of income for surgeons, while patients end up broke and no healthier than they were before the procedure. And considering coronary artery bypass surgery comes with serious potential complications like impotence,[13] brain damage, organ dysfunction,[14] or even death, the evidence suggests far more harm is being done than good.

Now, how about cancer surgery?

SURGERY VS. CANCER

The most comprehensive study ever undertaken on the efficacy of cancer surgery, to date, was conducted in 1844 by Dr. Leroy d'Etoilles of Paris, France and published in *The French Academy of Science*. After studying 2,781 cancer patients over a 30-year period who had undergone either surgery, caustics (application of a chemical that destroys tissue) or no treatment at all, Dr. d'Etoilles found that the average survival of patients following surgery was one year and five months. Remarkably, two years after cancer diagnosis, those who refused both surgery and caustics had a 50% higher rate of survival.[15]

Recent research has validated Dr. d'Etoilles pioneering work, showing that cutting out a tumor either provides no benefit to patients,[16,18] or increases mortality.[17,143,144] The more the body is cut, the worse the outcome appears to be.

CANCER SURGERY PROMOTES METASTASIS

Cancer metastasis is the primary cause of most cancer deaths,[20-22] and yet the public remains almost completely unaware that surgical removal of a tumor has been known to cause cancer metastasis for over 100 years.

In 1910, researchers implanted tumors into mice and found when they left the tumors alone, cancer metastasis almost never occurred. But when they incompletely cut out the tumors, metastasis frequently occurred.[23] A few years later a similar experiment was conducted using highly metastasizing tumors, and the results were the same - tumor resection increased cancer metastasis compared to control mice whose tumors were left untouched.[24]

This same phenomenon was demonstrated in humans by Dr. Warren Cole of the University of Illinois in 1974. In a series of experiments published in the *Annals of the New York Academy of Sciences,* Dr. Cole wrote, "Ten of our patients underwent an unsuccessful attempt by a surgeon to remove the tumor. All surgeons know that this procedure is usually followed by an increased growth of the tumor...metastasis develops so commonly after excision of the primary."[25]

German professor of Radiology Dr. Ernst H. Krokowski provided further evidence that surgery, and even tumor palpation and biopsy promote the spread of cancer. In a 1979 study, Dr. Krokowski wrote, "... manipulation of the tumor, such as severe palpation, biopsy or surgery, results in a sudden increase of the number of tumor cells released into the blood circulation." Dr. Krokowski also stated that about 90% of patients die from metastasis or secondary tumors and "Therefore it should be of great concern to therapists as well as patients that already more than 30 years ago it was conclusively shown that cancer surgery is the main cause of metastasis. However, this research was completely ignored by the profession, it was just too awful to contemplate, and patients never got to know about it."[26]

Since 1996, Dr. Michael Retsky of Harvard University and his international team of colleagues have been investigating the physiological mechanisms behind surgically-induced cancer metastasis. In a 2010 review of their work, they stated that tumors aren't in continuous growth as it was once thought. Instead, they undergo periods of dormancy, where they are sitting harmlessly and "surgery to remove the primary tumor often terminates dormancy resulting in accelerated relapses."[27]

Studies worldwide have demonstrated consistently and repeatedly that surgical removal of a tumor often terminates dormancy and leads to cancer metastasis.[28-34] Furthermore, surgical removal of lymph nodes (lymphadenectomy), which is standard practice following tumor removal for breast and skin cancer, was found in 2015 to increase "the growth of the primary tumor and associated blood vessels as well as promoted cancer cell survival and dissemination."[19]

5

Even the former director of the National Cancer Institute Vincent J. Davita Jr. wrote about surgically-induced cancer metastasis in the world's definitive, standard-setting oncology textbook *Cancer: Principles and Practise of Oncology* in 1982. "There seems to be little doubt that cancer can be spread from the primary site to distant tissues. There are numerous ways that surgical manipulation could be responsible for this."

THE STRESS OF SURGERY

Few people but surgeons are aware that the stress induced by surgery can result in serious, potentially fatal complications. Like all forms of stress, surgery activates the sympathetic 'flight or fight' nervous system,[35] which elevates stress hormones to liberate glucose from the liver and breakdown fat and muscle as additional energy sources to meet the demands of the upcoming fight.[36]

Even when a surgeon performs an operation successfully with no errors, the stress caused by being cut in one area of the body can lead to damage in another. Complications of surgical stress include, but are not limited to:

Blood Health:

- Surgical stress causes a loss of blood albumin[37]

Bone Health:

- Surgical stress causes bone loss (osteoporosis)[38,39]

Brain Health:

- Surgical stress causes delirium[40]
- Surgical stress causes cognitive dysfunction[41]
- Surgical stress causes memory impairment[42,78]
- Surgical stress causes nerve damage[44]
- Surgical stress causes stroke[45]
- Surgical stress causes seizures[46]
- Surgical stress causes paralysis[47]

Dental Health:

- Surgical stress causes dental caries (cavities)[48]

Depression:

- Surgical stress causes anxiety and depression[43,49]

Diabetes:

- Surgical stress causes insulin-resistance[50]

Digestive Health:

- Surgical stress increases intestinal permeability[51]
- Surgical stress reduces blood supply (ischemia) to the colon[47]
- Surgical stress causes gastric ulcers[52]
- Surgical stress causes gastric bleeding[53]

Exercise:

- Surgical stress causes loss of muscle mass and strength[54]

Eye Health:

- Surgical stress causes vision loss[55]

Hair Health:

- Surgical stress causes hair loss (alopecia)[56]

Healing:

- Surgical stress impairs wound healing[57]

Hearing:

- Surgical stress causes hearing loss[58]

Heart Health:

- Surgical stress causes heart attack[59,60]
- Surgical stress causes heart failure[61,62]

Immune System:

- Surgical stress impairs the immune system[63]
- Surgical stress suppresses anti-tumor immunity[64]
- Surgical stress increases risk of infection[65]

Kidney Health:

- Surgical stress causes kidney dysfunction[47]

Liver Health:

- Surgical stress causes liver dysfunction[66]
- Surgical stress causes multiple organ failure[53]

Lung Health:

- Surgical stress causes collapsed lung (atelectasis)[67]

Sexual Health:

- Surgical stress causes erectile dysfunction[68]
- Surgical stress significantly decreases blood testosterone levels[69]

Sleep:

- Surgical stress reduces sleep quality[70]

Thyroid Health:

- Surgical stress lowers thyroid function[71]

Tumor Microenvironment:

The area surrounding a tumor, commonly referred to as the tumor microenvironment, is one of the most important areas of cancer research. Its significance stems from the fact that substances present within it are in constant interaction with cancer cells and can determine the fate of a tumor.

Listed below are many of the changes that occur within the tumor microenvironment as a result of surgery.

- Surgical stress increases free radicals[89]
- Surgical stress increases high mobility group box 1 protein[73]
- Surgical stress increases tumor necrosis factor-alpha[75]

- Surgical stress increases interleukin-1beta[77]
- Surgical stress increases interleukin-4[74]
- Surgical stress increases interleukin-6[75,76]
- Surgical stress increases interleukin-8[75]
- Surgical stress increases nuclear factor-kappa b[72]
- Surgical stress increases cortisol[78]
- Surgical stress increases adrenaline[122]
- Surgical stress increases prolactin[35]
- Surgical stress increases vascular endothelial growth factor[79]
- Surgical stress increases epidermal growth factor[80]
- Surgical stress increases nitric oxide[82]
- Surgical stress increases lactic acid[100]
- Surgical stress increases estrogen[101]
- Surgical stress increases prostaglandins[102]
- Surgical stress increases serotonin[103]
- Surgical stress increases histamine[103]

16 WAYS SURGERY CAUSES CANCER

By investigating each individual factor found within the tumor microenvironment, we can pinpoint many of the ways cancer surgery promotes the growth and spread of cancer.

1. Nitric Oxide - Anytime a tissue has been injured, nitric oxide and other growth factors are released to signal cells to grow and divide to replace lost cells.[83] In a person with cancer, tumor cells caught in the crossfire of nitric oxide signaling will also be signaled to grow, which is why nitric oxide is a well-known promoter of angiogenesis and tumor progression.[84-87]

2. Nitric Oxide - Nitric oxide has also been demonstrated to trigger the adhesion of circulating tumor cells (like the ones released during cancer surgery) onto body tissues, which is the first step in new tumor formation.[88]

3. Vascular Endothelial Growth Factor – Similar to nitric oxide, VEGF is a protein that signals growth to help repair injured tissues.[124] Elevated blood levels of VEGF have been associated with the growth and progression of cancer.[125]

4. Epidermal Growth Factor – EGF, like nitric oxide and VEGF, enhances the growth, invasion and metastasis of tumors.[126] High levels of EGF are associated with poor prognosis in cancer patients.[127]

5. Free Radicals – Free radicals are highly-reactive molecules that are balanced by the body's antioxidant system. In excess, the oxidative damage caused by free radicals results in aging, cardiovascular disease, cancer and other chronic diseases.[148]

6. Adrenaline – The stress hormone adrenaline is one of the primary triggers of the breakdown of fat for energy (lipolysis).[123] Anytime unsaturated fatty acids enter the bloodstream, prostaglandins are formed,[90] which are carcinogenic.[91]

7. Cortisol - People with cancer have higher cortisol levels than people without cancer,[92] and a number of studies have shown that cancer patients with the highest levels of cortisol have the greatest risk of dying from the disease.[93,94]

8. Estrogen - The presence of cortisol in the bloodstream leads to increased production of the hormone estrogen.[95-97] The famous 1990's Women's Health Initiative study tested the effects of supplemental estrogen on women, but was forced to stop early after participants began developing cardiovascular disease, stroke, dementia and cancer.[98]

9. Serotonin - Since cortisol's basic action is to catabolize muscle tissue and muscle meat contains high levels of the amino acid tryptophan (a precursor for serotonin), stress increases serotonin production.[104] While most people think of serotonin as a 'happy hormone,' this cultural belief appears misguided, since serotonin is not a hormone and lowering it can alleviate depression.[120] Serotonin is part of the body's stress response and has been shown in numerous studies to promote tumor growth.[104-108]

10. Histamine - Histamine is an inflammatory mediator commonly known for its role in allergic reactions.[109,110] Substances that inhibit histamine prevent cancer growth and progression.[111-113]

11. Lactic Acid - Lactic acid is produced by cells that aren't getting what they need to produce energy efficiently. Lactic acid suppresses the immune system,[114] promotes cancer growth and metastasis[115] and also triggers the release of cortisol,[116] perpetuating the cycle of stress.

12. Prolactin - Elevated blood concentrations of the hormone prolactin trigger inflammation by amplifying the production of inflammatory cytokines,[117] and promote the formation and progression of numerous types of cancer. [118,119,121]

13. Tumor Necrosis Factor alpha – TNFalpha is an inflammatory cytokine released by macrophages in response to toxins or other stressors.[129] Due to its extreme toxicity, TNFalpha has been shown to kill cancer cells,[130] but the rest of the body is severely damaged in the process.[131-133] TNFalpha promotes inflammation, is involved in cancer growth and metastasis, and its presence in the body increases with age,[134] like cancer's.[135]

14. Nuclear Factor Kappa b – TNFalpha triggers the production of NFKB,[136] which is a protein that signals inflammation[137] and plays a key role in tumor formation, growth and spread.[138,139] Many ancient natural medicines found to be effective against cancer inhibit NFKB.[140]

15. Interleukin 6 – IL-6 is a highly-toxic pro-inflammatory cytokine[141,142] that plays a key role in the formation of numerous types of cancer, including colorectal,[128] pancreatic,[146] liver[147] and prostate.[81]

16. High-Mobility Group Box 1 Protein – HMGB1 is a pro-inflammatory protein that signals immune system activation in response to injury.[149] Overexpression of HMGB1 promotes inflammation, carcinogenesis, angiogenesis and metastasis. "Our studies and those of our colleagues suggest that HMGB1 is central to cancer."[145]

Surgical removal of a tumor triggers the release of an assortment of substances that each play important roles in cancer growth, progression and metastasis; and therefore, not only does cancer surgery promote the growth and spread of cancer, but *all forms of surgery* promote the growth and spread of cancer - even in people who don't have cancer.[99]

TIMELESS QUOTES

"Modern cancer surgery someday will be regarded with the same kind of horror that we now regard the use of leeches in George Washington's time."
- Dr. Robert Mendelsohn

"The disease always returns after removal, and operation only accelerates its growth and fatal termination."
- Alfred-Armand-Louis-Marie Velpeau, Surgeon (1795-1867)

"I do not despair of carcinoma being cured somewhere in the future, but this blessed achievement will, I believe, never be wrought by the knife of the surgeon."
- Dr. Hayes Agnew (1818-1892)

REFERENCES

1.   Leape LL. Unnecessary surgery. Health Serv Res. 1989;24(3):351-407.

2.   Rondberg, T.A. 1998. *Under the Influence of Modern Medicine.* Chiropractic Journal, 156 pps.

3.   Mendelsohn, R.S. 1979. *Confessions of a Medical Heretic.* McGraw-Hill Education, New York City, NY, 197 pps.

4.   Leape LL. Unnecessary surgery. Annu Rev Public Health. 1992;13:363-83.

5.   Eisler, P. and Hansen, B. (2013). *Doctors Perform Thousands of Unnecessary Surgeries.* USA Today. [Online.] Available: http://www.usatoday.com/story/news/nation/2013/06/18/unnecessary-surgery-usa-today-investigation/2435009 [December 1, 2016].

6.   Tayade MC, Dalvi SD. Fundamental Ethical Issues in Unnecessary Surgical Procedures. J Clin Diagn Res. 2016;10(4):JE01-4.

7.   Chisholm, D. (2016). *Many operations are no better than placebo, says top surgeon.* The Listener. [Online]. Available: http://www.noted.co.nz/health/health/many-operations-are-no-better-than-placebo-says-top-surgeon [December 1, 2016].

8.   Detre K, Murphy ML, Hultgren H. Effect of coronary bypass surgery on longevity in high and low risk patients. Report from the V.A. Cooperative Coronary Surgery Study. Lancet. 1977;2(8051):1243-5.

9.   Myocardial infarction and mortality in the coronary artery surgery study (CASS) randomized trial. N Engl J Med. 1984;310(12):750-8.

10.   Hueb W, Lopes NH, Gersh BJ, et al. Five-year follow-up of the Medicine, Angioplasty, or Surgery Study (MASS II): a randomized controlled clinical trial of 3 therapeutic strategies for multivessel coronary artery disease. Circulation. 2007;115(9):1082-9.

11.   Texas Heart Institute (2016). *Limited-Access Heart Surgery.* [Online]. Available: [December 1, 2016].

12.   Giacomino BD, Cram P, Vaughan-sarrazin M, Zhou Y, Girotra S. Association of Hospital Prices for Coronary Artery Bypass Grafting With Hospital Quality and Reimbursement. Am J Cardiol. 2016;117(7):1101-6.

13.   Heaton JP, Evans H, Adams MA, Smith K, Morales A. Coronary artery bypass graft surgery and its impact on erectile function: a preliminary retrospective study. Int J Impot Res. 1996;8(1):35-9.

14.   Dhein S, Grassl M, Gerdom M, et al. Organ-protective effects on the liver and kidney by minocycline in small piglets undergoing cardiopulonary bypass. Naunyn Schmiedebergs Arch Pharmacol. 2015;388(6):663-76.

15.   Walter H. Walshe, The Anatomy, Physiology, Pathology and Treatment of Cancer, (Boston: Ticknor & Co., 1844).

16.   Wilt TJ, Brawer MK, Jones KM, et al. Radical prostatectomy versus observation for localized prostate cancer. N Engl J Med. 2012;367(3):203-13.

17.   Jacobson JA, Danforth DN, Cowan KH, et al. Ten-year results of a comparison of conservation with mastectomy in the treatment of stage I and II breast cancer. N Engl J Med. 1995;332(14):907-11.

18.   Vila J, Gandini S, Gentilini O. Overall survival according to type of surgery in young (≤40 years) early breast cancer patients: A systematic meta-analysis comparing breast-conserving surgery versus mastectomy. Breast. 2015;24(3):175-81.

19.   Pin YK, Khoo K, Tham M, et al. Lymphadenectomy promotes tumor growth and cancer cell dissemination in the spontaneous RET mouse model of human uveal melanoma. Oncotarget. 2015;6(42):44806-18.

20. Langley RR, Fidler IJ. Tumor cell-organ microenvironment interactions in the pathogenesis of cancer metastasis. Endocr Rev. 2007;28(3):297-321.

21. Langley RR, Fidler IJ. The seed and soil hypothesis revisited--the role of tumor-stroma interactions in metastasis to different organs. Int J Cancer. 2011;128(11):2527-35.

22. Chen LL, Blumm N, Christakis NA, Barabási AL, Deisboeck TS. Cancer metastasis networks and the prediction of progression patterns. Br J Cancer. 2009;101(5):749-58.

23. Marie P, Clunet J. Fréquences des métastases viscérales chez les souris cancéreuses après ablation chirurgicale de leur tumeur. *Bull Assoc Franç pour l'étude du cancer* 1910;3:19-23.

24. Tyzzer EE. Factors in the production and growth of tumor metastases. J Med Res 1913;23:309-332.

25. Cole WH. Spontaneous regression of cancer: the metabolic triumph of the host?. Ann N Y Acad Sci. 1974;230:111-41.

26. Krokowski, E.H.: Is the Current Treatment of Cancer Self-Limiting in the Extent of its Success? J Int Acad Preventive Medicine, 6 (1) 23 – 39, 1979.

27. Retsky M, Demicheli R, Hrushesky W, Baum M, Gukas I. Surgery triggers outgrowth of latent distant disease in breast cancer: an inconvenient truth?. Cancers (Basel). 2010;2(2):305-37.

28. Lange PH, Hekmat K, Bosl G, Kennedy BJ, Fraley EE. Acclerated growth of testicular cancer after cytoreductive surgery. Cancer. 1980;45(6):1498-506.

29. Demicheli R, Retsky MW, Hrushesky WJ, Baum M. Tumor dormancy and surgery-driven interruption of dormancy in breast cancer: learning from failures. Nat Clin Pract Oncol. 2007;4(12):699-710.

30. Retsky MW, Demicheli R, Hrushesky WJ, Baum M, Gukas ID. Dormancy and surgery-driven escape from dormancy help explain some clinical features of breast cancer. APMIS. 2008;116(7-8):730-41.

31. Goldstein MR, Mascitelli L. Surgery and cancer promotion: are we trading beauty for cancer?. QJM. 2011;104(9):811-5.

32. Hanin L, Bunimovich-mendrazitsky S. Reconstruction of the natural history of metastatic cancer and assessment of the effects of surgery: Gompertzian growth of the primary tumor. Math Biosci. 2014;247:47-58.

33. Hanin L, Pavlova L. A quantitative insight into metastatic relapse of breast cancer. J Theor Biol. 2016;394:172-81.

34. Sano F, Ueda K, Murakami J, Hayashi M, Nishimoto A, Hamano K. Enhanced tumor growth in the remaining lung after major lung resection. J Surg Res. 2016;202(1):1-7.

35. Desborough JP. The stress response to trauma and surgery. Br J Anaesth. 2000;85(1):109-17.

36. Hooli 1 RS, Gavimath CC, Ravishankera BE. Study to assess stress among cardiac surgical patients. International Journal of Pharmaceutical Applications. 2012; Vol 3, Issue 1, 2012, pp 282-288.

37. Gibbs J, Cull W, Henderson W, Daley J, Hur K, Khuri SF. Preoperative Serum Albumin Level as a Predictor of Operative Mortality and MorbidityResults From the National VA Surgical Risk Study. *Arch Surg.* 1999;134(1):36-42.

38. Kim WK, Ke K, Sul OJ, et al. Curcumin protects against ovariectomy-induced bone loss and decreases osteoclastogenesis. J Cell Biochem. 2011;112(11):3159-66.

39. Yu EW, Bouxsein ML, Roy AE, et al. Bone loss after bariatric surgery: discordant results between DXA and QCT bone density. J Bone Miner Res. 2014;29(3):542-50.

40. Kronzer VL, Avidan MS. Preventing postoperative delirium: all that glisters is not gold. Lancet. 2016;388(10054):1854-1856.

41. Benson RA, Ozdemir BA, Matthews D, Loftus IM. A systematic review of postoperative cognitive decline following open and endovascular aortic aneurysm surgery. Ann R Coll Surg Engl. 2016;:1-4.

42. Fidalgo AR, Cibelli M, White JP, Nagy I, Maze M, Ma D. Systemic inflammation enhances surgery-induced cognitive dysfunction in mice. Neurosci Lett. 2011;498(1):63-6.

43. Kumar N, Singh JG. A study of surgical stress in female patients. Available: https://www.researchgate.net/publication/279471510_A_study_of_Surgical_Stress_in_Female_patie nts [December 1, 2016].

44. Staff NP, Engelstad J, Klein CJ, et al. Post-surgical inflammatory neuropathy. Brain. 2010;133(10):2866-80.

45. Egido JA, Castillo O, Roig B, et al. Is psycho-physical stress a risk factor for stroke? A case-control study. J Neurol Neurosurg Psychiatr. 2012;83(11):1104-10.

46. Schachter SC. Iatrogenic seizures. Neurol Clin. 1998;16(1):157-70.

47. Perdrizet GA, Lena CJ, Shapiro DS, Rewinski MJ. Preoperative stress conditioning prevents paralysis after experimental aortic surgery: increased heat shock protein content is associated with ischemic tolerance of the spinal cord. J Thorac Cardiovasc Surg. 2002;124(1):162-70.

48. Fukuda M, Hirota M, Sato S. Bone lesions and dental caries after gastrectomy--evaluation of milk intolerance and operative procedure. Jpn J Surg. 1986;16(1):36-41.

49. Carr EC, Nicky thomas V, Wilson-barnet J. Patient experiences of anxiety, depression and acute pain after surgery: a longitudinal perspective. Int J Nurs Stud. 2005;42(5):521-30.

50. Thorell A, Nygren J, Ljungqvist O. Insulin resistance: a marker of surgical stress. Curr Opin Clin Nutr Metab Care. 1999;2(1):69-78.

51. Ramachandran A, Balasubramanian KA. Protease activation during surgical stress in the rat small intestine. J Surg Res. 2000;92(2):283-90.

52. Briusov PG, Osipov IS. [Stress ulcers of the gastrointestinal tract in surgical patients]. Voen Med Zh. 1998;319(1):30-8.

53. Martin LF, Booth FV, Reines HD, et al. Stress ulcers and organ failure in intubated patients in surgical intensive care units. Ann Surg. 1992;215(4):332-7.

54. Watters JM, Clancey SM, Moulton SB, Briere KM, Zhu JM. Impaired recovery of strength in older patients after major abdominal surgery. Ann Surg. 1993;218(3):380-90.

55. Pierce V, Kendrick P. Ischemic optic neuropathy after spine surgery. AANA J. 2010;78(2):141-5.

56. Wiener DJ, Rüfenacht S, Koch HJ, Mauldin EA, Mayer U, Welle MM. Estradiol-induced alopecia in five dogs after contact with a transdermal gel used for the treatment of postmenopausal symptoms in women. Vet Dermatol. 2015;26(5):393-6, e90-1.

57. West JM. Wound healing in the surgical patient: influence of the perioperative stress response on perfusion. AACN Clin Issues Crit Care Nurs. 1990;1(3):595-601.

58. Reversible sensorineural hearing loss after non-otological surgery under general anaesthetic. Postgraduate Medical Journal. 2000;76(895):304.

59. Badner NH, Knill RL, Brown JE, Novick TV, Gelb AW. Myocardial infarction after noncardiac surgery. Anesthesiology. 1998;88(3):572-8.

60. Nito I, Waspadji S, Harun S, Markum HM. Correlation between cortisol levels and myocardial infarction mortality among intensive coronary care unit patients during first seven days in hospital. Acta Med Indones. 2004;36(1):8-14.

61. Gallerani M, Maida G, Boari B, Galeotti R, Rocca T, Gasbarro V. High output heart failure due to an iatrogenic arterio-venous fistula after lumbar disc surgery. Acta Neurochir (Wien). 2007;149(12):1243-7.

62. Güder G, Bauersachs J, Frantz S, et al. Complementary and incremental mortality risk prediction by cortisol and aldosterone in chronic heart failure. Circulation. 2007;115(13):1754-61.

63. Xie ZB, Zhu SL, Peng YC, et al. Postoperative hepatitis B virus reactivation and surgery-induced immunosuppression in patients with hepatitis B-related hepatocellular carcinoma. J Surg Oncol. 2015;112(6):634-42.

64. Xu P, Zhang P, Sun Z, Wang Y, Chen J, Miao C. Surgical trauma induces postoperative T-cell dysfunction in lung cancer patients through the programmed death-1 pathway. Cancer Immunol Immunother. 2015;64(11):1383-92.

65. Goldfarb Y, Sorski L, Benish M, Levi B, Melamed R, Ben-eliyahu S. Improving postoperative immune status and resistance to cancer metastasis: a combined perioperative approach of immunostimulation and prevention of excessive surgical stress responses. Ann Surg. 2011;253(4):798-810.

66. Nakatani T, Kobayashi K. [Surgical stress and organ dysfunction: liver]. Nihon Geka Gakkai Zasshi. 1996;97(9):752-8.

67. Massard G, Wihlm JM. Postoperative atelectasis. Chest Surg Clin N Am. 1998;8(3):503-28, viii.

68. Mogos V, Mogos S. Iatrogenic erectile dysfunction after pelvic surgery: prostatectomy, colonic and rectal surgery. Available: https://www.researchgate.net/publication/267398060_IATROGENIC_ERECTILE_DYSFUNCTIO N_AFTER_PELVIC_SURGERY_PROSTATECTOMY_COLONIC_AND_RECTAL_SURGERY. [December 1, 2016].

69. Canbaz S, Ege T, Sunar H, Cikirikcioglu M, Acipayam M, Duran E. The effects of cardiopulmonary bypass on androgen hormones in coronary artery bypass surgery. J Int Med Res. 2002;30(1):9-14.

70. Yasuma F, Okada T. [Sleep disturbances complicated by surgical stress; a questionnaire survey of 50 patients]. Masui. 1989;38(1):66-70.

71. Gejrot T, Notter G. Effects of surgical stress on thyroid function in man. Acta Otolaryngol. 1962;55:1-10.

72. Li RL, Zhang ZZ, Peng M, et al. Postoperative impairment of cognitive function in old mice: a possible role for neuroinflammation mediated by HMGB1, S100B, and RAGE. J Surg Res. 2013;185(2):815-24.

73. Terrando N, Yang T, Wang X, et al. Systemic HMGB1 Neutralization Prevents Postoperative Neurocognitive Dysfunction in Aged Rats. Front Immunol. 2016;7:441.

74. Helmy SA, Wahby MA, El-nawaway M. The effect of anaesthesia and surgery on plasma cytokine production. Anaesthesia. 1999;54(8):733-8.

75. Hildebrand F, Pape HC, Krettek C. [The importance of cytokines in the posttraumatic inflammatory reaction]. Unfallchirurg. 2005;108(10):793-4, 796-803.

76. Thaeter M, Knobe M, Vande kerckhove M, et al. Perioperative inflammatory response in major fracture: do geriatric patients behave differently?. Eur J Trauma Emerg Surg. 2016;42(5):547-551.

77. Cibelli M, Fidalgo AR, Terrando N, et al. Role of interleukin-1beta in postoperative cognitive dysfunction. Ann Neurol. 2010;68(3):360-8.

78. Sun L, Jia P, Zhang J, et al. Production of inflammatory cytokines, cortisol, and Aβ1-40 in elderly oral cancer patients with postoperative delirium. Neuropsychiatr Dis Treat. 2016;12:2789-2795.

79. Maniwa Y, Okada M, Ishii N, Kiyooka K. Vascular endothelial growth factor increased by pulmonary surgery accelerates the growth of micrometastases in metastatic lung cancer. Chest. 1998;114(6):1668-75.

80. Tagliabue E, Agresti R, Carcangiu ML, et al. Role of HER2 in wound-induced breast carcinoma proliferation. Lancet. 2003;362(9383):527-33.

81.   Nguyen DP, Li J, Tewari AK. Inflammation and prostate cancer: the role of interleukin 6 (IL-6). BJU Int. 2014;113(6):986-92.

82.   Kooguchi K, Kobayashi A, Kitamura Y, et al. Elevated expression of inducible nitric oxide synthase and inflammatory cytokines in the alveolar macrophages after esophagectomy. Crit Care Med. 2002;30(1):71-6.

83.   Morbidelli L, Donnini S, Ziche M. Role of nitric oxide in the modulation of angiogenesis. Curr Pharm Des. 2003;9(7):521-30.

84.   Morbidelli L, Donnini S, Ziche M. Role of nitric oxide in tumor angiogenesis. Cancer Treat Res. 2004;117:155-67.

85.   Ziche M, Morbidelli L. Nitric oxide and angiogenesis. J Neurooncol. 2000;50(1-2):139-48.

86.   Morbidelli L, Donnini S, Ziche M. Role of nitric oxide in tumor angiogenesis. Cancer Treat Res. 2004;117:155-67.

87.   Gallo O, Masini E, Morbidelli L, et al. Role of nitric oxide in angiogenesis and tumor progression in head and neck cancer. J Natl Cancer Inst. 1998;90(8):587-96.

88.   Vidal MJ, Zocchi MR, Poggi A, Pellegatta F, Chierchia SL. Involvement of nitric oxide in tumor cell adhesion to cytokine-activated endothelial cells. J Cardiovasc Pharmacol. 1992;20 Suppl 12:S155-9.

89.   Klaunig JE, Kamendulis LM, Hocevar BA. Oxidative stress and oxidative damage in carcinogenesis. Toxicol Pathol. 2010;38(1):96-109.

90.   Shavit Y, Weidenfeld J, Dekeyser FG, et al. Effects of surgical stress on brain prostaglandin E2 production and on the pituitary-adrenal axis: attenuation by preemptive analgesia and by central amygdala lesion. Brain Res. 2005;1047(1):10-7.

91.   Wolfle D. Enhancement of carcinogen-induced malignant cell transformation by prostaglandin F2a. 2003; Volume 188, Issues 2-3, pages 139-147.

92.   Fabre B, Grosman H, Gonzalez D, et al. Prostate Cancer, High Cortisol Levels and Complex Hormonal Interaction. Asian Pac J Cancer Prev. 2016;17(7):3167-71.

93.   Kim HM, Ha KS, Hwang IC, Ahn HY, Youn CH. Random Serum Cortisol as a Predictor for Survival of Terminally Ill Patients With Cancer: A Preliminary Study. Am J Hosp Palliat Care. 2016;33(3):281-5.

94.   Cohen L, Cole SW, Sood AK, et al. Depressive symptoms and cortisol rhythmicity predict survival in patients with renal cell carcinoma: role of inflammatory signaling. PLoS ONE. 2012;7(8):e42324.

95.   Schmidt M, Löffler G. Induction of aromatase in stromal vascular cells from human breast adipose tissue depends on cortisol and growth factors. FEBS Lett. 1994;341(2-3):177-81.

96.   Wang WS, Liu C, Li WJ, Zhu P, Li JN, Sun K. Involvement of CRH and hCG in the induction of aromatase by cortisol in human placental syncytiotrophoblasts. Placenta. 2014;35(1):30-6.

97.   Wang W, Li J, Ge Y, et al. Cortisol induces aromatase expression in human placental syncytiotrophoblasts through the cAMP/Sp1 pathway. Endocrinology. 2012;153(4):2012-22.

98.   Women's Health Initiative. Available: https://www.nhlbi.nih.gov/whi/estro_alone.htm. [December 1, 2016].

99.   Goldstein MR, Mascitelli L. Surgery and cancer promotion: are we trading beauty for cancer?. QJM. 2011;104(9):811-5.

100.   Waters JH, Miller LR, Clack S, Kim JV. Cause of metabolic acidosis in prolonged surgery. Crit Care Med. 1999;27(10):2142-6.

101.   Macniven E, Decatanzaro D, Younglai EV. Chronic stress increases estrogen and other steroids in inseminated rats. Physiol Behav. 1992;52(1):159-62.

102. Shavit Y, Weidenfeld J, Dekeyser FG, et al. Effects of surgical stress on brain prostaglandin E2 production and on the pituitary-adrenal axis: attenuation by preemptive analgesia and by central amygdala lesion. Brain Res. 2005;1047(1):10-7.

103. Singh, M. Stress response and anesthesia: Altering the peri and post-operative management. Indian J. Anaesth. 2003; 47 (6): 427-434.

104. Soll C, Jang JH, Riener MO, et al. Serotonin promotes tumor growth in human hepatocellular cancer. Hepatology. 2010;51(4):1244-54.

105. Gurbuz N, Ashour AA, Alpay SN, Ozpolat B. Down-regulation of 5-HT1B and 5-HT1D receptors inhibits proliferation, clonogenicity and invasion of human pancreatic cancer cells. PLoS ONE. 2014;9(8):e105245.

106. Pai VP, Marshall AM, Hernandez LL, Buckley AR, Horseman ND. Altered serotonin physiology in human breast cancers favors paradoxical growth and cell survival. Breast Cancer Res. 2009;11(6):R81.

107. Siddiqui EJ, Shabbir MA, Mikhailidis DP, Mumtaz FH, Thompson CS. The effect of serotonin and serotonin antagonists on bladder cancer cell proliferation. BJU Int. 2006;97(3):634-9.

108. Sui H, Xu H, Ji Q, et al. 5-hydroxytryptamine receptor (5-HT1DR) promotes colorectal cancer metastasis by regulating Axin1/β-catenin/MMP-7 signaling pathway. Oncotarget. 2015;6(28):25975-87.

109. Koh KJ, Pearce AL, Marshman G, Finlay-jones JJ, Hart PH. Tea tree oil reduces histamine-induced skin inflammation. Br J Dermatol. 2002;147(6):1212-7.

110. Adlesic M, Verdrengh M, Bokarewa M, Dahlberg L, Foster SJ, Tarkowski A. Histamine in rheumatoid arthritis. Scand J Immunol. 2007;65(6):530-7.

111. Lefranc F, Yeaton P, Brotchi J, Kiss R. Cimetidine, an unexpected anti-tumor agent, and its potential for the treatment of glioblastoma (review). Int J Oncol. 2006;28(5):1021-30.

112. Hsieh HY, Shen CH, Lin RI, et al. Cyproheptadine exhibits antitumor activity in urothelial carcinoma cells by targeting GSK3β to suppress mTOR and β-catenin signaling pathways. Cancer Lett. 2016;370(1):56-65.

113. Harris AL, Smith IE. Regression of carcinoid tumour with cyproheptadine. Br Med J (Clin Res Ed). 1982;285(6340):475.

114. Choi SY, Collins CC, Gout PW, Wang Y. Cancer-generated lactic acid: a regulatory, immunosuppressive metabolite?. J Pathol. 2013;230(4):350-5.

115. Dhup S, Dadhich RK, Porporato PE, Sonveaux P. Multiple biological activities of lactic acid in cancer: influences on tumor growth, angiogenesis and metastasis. Curr Pharm Des. 2012;18(10):1319-30.

116. Wahl P, Zinner C, Achtzehn S, Bloch W, Mester J. Effect of high- and low-intensity exercise and metabolic acidosis on levels of GH, IGF-I, IGFBP-3 and cortisol. Growth Horm IGF Res. 2010;20(5):380-5.

117. Brand JM, Frohn C, Cziupka K, Brockmann C, Kirchner H, Luhm J. Prolactin triggers pro-inflammatory immune responses in peripheral immune cells. Eur Cytokine Netw. 2004;15(2):99-104.

118. Tworoger SS, Eliassen AH, Zhang X, et al. A 20-year prospective study of plasma prolactin as a risk marker of breast cancer development. Cancer Res. 2013;73(15):4810-9.

119. Clevenger, C.V. Role of Prolactin/Prolactin Receptor Signaling in Human Breast Cancer. Breast Disease. 18(1):75.

120. Recchione C, Galante E, Secreto G, Cavalleri A, Dati V. Abnormal serum hormone levels in lung cancer. Tumori. 1983;69(4):293-8.

121. Capuron L, Ravaud A, Neveu PJ, Miller AH, Maes M, Dantzer R. Association between decreased serum tryptophan concentrations and depressive symptoms in cancer patients undergoing cytokine therapy. Mol Psychiatry. 2002;7(5):468-73.

122. Håkanson E, Rutberg H, Jorfeldt L. Effect of adrenaline on exchange of free fatty acids in leg tissues and splanchnic area. A comparison with the metabolic response to surgical stress. Clin Physiol. 1986;6(5):453-63.

123. Coppack SW, Jensen MD, Miles JM. In vivo regulation of lipolysis in humans. J Lipid Res. 1994;35(2):177-93.

124. Lee CG, Link H, Baluk P, et al. Vascular endothelial growth factor (VEGF) induces remodeling and enhances TH2-mediated sensitization and inflammation in the lung. Nat Med. 2004;10(10):1095-103.

125. Manzoor H, Qadir MI, Abbas K, et al. Vascular endothelial growth factor (VEGF) in cancer. African journal of pharmacy and pharmacology. 2014;8(37):917-923.

126. Sasaki T, Hiroki K, Yamashita Y. The role of epidermal growth factor receptor in cancer metastasis and microenvironment. Biomed Res Int. 2013;2013:546318.

127. Koenders PG, Beex LV, Kienhuis CB, Kloppenborg PW, Benraad TJ. Epidermal growth factor receptor and prognosis in human breast cancer: a prospective study. Breast Cancer Res Treat. 1993;25(1):21-7.

128. Waldner MJ, Foersch S, Neurath MF. Interleukin-6--a key regulator of colorectal cancer development. Int J Biol Sci. 2012;8(9):1248-53.

129. Lentz EK, Cherla RP, Jaspers V, Weeks BR, Tesh VL. Role of tumor necrosis factor alpha in disease using a mouse model of Shiga toxin-mediated renal damage. Infect Immun. 2010;78(9):3689-99.

130. Mocellin S, Rossi CR, Pilati P, Nitti D. Tumor necrosis factor, cancer and anticancer therapy. Cytokine Growth Factor Rev. 2005;16(1):35-53.

131. Ulich TR, Del castillo J, Ni RX, Bikhazi N, Calvin L. Mechanisms of tumor necrosis factor alpha-induced lymphopenia, neutropenia, and biphasic neutrophilia: a study of lymphocyte recirculation and hematologic interactions of TNF alpha with endogenous mediators of leukocyte trafficking. J Leukoc Biol. 1989;45(2):155-67.

132. Clark GC, Taylor MJ. Tumor necrosis factor involvement in the toxicity of TCDD: the role of endotoxin in the response. Exp Clin Immunogenet. 1994;11(2-3):136-41.

133. Degasperi GR, Romanatto T, Denis RG, et al. UCP2 protects hypothalamic cells from TNF-alpha-induced damage. FEBS Lett. 2008;582(20):3103-10.

134. Han D, Hosokawa T, Aoike A, Kawai K. Age-related enhancement of tumor necrosis factor (TNF) production in mice. Mech Ageing Dev. 1995;84(1):39-54.

135. Schmidlin K, Spoerri A, Egger M, et al. Cancer, a disease of aging (part 1) - trends in older adult cancer mortality in Switzerland 1991-2008. Swiss Med Wkly. 2012;142:w13637.

136. Pinna F, Sahle S, Beuke K, et al. A Systems Biology Study on NFκB Signaling in Primary Mouse Hepatocytes. Front Physiol. 2012;3:466.

137. Wang S, Liu Z, Wang L, Zhang X. NF-kappaB signaling pathway, inflammation and colorectal cancer. Cell Mol Immunol. 2009;6(5):327-34.

138. Sakamoto K, Maeda S, Hikiba Y, et al. Constitutive NF-kappaB activation in colorectal carcinoma plays a key role in angiogenesis, promoting tumor growth. Clin Cancer Res. 2009;15(7):2248-58.

139.   Bharti AC, Aggarwal BB. Nuclear factor-kappa B and cancer: its role in prevention and therapy. Biochem Pharmacol. 2002;64(5-6):883-8.

140.   Olivier S, Robe P, Bours V. Can NF-kappaB be a target for novel and efficient anti-cancer agents?. Biochem Pharmacol. 2006;72(9):1054-68.

141.   Weber J, Yang JC, Topalian SL, et al. Phase I trial of subcutaneous interleukin-6 in patients with advanced malignancies. J Clin Oncol. 1993;11(3):499-506.

142.   Weiss GR, Margolin KA, Sznol M, et al. A phase II study of the continuous intravenous infusion of interleukin-6 for metastatic renal cell carcinoma. J Immunother Emphasis Tumor Immunol. 1995;18(1):52-6.

143.   Shalowitz DI, Epstein AJ, Buckingham L, Ko EM, Giuntoli RL. Survival implications of time to surgical treatment of endometrial cancers. Am J Obstet Gynecol. 2016.

144.   Bethune R, Sbaih M, Brosnan C, Arulampalam T. What happens when we do not operate? Survival following conservative bowel cancer management. Ann R Coll Surg Engl. 2016;98(6):409-12.

145.   Tang D, Kang R, Zeh HJ, Lotze MT. High-mobility group box 1 and cancer. Biochim Biophys Acta. 2010;1799(1-2):131-40.

146.   Okada S, Okusaka T, Ishii H, et al. Elevated serum interleukin-6 levels in patients with pancreatic cancer. Jpn J Clin Oncol. 1998;28(1):12-5.

147.   Tian G, Mi J, Wei X, et al. Circulating interleukin-6 and cancer: A meta-analysis using Mendelian randomization. Sci Rep. 2015;5:11394.

148.   Lobo V, Patil A, Phatak A, Chandra N. Free radicals, antioxidants and functional foods: Impact on human health. Pharmacogn Rev. 2010;4(8):118-26.

149.   Chen Q, Guan X, Zuo X, Wang J, Yin W. The role of high mobility group box 1 (HMGB1) in the pathogenesis of kidney diseases. Acta Pharm Sin B. 2016;6(3):183-8

CHAPTER 2

CHEMOTHERAPY

CHEMOTHERAPY IS A cancer treatment where highly-toxic chemicals are injected into patients in an attempt to kill cancer cells. The first chemotherapeutic agent ever used, which is still being administered to this day, is a derivative of the chemical weapon mustard gas, called mustargen.

The United States learned a lot about mustard gas during World War II, where damaged bone marrow and lymph tissues seen in autopsies of exposed soldiers revealed the weapon's prime target: the immune system.[1] Even more was learned about the effects of mustard gas when the US government conducted a series of secret tests on 60,000 of its own troops. *National Public Radio* broke the story in 2015,

"Sixty-thousand American troops served as test subjects, and about 4,000 were used in extreme tests that government studies have linked to illnesses including skin cancer, leukemia and chronic breathing problems. The test subjects were sworn to secrecy until the program was formally declassified in 1993. By then, the youngest World War II veterans were in their 60s and 70s. Many of the men in the experiments never shared the details with their families."[2]

FROM BATTLEFIELD TO CANCER CLINIC

What do you do after discovering a chemical weapon that knocks out the immune system, causes cancer and makes exposed skin literally slough off the body? Naturally you dispose of it – as safely as possible – and stop its production forever. But while mustard gas has been banned on the battlefield by international treaties,[3] instead of leaving this devastating poison behind us as a dark remnant of our past to be revisited only in history books – the government decided to begin injecting it into sick people with cancer.

After World War II ended, the US Department of Defense funded Dr. Goodman and Dr. Gilman of Yale University to administer mustard gas to rats and observe its effects on tumors. Their tumors regressed. They tested it on a lymphoma patient with advanced cancer and their tumors also regressed.[4-6] So amazed was the medical community that a drug could cause tumor regression, that it didn't seem to matter the patient died within a couple of months.

Interestingly, around this same time Dr. Gerson – an American physician famous for his nutritional approach to cancer, which included fresh fruit and vegetable juices, liver extract injections, thyroid hormone, coffee enemas and other nutrients – presented cases to US congress of cancer patients he had cured using his nutritional therapy.[7] The world of medicine was at a fork in the road, Dr. Nicholas Gonzales explains, "it could have gone toward natural treatments, it could have gone toward synthetic. But because of that extraordinary response in a single patient that lasted a few weeks, the entire chemo industry came into fruition."[8]

WARNING LABEL FOR MUSTARGEN

"This drug is HIGHLY TOXIC and both powder and solution must be handled and administered with care. Inhalation of dust or vapors and contact with skin or mucous membranes, especially those of the eyes, must be avoided. Avoid exposure during pregnancy. Due to the toxic properties of mechlorethamine (e.g., corrosivity, carcinogenicity, mutagenicity, teratogenicity), special handling procedures should be reviewed prior to handling and followed diligently. Extravasation of the drug into subcutaneous tissues results in a painful inflammation. The area usually becomes indurated and sloughing may occur."[18]

CHEMOTHERAPY VS. CANCER

It doesn't take more than common sense to reason that injecting poison into the veins of a sick person will 1) not cure them and 2) probably make their health worse. A study published in *The Lancet* in 1980 found that of 78 patients who received chemotherapy, survival "was no better than that of the 80 who did not receive chemotherapy." Furthermore, regression of tumors was found to have no impact on survival and, "survival may even have been shortened in some patients given chemotherapy," the study reports.[9]

The most comprehensive review ever conducted on the efficacy of chemotherapy was completed by German epidemiologist and biostatistician Dr. Ulrich Abel. Europe's most popular news magazine *Der Spiegel*, which sells over 1-million copies per week, featured Dr. Abel's publication in a 2004 article titled *Useless Poisonous Cures* (*Giftkur ohne Nutzen*).[10] In order to obtain every study and clinical trial ever published on chemotherapy, Dr. Abel sent letters to over 350 medical centers across the world; his review consisted of thousands of studies and took two years to complete.

Dr. Abel pronounced that despite new and increasingly expensive poisons being used during chemotherapy, "patients do not live a day longer" than they did 25 years prior. Overall worldwide chemotherapy success rates he said were "appalling," and that "for most internal cancers no proof exists that chemotherapy, especially the increasingly high dose variety, increases life expectancy or improves quality of life." Dr. Abel estimated at least 80% of chemotherapy administered throughout the world is completely worthless.[11]

A group of Australian scientists published a study in 2004 suggesting that *far more* than just 80% of chemotherapy administered is worthless. During a follow-up with cancer patients 5-years after receiving chemotherapy, the researchers determined that only 2.1% of patients in the US and 2.3% of patients in Australia were still alive – exposing chemotherapy's astonishing 98% failure rate.[12] *I wonder how many of these patients would have been alive at 5-years if they hadn't received chemotherapy.*

Seeking a greater understanding of what happens inside the body after an injection of chemotherapy, scientists from Harvard Medical School and the University of Massachusetts tested 88 currently-used chemotherapeutic drugs on fruit flies in 2013. Michelle Markstein, molecular biologist and co-author of the study reported, "...several chemotherapeutics that stop fast growing tumors have the opposite effect on stem cells in the same animal, causing them to divide too rapidly."[13] By shrinking the initial tumor mass, chemotherapy deceives doctors into thinking patients are benefitting from the treatment, when in actuality, the growth and spread of cancer are being accelerated by it.

Another way of analyzing the effects of chemotherapy on human health is to look at people who were involved in producing it during times of war. Retired Japanese poison gas factory workers were evaluated 57-years after they had been manufacturing mustard gas during World War II. The study found that exposure to mustard gas "significantly increases the long-term risk of death from respiratory cancer and chronic bronchitis/emphysema."[84]

For the first time ever, researchers investigated chemotherapy-induced death at a number of hospitals in the UK. Published in the esteemed journal *Lancet Oncology* in 2016, the study found that 8.4% of people undergoing chemotherapy for lung cancer and 2.4% of people treated for breast cancer nationwide were killed by the treatment within 30-days of administration. When they looked at the numbers from the Milton Keynes Hospital they discovered an even more startling figure: 50.9% of lung cancer patients were killed by chemotherapy within 30-days of treatment.[14]

SUCCESS STORIES?

One Cancer Patient's Experience with Chemotherapy

"This highly toxic fluid was being injected into my veins. The nurse administering it was wearing protective gloves because it would burn her skin if just a tiny drip came into contact with it. I couldn't help asking myself 'If such precautions are needed to be taken on the outside, what is it doing to me on the inside?' From 7 pm that evening, I vomited solidly for two and a half days. During my treatment, I lost my hair by the handful, I lost my appetite, my skin colour, my zest for life. I was death on legs," described a cancer patient in the book *Now and Then* by Bob Madison.

Women Struggling to Live Normal Lives Following Chemotherapy

Thousands of women who have received chemotherapy for breast cancer are struggling to live normal lives, reports a 2016 study published in the journal *Cancer*.

Just one year after treatment, 20% of women above the age of 65 were so debilitated that they couldn't carry out basic daily tasks like walking across the room, light housework, shopping, kneeling or standing long enough to shower.[15]

Cancer Patient Survives Decades Until Chemotherapy

The longest-surviving breast cancer patient of all-time was diagnosed at age 45 and lived until she was 93-years-old. Following her diagnosis, she received no treatment for 22 years, at which point doctors discovered metastatic cancer in her lungs and put her on estrogen-inhibiting drugs.

14 years later, they found cancer on her spine and put her on a different estrogen inhibitor. Years later, doctors found cancer in her liver and finally decided to try chemotherapy.

After receiving two cycles of the chemotherapy drug capecitabine, she refused further treatment due to intolerable side effects, and was dead within two years.[16]

ADDITIONAL HEALTH EFFECTS

Despite careful adherence to a strict set of safety protocols for handling chemotherapy drugs, including the use of personal protective equipment, more than half of nursing and pharmacy workers in a 2016 study reported complaints of dizziness simply from working with chemotherapy drugs.[17]

Side effects of chemotherapy include, but are not limited to:

Blood Health:

- Chemotherapy decreases red blood cells (anemia)[19]
- Chemotherapy decreases white blood cells (leukopenia)[20]
- Chemotherapy decreases blood platelets (thrombocytopenia)[21]

Bone Health:

- Chemotherapy causes bone death (osteonecrosis)[22]
- Chemotherapy causes loss of bone mineral density (osteoporosis)[23,24]

Brain Health:

- Chemotherapy is toxic to the brain (neurotoxic)[25]
- Chemotherapy causes long-lasting impairment of concentration, forgetfulness and slower thinking; termed "chemobrain" [26,27]
- Chemotherapy causes altered consciousness[28]
- Chemotherapy causes degeneration of white matter in the brain (leukoencephalopathy) [28]
- Chemotherapy causes nerve damage (neuropathy) [28]
- Chemotherapy causes seizures[28]
- Chemotherapy causes paralysis[28]
- Chemotherapy causes stroke (cerebral infarction) [28]

Digestive Health:

- Chemotherapy causes diarrhea[36]
- Chemotherapy causes painful inflammation and ulceration in the digestive tract (intestinal mucositis)[41]
- Chemotherapy causes "significant intestinal damage in both jejunum and colon"[37]

Exercise:

- Chemotherapy reduces grip strength[38]
- Chemotherapy causes muscle dysfunction and a loss of overall strength[39]

Eye Health:

- Chemotherapy causes severe vision loss and altered color vision[40]
- Chemotherapy causes complete blindness[41]

Hair Health:

- Chemotherapy causes hair loss[50]

Healing:

- Chemotherapy impairs wound healing[51]

Hearing:

- Chemotherapy causes "severe to profound hearing loss"[52]
- Chemotherapy causes chronic ringing of the ears (tinnitus)[52]

Heart Health:

- Chemotherapy damages the heart[53]
- Chemotherapy causes heart disease[54]
- Chemotherapy causes heart failure[55]
- Chemotherapy causes heart attacks (myocardial infarction)[56]

Immune System:

- Chemotherapy causes long-term immune system damage[57,58]
- Chemotherapy exacerbates existing hepatitis C infections[59]
- Chemotherapy reactivates hepatitis B virus[60]
- Chemotherapy impairs anti-tumor immune response[61]

Kidney Health:

- Chemotherapy causes kidney failure[65]

Liver Health:

- Chemotherapy causes liver injury[66]

Lung Health:

- Chemotherapy causes lung disease[67]

Mental Health:

- Chemotherapy "decreased emotional and social function and increased distress"[29]
- Chemotherapy causes depression[30]
- Chemotherapy causes anxiety[31]

Oral Health:

- Chemotherapy causes severe dental caries[32]
- Chemotherapy causes dry mouth (xerostomia), ulcers and mouth sores[68]
- Chemotherapy causes oral candida (fungal) infection[33]
- Chemotherapy causes painful inflammation and ulceration in the mouth (oral mucositis)[34]
- Chemotherapy causes "a diverse spectrum of oral changes that generally are attributed to immunosuppression and bleeding tendencies"[35]

Pain:

- Chemotherapy causes neuropathic pain; burning or coldness, "pins and needles" sensations, numbness and itching[69]
- Chemotherapy pain remains one-year after treatment[70]

Quality of Life:

- Chemotherapy causes difficulty swallowing (dysphagia)[71]
- Chemotherapy causes nausea and vomiting (emesis)[72,73]
- Chemotherapy causes altered taste sensation[74]
- Chemotherapy causes migraine headaches[75]

Sexual Health:

- Chemotherapy causes infertility and premature ovarian failure;[42,43] in up to 66% of women[44]
- Chemotherapy causes absence of menstrual period (amenorrhea)[45]
- Chemotherapy causes menopausal symptoms[45]
- Chemotherapy damages sperm and testicular tissue"[46,47]
- Chemotherapy reduces reproductive organ weight, sperm count and sperm motility[46]
- Chemotherapy causes "a significant decline in serum testosterone" [46]
- Chemotherapy causes erectile dysfunction[48,49]

Skin:

- Chemotherapy causes dermatitis: itchiness, red skin, or a rash[76]

Sleep:

- Chemotherapy reduces sleep quality[77]

Thyroid Health:

- Chemotherapy "blunts thyroid function"[78]
- Chemotherapy impairs thyroid hormone synthesis and secretion from the thyroid gland[79]
- Thyroid hormones "…were remarkably altered after each cycle of chemotherapy leading to decline in thyroid function…"[80]

Tumor Microenvironment:

- Chemotherapy increases free radicals[85]
- Chemotherapy increases cortisol[85]
- Chemotherapy increases adrenaline[93]
- Chemotherapy increases prolactin[94]
- Chemotherapy increases estrogen[64]
- Chemotherapy increases tumor necrosis factor-alpha[62]
- Chemotherapy increases interleukin 1- beta[62]
- Chemotherapy increases interleukin-6[91]
- Chemotherapy increases interleukin-8[92]
- Chemotherapy increases nuclear factor-kappa b[62]
- Chemotherapy increases prostaglandins[86]
- Chemotherapy increases nitric oxide[46]
- Chemotherapy increases vascular endothelial growth factor[95]
- Chemotherapy increases epidermal growth factor[96]
- Chemotherapy increases lactic acid[87]
- Chemotherapy increases serotonin[88]
- Chemotherapy increases histamine[89]
- Chemotherapy increases high-mobility group box 1 protein[90]

Urinary Health:

- Chemotherapy causes blood in the urine (hematuria)[81]
- Chemotherapy causes painful urination (dysuria)[81]

Weight Loss:

- Chemotherapy causes muscle-wasting (cachexia)[82]

- "Severe loss of body weight (cachexia) is a frequent cause of death in cancer patients and is exacerbated by chemotherapy"[83]

TIMELESS QUOTES

"Most cancer patients in this country die of chemotherapy. Chemotherapy does not eliminate breast, colon, or lung cancers. This fact has been documented for over a decade, yet doctors still use chemotherapy for these tumors."
- Dr. Allen Levin, The Healing of Cancer

"As a chemist trained to interpret data, it is incomprehensible to me that physicians can ignore the clear evidence that chemotherapy does much, much more harm than good."
- Alan Nixon, Ph.D., Past President of The American Chemical Society

"Chemotherapy and radiotherapy will make the ancient method of drilling holes in a patient's head to permit the escape of demons look relatively advanced. Toxic chemotherapy is a hoax. The doctors who use it are guilty of pre-meditated murder, and the use of cobalt and other methods of cancer treatment popular today effectively closes the door on cure."
- Ernst T. Krebs Jr., American Biochemist (1911-1996)

"To sell chemotherapy as a 'therapy' is most likely the biggest deceit in the history of medicine. Whoever masterminded this chemo-torture deserves a monument in hell."
- Dr. Ryke Geerd Hamer, M.D.

REFERENCES

1.	(2014). Evolution of Cancer Treatments: Chemotherapy. [Online] Available: http://www.cancer.org/cancer/cancerbasics/thehistoryofcancer/the-history-of-cancer-cancer-treatment-chemo. [November 28, 2016].

2.	Dickerson, C. (2015). *Families React To NPR's Reporting Of Secret Mustard Gas Testing.* [Online]. Available: http://www.npr.org/2015/11/03/453962074/families-react-to-nprs-reporting-of-secret-mustard-gas-testing. [November 28, 2016].

3.	(2011). Chemical Weapons Specialist Helps WWII Veteran Find Effective Treatment For Mustard Gas Symptoms. [Online]. Available: http://www.cdc.gov/nceh/stories/mustard_gas.html. [November 28, 2016].

4.	Gilman A. Therapeutic applications of chemical warfare agents. Fed Proc. 1946;5:285-92.

5.	Goodman LS, Wintrobe MM. Nitrogen mustard therapy; use of methyl-bis (beta-chloroethyl) amine hydrochloride and tris (beta-chloroethyl) amine hydrochloride for Hodgkin's disease, lymphosarcoma, leukemia and certain allied and miscellaneous disorders. J Am Med Assoc. 1946;132:126-32.

6.	Gilman A, Philips FS. The Biological Actions and Therapeutic Applications of the B-Chloroethyl Amines and Sulfides. Science. 1946;103(2675):409-36.

7.	The Gerson Institute. *Dr. Gerson's Suppressed 1946 Congressional Testimony.* [Online]. Available: http://whale.to/cancer/dr_gerson.html. [November 28, 2016].

8.	iHealthTube.com, Gonzales, N. (2012). *The Shocking History of Chemotherapy.* [YouTube]. Available: https://www.youtube.com/watch?v=_TptKbxQJr4. [November 28, 2016].

9.	Powles TJ, Coombes RC, Smith IE, Jones JM, Ford HT, Gazet JC. Failure of chemotherapy to prolong survival in a group of patients with metastatic breast cancer. Lancet. 1980;1(8168 Pt 1):580-2.

10.	Blech, Jorg. (2004). *Giftkur ohne Nutzen.* [Online]. Available: http://www.spiegel.de/spiegel/print/d-32362278.html [November 28, 2016].

11.	Abel, Ulrich, PhD "Cytostatic Therapy of Advanced Epithelial Tumors – A Critique" Lancet 10 Aug 1991.

12.	Morgan G, Ward R, Barton M. The contribution of cytotoxic chemotherapy to 5-year survival in adult malignancies. Clin Oncol (R Coll Radiol). 2004;16(8):549-60.

13.	Markstein M, Dettorre S, Cho J, Neumüller RA, Craig-müller S, Perrimon N. Systematic screen of chemotherapeutics in Drosophila stem cell tumors. Proc Natl Acad Sci USA. 2014;111(12):4530-5.

14.	Wallington M, Saxon EB, Bomb M, et al. 30-day mortality after systemic anticancer treatment for breast and lung cancer in England: a population-based, observational study. Lancet Oncol. 2016;17(9):1203-16.

15.	Owusu C, Margevicius S, Schluchter M, Koroukian SM, Schmitz KH, Berger NA. Vulnerable elders survey and socioeconomic status predict functional decline and death among older women with newly diagnosed nonmetastatic breast cancer. Cancer. 2016;122(16):2579-86.

16.	Bayraktar S, Garcia-buitrago MT, Hurley E, Gluck S. Surviving metastatic breast cancer for 18 years: a case report and review of the literature. Breast J. 2011;17(5):521-4.

17.	Fernandes NM, Pelissari IG, Cogo LA, Santos filha VA. Workplace Activity in Health Professionals Exposed to Chemotherapy Drugs: An Otoneurological Perspective. Int Arch Otorhinolaryngol. 2016;20(4):331-338.

18.	Drugs.com. (2013). *Mustargen.* [Online]. Available: https://www.drugs.com/pro/mustargen.html [November 28, 2016].

19.	Mountzios G, Aravantinos G, Alexopoulou Z, et al. Lessons from the past: Long-term safety and survival outcomes of a prematurely terminated randomized controlled trial on prophylactic vs.

hemoglobin-based administration of erythropoiesis-stimulating agents in patients with chemotherapy-induced anemia. Mol Clin Oncol. 2016;4(2):211-220.

20. Li DY, Yu TT, Bai H, Chen XY. [Clinical study on effect of compound granule prescription of thunberg fritillary bulb in relieving post-chemotherapy bone marrow suppression in RAL patients]. Zhongguo Zhong Yao Za Zhi. 2012;37(20):3155-7.

21. Tamamyan G, Danielyan S, Lambert MP. Chemotherapy induced thrombocytopenia in pediatric oncology. Crit Rev Oncol Hematol. 2016;99:299-307.

22. Antonuzzo L, Lunghi A, Giommoni E, Brugia M, Di costanzo F. Regorafenib Also Can Cause Osteonecrosis of the Jaw. J Natl Cancer Inst. 2016;108(4).

23. Bordbar MR, Haghpanah S, Dabbaghmanesh MH, Omrani GR, Saki F. Bone mineral density in children with acute leukemia and its associated factors in Iran: a case-control study. Arch Osteoporos. 2016;11(1):36.

24. Lee SW, Yeo SG, Oh IH, Yeo JH, Park DC. Bone mineral density in women treated for various types of gynecological cancer. Asia Pac J Clin Oncol. 2016;

25. Matsuoka A, Mitsuma A, Maeda O, et al. Quantitative assessment of chemotherapy-induced peripheral neurotoxicity using a point-of-care nerve conduction device. Cancer Sci. 2016;107(10):1453-1457.

26. Iarkov A, Appunn D, Echeverria V. Post-treatment with cotinine improved memory and decreased depressive-like behavior after chemotherapy in rats. Cancer Chemother Pharmacol. 2016;78(5):1033-1039.

27. Rendeiro C, Sheriff A, Bhattacharya TK, et al. Long-lasting impairments in adult neurogenesis, spatial learning and memory from a standard chemotherapy regimen used to treat breast cancer. Behav Brain Res. 2016;315:10-22.

28. Reddy AT, Witek K. Neurologic complications of chemotherapy for children with cancer. Curr Neurol Neurosci Rep. 2003;3(2):137-42.

29. Dunn J, Watson M, Aitken JF, Hyde MK. Systematic Review of Psychosocial Outcomes for Patients with Advanced Melanoma. Psychooncology. 2016;

30. Oh PJ, Lee JR. [Effect of Cancer Symptoms and Fatigue on Chemotherapy-related Cognitive Impairment and Depression in People with Gastrointestinal Cancer]. J Korean Acad Nurs. 2016;46(3):420-30.

31. Baek Y, Yi M. [Factors Influencing Quality of Life during Chemotherapy for Colorectal Cancer Patients in South Korea]. J Korean Acad Nurs. 2015;45(4):604-12.

32. Peretz B, Sarnat H, Kharouba J. Chemotherapy induced dental changes in a child with medulloblastoma: a case report. J Clin Pediatr Dent. 2014;38(3):251-4.

33. Alt-epping B, Nejad RK, Jung K, Gross U, Nauck F. Symptoms of the oral cavity and their association with local microbiological and clinical findings--a prospective survey in palliative care. Support Care Cancer. 2012;20(3):531-7.

34. Dreizen S, Mccredie KB, Keating MJ. Chemotherapy-induced oral mucositis in adult leukemia. Postgrad Med. 1981;69(2):103-8, 111-2.

35. Farsi DJ. Children Undergoing Chemotherapy: Is It Too Late for Dental Rehabilitation?. J Clin Pediatr Dent. 2016;40(6):503-505.

36. Abalo R, Uranga JA, Pérez-garcía I, et al. May cannabinoids prevent the development of chemotherapy-induced diarrhea and intestinal mucositis? Experimental study in the rat. Neurogastroenterol Motil. 2016.

37. Forsgård RA, Korpela R, Holma R, et al. Intestinal permeability to iohexol as an in vivo marker of chemotherapy-induced gastrointestinal toxicity in Sprague-Dawley rats. Cancer Chemother Pharmacol. 2016;78(4):863-74.

38. Klepin HD, Tooze JA, Pardee TS, et al. Effect of Intensive Chemotherapy on Physical, Cognitive, and Emotional Health of Older Adults with Acute Myeloid Leukemia. J Am Geriatr Soc. 2016;64(10):1988-1995.

39. Gilliam LA, Lark DS, Reese LR, et al. Targeted overexpression of mitochondrial catalase protects against cancer chemotherapy-induced skeletal muscle dysfunction. Am J Physiol Endocrinol Metab. 2016;311(2):E293-301.

40. Giralt J, Rey A, Villanueva R, Alforja S, Casaroli-marano RP. Severe visual loss in a breast cancer patient on chemotherapy. Med Oncol. 2012;29(4):2567-9.

41. Cloutier AO. Ocular side effects of chemotherapy: nursing management. Oncol Nurs Forum. 1992;19(8):1251-9.

42. Batchvarov IS, Taylor RW, Bustamante-marín X, et al. A grafted ovarian fragment rescues host fertility after chemotherapy. Mol Hum Reprod. 2016.

43. Clowse ME, Behera MA, Anders CK, et al. Ovarian preservation by GnRH agonists during chemotherapy: a meta-analysis. J Womens Health (Larchmt). 2009;18(3):311-9.

44. Garrido-oyarzún MF, Castelo-branco C. Controversies over the use of GnRH agonists for reduction of chemotherapy-induced gonadotoxicity. Climacteric. 2016;19(6):522-525.

45. Li CY, Chen ML. [Chemotherapy-Induced Amenorrhea and Menopause Symptoms in Women With Breast Cancer]. Hu Li Za Zhi. 2016;63(5):19-26.

46. Eid AH, Abdelkader NF, Abd el-raouf OM, Fawzy HM, El-denshary ES. Carvedilol alleviates testicular and spermatological damage induced by cisplatin in rats via modulation of oxidative stress and inflammation. Arch Pharm Res. 2016.

47. Levi M, Popovtzer A, Tzabari M, et al. Cetuximab intensifies cisplatin-induced testicular toxicity. Reprod Biomed Online. 2016;33(1):102-10.

48. Huang M, Lin J, Yu X, et al. Erectile and urinary function in men with rectal cancer treated by neoadjuvant chemoradiotherapy and neoadjuvant chemotherapy alone: a randomized trial report. Int J Colorectal Dis. 2016;31(7):1349-57.

49. Annam K, Voznesensky M, Kreder KJ. Understanding and Managing Erectile Dysfunction in Patients Treated for Cancer. J Oncol Pract. 2016;12(4):297-304.

50. Trüeb RM. Chemotherapy-induced alopecia. Semin Cutan Med Surg. 2009;28(1):11-4.

51. Tanaka S, Hayek G, Jayapratap P, et al. The Impact of Chemotherapy on Complications Associated with Mastectomy and Immediate Autologous Tissue Reconstruction. Am Surg. 2016;82(8):713-7.

52. Frisina RD, Wheeler HE, Fossa SD, et al. Comprehensive Audiometric Analysis of Hearing Impairment and Tinnitus After Cisplatin-Based Chemotherapy in Survivors of Adult-Onset Cancer. J Clin Oncol. 2016;34(23):2712-20.

53. Truong J, Yan AT, Cramarossa G, Chan KK. Chemotherapy-induced cardiotoxicity: detection, prevention, and management. Can J Cardiol. 2014;30(8):869-78.

54. Granger CB. Prediction and prevention of chemotherapy-induced cardiomyopathy: can it be done?. Circulation. 2006;114(23):2432-3.

55. Smith SA, Auseon AJ. Chemotherapy-induced takotsubo cardiomyopathy. Heart Fail Clin. 2013;9(2):233-42.

56. Sakka S, Kawai K, Tsujimoto I, et al. [Severe Acute Myocardial Infarction during Induction Chemotherapy for Retroperitoneal Germ Cell Tumor : A Case Report]. Hinyokika Kiyo. 2016;62(9):483-487.

57. Perkins JL, Harris A, Pozos TC. Immune Dysfunction After Completion of Childhood Leukemia Therapy. J Pediatr Hematol Oncol. 2016.

58. Verma R, Foster RE, Horgan K, et al. Lymphocyte depletion and repopulation after chemotherapy for primary breast cancer. Breast Cancer Res. 2016;18(1):10.

59. Lin JW, Chang ML, Hsu CW, et al. Acute exacerbation of hepatitis C in hepatocellular carcinoma patients receiving chemotherapy. J Med Virol. 2017;89(1):153-160.

60. Qin L, Wang F, Zou BW, Ding ZY. Chemotherapy-induced fatal hepatitis B virus reactivation in a small-cell lung cancer patient. Mol Clin Oncol. 2016;5(4):382-384.

61. Wu Y, Deng Z, Wang H, Ma W, Zhou C, Zhang S. Repeated cycles of 5-fluorouracil chemotherapy impaired anti-tumor functions of cytotoxic T cells in a CT26 tumor-bearing mouse model. BMC Immunol. 2016;17(1):29.

62. Li W, Yan MH, Liu Y, et al. Ginsenoside Rg5 Ameliorates Cisplatin-Induced Nephrotoxicity in Mice through Inhibition of Inflammation, Oxidative Stress, and Apoptosis. Nutrients. 2016;8(9).

63. El-naga RN. Pre-treatment with cardamonin protects against cisplatin-induced nephrotoxicity in rats: impact on NOX-1, inflammation and apoptosis. Toxicol Appl Pharmacol. 2014;274(1):87-95.

64. Tiong V, Rozita AM, Taib NA, Yip CH, Ng CH. Incidence of chemotherapy-induced ovarian failure in premenopausal women undergoing chemotherapy for breast cancer. World J Surg. 2014;38(9):2288-96.

65. Dugbartey GJ, Peppone LJ, De graaf IA. An integrative view of cisplatin-induced renal and cardiac toxicities: Molecular mechanisms, current treatment challenges and potential protective measures. Toxicology. 2016;371:58-66.

66. Hiroshima Y, Shuto K, Yamazaki K, et al. Fractal Dimension of Tc-99m DTPA GSA Estimates Pathologic Liver Injury due to Chemotherapy in Liver Cancer Patients. Ann Surg Oncol. 2016;23(13):4384-4391.

67. Limper AH. Chemotherapy-induced lung disease. Clin Chest Med. 2004;25(1):53-64.

68. Berger velten D, Zandonade E, Monteiro de barros miotto MH. Prevalence of oral manifestations in children and adolescents with cancer submitted to chemotherapy. BMC Oral Health. 2016;16(1):107.

69. Gong SS, Li YX, Zhang MT, et al. Neuroprotective Effect of Matrine in Mouse Model of Vincristine-Induced Neuropathic Pain. Neurochem Res. 2016;41(11):3147-3159.

70. Hellerstedt-börjesson S, Nordin K, Fjällskog ML, Holmström IK, Arving C. Women Treated for Breast Cancer Experiences of Chemotherapy-Induced Pain: Memories, Any Present Pain, and Future Reflections. Cancer Nurs. 2016;39(6):464-472.

71. Mcnamara MJ, Adelstein DJ, Allende DS, et al. Persistent Dysphagia After Induction Chemotherapy in Patients with Esophageal Adenocarcinoma Predicts Poor Post-Operative Outcomes. J Gastrointest Cancer. 2016.

72. Fakhfouri G, Mousavizadeh K, Mehr SE, et al. From Chemotherapy-Induced Emesis to Neuroprotection: Therapeutic Opportunities for 5-HT3 Receptor Antagonists. Mol Neurobiol. 2015;52(3):1670-9.

73. Thamlikitkul L, Srimuninnimit V, Akewanlop C, et al. Efficacy of ginger for prophylaxis of chemotherapy-induced nausea and vomiting in breast cancer patients receiving adriamycin-cyclophosphamide regimen: a randomized, double-blind, placebo-controlled, crossover study. Support Care Cancer. 2016.

74. Sozeri E, Kutluturkan S. The Validity and Reliability of Turkish Version of the Chemotherapy-induced Taste Alteration Scale (CiTAS). Clin Nurs Res. 2016.

75. Rajasekhar A, George TJ. Gemcitabine-induced reversible posterior leukoencephalopathy syndrome: a case report and review of the literature. Oncologist. 2007;12(11):1332-5.

76. Esquirol caussa J, Herrero vila E. [Epidermal growth factor, innovation and safety]. Med Clin (Barc). 2015;145(7):305-12.

77. Bagheri-nesami M, Goudarzian AH, Jan babaei G, Badiee M, Mousavi M, Sadegh sharifi M. Sleep Quality and Associated Risk Factors in Leukemia Patients Undergoing Chemotherapy in Iran. Asian Pac J Cancer Prev. 2016;17 Spec No.:107-11.

78. De groot S, Janssen LG, Charehbili A, et al. Thyroid function alters during neoadjuvant chemotherapy in breast cancer patients: results from the NEOZOTAC trial (BOOG 2010-01). Breast Cancer Res Treat. 2015;149(2):461-6.

79. Anker GB, Lønning PE, Aakvaag A, Lien EA. Thyroid function in postmenopausal breast cancer patients treated with tamoxifen. Scand J Clin Lab Invest. 1998;58(2):103-7.

80. Khan MA, Bhurani D, Agarwal NB. Alteration of Thyroid Function in Indian HER 2-Negative Breast Cancer Patients Undergoing Chemotherapy. Asian Pac J Cancer Prev. 2015;16(17):7701-5.

81. Degener S, Pohle A, Strelow H, et al. Long-term experience of hyperbaric oxygen therapy for refractory radio- or chemotherapy-induced haemorrhagic cystitis. BMC Urol. 2015;15:38.

82. Nissinen TA, Degerman J, Räsänen M, et al. Systemic blockade of ACVR2B ligands prevents chemotherapy-induced muscle wasting by restoring muscle protein synthesis without affecting oxidative capacity or atrogenes. Sci Rep. 2016;6:32695.

83. Klose R, Krzywinska E, Castells M, et al. Targeting VEGF-A in myeloid cells enhances natural killer cell responses to chemotherapy and ameliorates cachexia. Nat Commun. 2016;7:12528.

84. Mukaida K, Hattori N, Iwamoto H, et al. Mustard gas exposure and mortality among retired workers at a poisonous gas factory in Japan: a 57-year follow-up cohort study. Occup Environ Med. 2016.

85. Limberaki E, Eleftheriou P, Gasparis G, Karalekos E, Kostoglou V, Petrou C. Cortisol levels and serum antioxidant status following chemotherapy. 2012; Available at: https://www.researchgate.net/publication/224943223_Cortisol_levels_and_serum_antioxidant_status_follo wing_chemotherapy. [December 1, 2016].

86. Lalla RV, Pilbeam CC, Walsh SJ, Sonis ST, Keefe DM, Peterson DE. Role of the cyclooxygenase pathway in chemotherapy-induced oral mucositis: a pilot study. Support Care Cancer. 2010;18(1):95-103.

87. Kondo K, Fujiwara M, Murase M, et al. Severe acute metabolic acidosis and Wernicke's encephalopathy following chemotherapy with 5-fluorouracil and cisplatin: case report and review of the literature. Jpn J Clin Oncol. 1996;26(4):234-6.

88. Cubeddu LX, Hoffmann IS, Fuenmayor NT, Malave JJ. Changes in serotonin metabolism in cancer patients: its relationship to nausea and vomiting induced by chemotherapeutic drugs. Br J Cancer. 1992;66(1):198-203.

89. Eschalier A, Lavarenne J, Burtin C, Renoux M, Chapuy E, Rodriguez M. Study of histamine release induced by acute administration of antitumor agents in dogs. Cancer Chemother Pharmacol. 1988;21(3):246-50.

90. Nguyen A, Bhavsar S, Riley E, Caponetti G, Agrawal D. Clinical Value of High Mobility Group Box 1 and the Receptor for Advanced Glycation End-products in Head and Neck Cancer: A Systematic Review. Int Arch Otorhinolaryngol. 2016;20(4):382-389.

91. Cheung YT, Ng T, Shwe M, et al. Association of proinflammatory cytokines and chemotherapy-associated cognitive impairment in breast cancer patients: a multi-centered, prospective, cohort study. Ann Oncol. 2015;26(7):1446-51.

92. Waugh DJ, Wilson C. The interleukin-8 pathway in cancer. Clin Cancer Res. 2008;14(21):6735-41.

93. Tiligada E. Chemotherapy: induction of stress responses. Endocr Relat Cancer. 2006;13 Suppl 1(Supplement 1):S115-24.

94. Hinterberger-fischer M, Ogris E, Kier P, et al. Elevation of plasma prolactin in patients undergoing autologous blood stem-cell transplantation for breast cancer: is its modulation a step toward posttransplant immunotherapy?. Am J Clin Oncol. 2000;23(4):325-9.

95. Fan F, Gray MJ, Dallas NA, et al. Effect of chemotherapeutic stress on induction of vascular endothelial growth factor family members and receptors in human colorectal cancer cells. Mol Cancer Ther. 2008;7(9):3064-70.

96. Wang F, Liu R, Lee SW, Sloss CM, Couget J, Cusack JC. Heparin-binding EGF-like growth factor is an early response gene to chemotherapy and contributes to chemotherapy resistance. Oncogene. 2007;26(14):2006-16.

CHAPTER 3

RADIOTHERAPY

RADIOTHERAPY, ALSO KNOWN as radiation therapy, is a treatment where ionizing x-ray and gamma ray radiation are directed at tumors and used to kill cancer cells. Blasting cells with radiation stops them from growing and multiplying, but it also damages every other cell in its path and sets in motion a cascade of negative physiological effects that can persist for multiple generations.

Today, up to 60% of cancer patients receive radiotherapy as a part of their treatment regimens[1] and yet most are never fully aware of the risks involved with exposure to ionizing radiation.

THE DISCOVERY OF X-RAYS

X-rays were first discovered in 1895 by German physics professor Wilhelm Röntgen. In 1901, Röntgen was awarded the Nobel Prize for his discovery and ironically, both he and his wife ended up dying from cancer caused by x-ray exposure.[2]

With the advent of a machine that could produce x-rays, suddenly the medical industry had an impressive new way to destroy cells other than cauterizing or burning with acid; and within a few years, ionizing radiation was put to use on cancer patients. However, a number of common side effects quickly became known, including burns, skin disease and the formation of tumors, but society failed to take these warnings seriously and by 1922, over 100 radiologists and many others working in the medical industry had died from cancer caused by x-rays.[3] And yet the ignorance continued...

SHOE-FITTING X-RAY FLUOROSCOPES

In the 1920's, portable x-ray devices became widely available in shoe stores so customers could see the bones in their feet to determine which shoes were the right fit - and kids loved them![4] At the peak of popularity in the United States, there were at least 10,000 shoe-fitting x-ray fluoroscopes in use, and despite the massive radiation exposure (equal to more than 1000 chest x-rays) and the significant amount of scatter radiation emitted from these "cancer boxes," the horrifying nature of the technology was largely brushed off by the government and medical community.

By the 1970's, the incidence of foot cancer spiked dramatically and the negative effects could no longer be denied.[5] The shoe-fitting fluoroscopes used in shoe stores for around 50-years had officially been banned.

FLUOROSCOPES AS ENTERTAINMENT

After World War II, every physician in America was urged to have an x-ray fluoroscope in their office and no examination was considered complete unless patients were fluoroscoped.[6] In the 1940's, some pediatricians used fluoroscopes on babies every single month during checkups for the first two years of life.[6] Doctors would flaunt their fancy fluoroscopes to patients as a source of entertainment, which Dr. Raymond Peat, endocrinologist, physiologist and science historian described as "a combination of ignorance and arrogance."[7] It seems society was obsessed with technology in much the same way we are today with computers, cell phones and other gadgets.

RADIOTHERAPY VS. CANCER

During the Chernobyl nuclear disaster in 1986, massive amounts of radioactive isotopes billowed up into the atmosphere before reigning down onto most of Europe – and nobody exposed to fallout from this catastrophe was cured of cancer. In fact, the largest and most comprehensive mortality study on the Chernobyl disaster to date, which included data from over 1000 published studies and over 5000 internet and printed publications, concluded that between the years 1986 and 2004, the radioactivity released by this event caused 985,000 deaths, mostly from cancer.[8]

RADIOTHERAPY ADMINISTERS 5X THE FATAL DOSE

Emeritus Professor of Physics at the University of Oxford Wade Allison briefly discussed radiotherapy in a 2012 report on Nuclear Technology.[9] Over the course of a month, he wrote, "the tumour gets more than 40,000 mSv [millisieverts] and the peripheral healthy tissue as much as 20,000 mSv – that is five times the fatal dose experienced by some Chernobyl workers." In other words, if radiotherapy doses weren't spread out over the course of a month or longer, every patient receiving it would die instantly.

RADIOTHERAPY AND BREAST CANCER

Since radiotherapy first came onto the scene, the standard of care for women with breast cancer was surgical breast removal (radical mastectomy) followed by radiotherapy. However, at the time this regimen was put into practice, scientific research hadn't even established that it was beneficial for patients; and up until 1960, a large amount of conflicting research had been published:

- Some studies indicated radiotherapy following radical mastectomy provided good results[10-14]
- Others reported no benefit from the treatment[15-23]
- And several suggested radiotherapy was harmful[24,25]

The National Cancer Institute responded to this uncertainty in 1961 by launching *The National Surgical Adjuvant Breast and Bowel Project* (NSABP). For the project, American scientist Bernard Fisher and his colleagues compared the efficacy of mastectomy alone with mastectomy followed by irradiation. Published in the *Annals of Surgery* in 1970, the study found that radiotherapy *decreased survival of all patients*. "Survival of patients was determined 3, 4 and 5 years following operation…At each time, survival of those irradiated was slightly less than in the control patients."[26]

In 1974, researchers from the Swiss Institute for Experimental Cancer Research examined survival rates of women from six clinical trials who received either radical mastectomy or radical mastectomy followed by irradiation for breast cancer. Published in *The Lancet*, scientists concluded, "An increased mortality in early breast cancer can be correlated to the routine use of local postoperative irradiation. The decreased survival is statistically significant. Of controlled clinical trials so far published, all six, including more than 3400 patients, demonstrate decreased survival of between 1 and 10% in irradiated patients when compared with those treated by mastectomy alone."[27]

In 1995, a meta-analysis of 64 randomized trials was conducted to find out if irradiation following either mastectomy or lumpectomy improves survival of patients with breast cancer. Published in *The New England Journal of Medicine*, the study reports, "The addition of radiotherapy to surgery resulted in…no significant difference in 10-year survival."[28]

So far the evidence suggests that at best, radiotherapy doesn't improve survival of breast cancer patients, and at worst, radiotherapy is killing cancer patients more quickly than they would have died without it. Couple these findings with similar findings about radiotherapy following lung cancer surgery and it seems likely that the latter is true.

RADIOTHERAPY AND LUNG CANCER

A 1998 review of nine randomized trials compared survival rates of 2,128 lung cancer patients who received radiotherapy following surgery with patients who received surgery alone. Published in *The Lancet*, results showed that patients who received radiotherapy following surgery had a 27%

increased risk of death. Researchers concluded that, "Postoperative radiotherapy is detrimental to patients with early-stage completely resected NSCLC [non-small-cell lung cancer] and should not be used routinely for such patients."[29]

Scientists from the United Kingdom conducted an extensive review in 2005 evaluating the efficacy of radiotherapy following surgery in patients with non-small-cell lung cancer. Published in the journal *Lung Cancer,* they wrote, "Results continue to show PORT [postoperative radiotherapy] to be detrimental, with an 18% relative increase in the risk of death."[30]

WHISTLEBLOWER EXPOSES CANCER MORTALITY STATISTICS

One of the most fascinating statements made by whistleblower Dr. Ralph Moss in his book *The Cancer Industry* is that official cancer mortality statistics are being intentionally manipulated in order to make it appear like cancer treatments are better than they actually are.

Since radiotherapy damages all organs and systems of the body, including the brain,[96-99] heart,[110-115] liver,[128-129] kidneys,[127] thyroid,[157] immune system,[116-125] and impairs the healing process,[103-105] there are endless ways that its side effects can eventually kill a person. One of the most common ways is heart disease;[110-115] so what Dr. Moss was referring to, was the fact that if a patient receives radiotherapy then has a heart attack and dies a week, month or even a few years later, their cause of death will be deemed a heart attack rather than a cancer death due to treatment failure; and consequently, the public never finds out just how unsuccessful radiotherapy actually is. Evidence of this can be seen in studies reporting decreased cancer deaths while simultaneously reporting increased non-cancer deaths following radiotherapy treatment.[28,32,33]

In 1993, Texas researchers from the Anderson Cancer Center in Houston questioned the validity of official government cancer mortality statistics by examining non-cancer deaths of 470,000 cancer patients. Published in the *Journal of the National Cancer Institute*, the study found that 27% of patients who were reported dead for reasons other than cancer had died within a year after diagnosis, suggesting they were probably killed by their treatments; "...it appears that this excess was caused by treatment of the cancer."[31] In other words, cancer treatments are less effective than we're told and the true death toll from cancer is actually much greater than we're told.

RADIOTHERAPY ELEVATES LIFETIME RISK OF CANCER

Whether radiotherapy treatment is used for acne, peptic ulcers, scalp ringworm or cancer, universally we see an elevated risk of cancer that lasts for the remainder of the patient's life.[34] For example, a 36-year-old male patient who was treated with radiotherapy and chemotherapy for Hodgkin's disease in 1972 developed colon cancer 18 years later.[35]

"Indeed, young patients treated with chemotherapy and especially radiation therapy are at high risk of developing secondary cancers. Chemo-radiotherapy appears to also increase more significantly the risk."[36] What's more, the risk of secondary cancers developing later in life is even greater for those treated during childhood; "Risks of radiation-related cancer are greatest for those exposed early in life, and these risks appear to persist throughout life."[37]

- Radiotherapy for scalp ringworm causes multiple basal cell carcinomas in about 40% of patients up to 50 years later.[38]
- Radiotherapy for acne is strongly associated with basal cell carcinoma arising within the radiation treatment field.[39]
- Radiotherapy for Hodgkin's lymphoma in children increases breast cancer risk 24-times.[40]
- Radiotherapy for Hodgkin's lymphoma increases stomach cancer risk 3.4-times[41]
- Radiotherapy for Hodgkin's lymphoma increases the risk of breast cancer, "…with risk increasing dramatically more than 15 years after therapy."[42]
- Radiotherapy for testicular cancer increases pancreatic cancer risk 2.9-times, persisting for over 20 years.[43]
- Radiotherapy for testicular cancer increases stomach cancer risk 5.9-times, persisting "for several decades."[44]

- Radiotherapy for breast cancer significantly increases cancer formation in the other (contralateral) breast[33]
- Radiotherapy for peptic ulcers increases risk of cancer; "Cancer mortality remained high for up to 50 years, indicating that radiation damage may persist to the end of life."[45]

What is happening inside the body as a result of exposure to ionizing radiation that causes lifelong damage?

RADIATION BYSTANDER EFFECTS

To this day, mainstream theory states that radiation kills cancer cells by directly damaging DNA.[46] However, in 1992, Harvard researchers discovered something that called the entire theory into question:[47] when a cell is irradiated, something is emitted by the injured cell that transfers the same damage to non-irradiated cells – a term called a 'bystander effect.'[48]

A colorful demonstration of bystander effects was performed by researchers at McMaster University in Ontario, Canada in 2006, where scientist Carmel E. Mothersill and her colleagues irradiated rainbow trout (0.5 Gy dose) and then placed them in water-filled containers with non-irradiated fish. Two days later, they discovered that the damage had been transferred from the irradiated fish to the non-irradiated fish – an effect that was said to be caused by the "secretion of a chemical messenger into the water."[49]

Bystander effects have also been demonstrated in animals,[50,51,52] in humans,[53,54] and even in plants.[55]

A CLOSER LOOK...

- Chinese researchers irradiated the roots of young Arabidopsis thaliana plants to determine if it would cause bystander effects. As the plant grew, researchers found evidence of radiation damage "in every true leaf over the course of rosette development." They even found damage in non-irradiated plants that were nearby.[55]
- In 2008, researchers from Alberta, Canada irradiated the heads of mice "while the remainder of the body was completely protected by a medical-

grade shield." They discovered DNA damage, altered cellular growth and cell death in shielded spleen cells.[52]

- Scientists from the University of Washington investigated the effects of dental x-rays on pregnant women and their offspring in 2004. Even though the women were entirely shielded with lead aprons during the X-ray images, irradiation damage was transferred to the fetus and many of the babies were born underweight.[54]

What is the chemical messenger released by irradiated cells that causes bystander effects?

Although at least one other factor is involved,[56] by far the major facilitator of bystander effects is nitric oxide (NO). Nitric oxide's effects include genomic instability,[57] genetic errors,[57] double-strand DNA breaks,[58] cell death (apoptosis),[59] inflammation,[59] and ultimately, carcinogenesis.[78,79] Lowering nitric oxide levels (for example, by supplementing with an inexpensive, medicinal blue dye called methylene blue[60]) can 'switch off' bystander effects and halt the self-perpetuating cycle of damage.[61]

Interestingly, the effects of ionizing radiation appear to be indistinguishable from estrogen,[62] and since estrogen rapidly elevates levels of nitric oxide in the body,[63,64] lowering estrogen is probably a more fundamental way to interrupt bystander effects.

When any part of the body is exposed to ionizing radiation, even at the low-doses commonly used during medical x-rays,[65] nitric oxide-mediated bystander effects transfer the damage to unexposed body parts - but it goes beyond that.

In 2010, researchers from Texas discovered that millimeter waves - a much less intense form of radiation that's often used at airport security checkpoints - can also induce bystander effects.[66]

Biochemist Martin Pall of Washington State University tested even lower frequencies to see if they could induce bystander effects in 2013. Published in the journal *Bioelectromagnetics*, Pall found that microwave and even extra-low frequency (ELF) radiation - the kind emitted from cell phones and other wireless devices - both induce nitric oxide synthesis.[67] This suggests that both non-ionizing microwave and ELF radiation will have some of the same effects as ionizing radiation. And indeed, there is abundant evidence within the scientific literature associating cell phone use with cancer; including brain tumors[68-73] mouth cancer,[74] lymphoma,[75] breast cancer[76] and eye cancer.[77]

SUCCESS STORIES?

Richard Wayman

One year after 59-year-old Richard Wayman received radiotherapy for cancer of the tonsils, he began feeling a "painful tingling" in his legs. Within weeks, he was struggling to walk and was admitted to the hospital for x-rays, scans and other tests.

"The scans revealed lesions on my lungs, which raised fears that the cancer had spread, so I was admitted to another hospital for a biopsy and, as a result, contracted MRSA [infection] and pneumonia."

During his time spent in the hospital to treat his conditions, Richard lost around 50 lbs. "I thought I was never going to get out of there," he remarked. Finally, doctors diagnosed his lung lesions as a side-effect of radiotherapy, but his problems continued.

After having a tooth pulled by his dentist, the bone around the extracted tooth "started to crumble and become infected."

Within a couple months he had an open wound running from his outer cheek through his jaw bone and into his mouth, called bone necrosis - another side effect of radiotherapy.[91]

Scott Jerome-Parks and Alexandra Jn-Charles

Anytime technology is involved there is the potential that it could malfunction. Although rare, errors during radiotherapy administration have occurred and the results have been disastrous.

Cancer patient Scott Jerome-Parks was overdosed with radiation that left him burnt, deaf, visually impaired, with ulcers in his mouth, teeth falling out, unable to swallow or breathe and dead several painful weeks later.

Another victim of technological failure was 32-year-old breast cancer patient Alexandra Jn-Charles, who received 27 days of radiation overdoses that burnt a hole in her chest and left a gaping wound so painful that it made her consider suicide. [93]

ADDITIONAL HEALTH EFFECTS

Here's a list of side effects of radiotherapy reported in the scientific literature.

Bone Health:

- Radiotherapy damages the spinal cord[93]
- Radiotherapy causes bone fractures[94]
- Radiotherapy causes bone and joint degeneration[95]

Brain Health:

- Radiotherapy lowers IQ[96]
- Radiotherapy impairs memory, attention, and executive function[97,98]
- Radiotherapy increases lifetime risk of having a stroke[99]

Eye Health:

- Radiotherapy causes vision loss[100]
- Radiotherapy causes complete blindness[101]

Hair Health:

- Radiotherapy causes complete hair loss (alopecia)[102]

Healing:

- Radiotherapy slows wound healing[103-105]

Hearing:

- Radiotherapy causes immediate partial or total deafness[106] in 45.71% of patients[107]
- Radiotherapy-induced hearing loss continues to worsen over time[108,109]

Heart Health:

- Radiotherapy causes micro-vascular damage to the heart[112]
- Radiotherapy weakens the heart, blood vessels surrounding the heart and narrows arteries[113]

- Radiotherapy significantly increases mortality from cardiovascular death more than 15 years later[110-115]

Immune System:

- Radiotherapy suppresses the immune system[116]
- Radiotherapy inhibits anti-tumor immunity[116]
- Radiotherapy significantly increases risk of infection[117-124]
- "Immunity in young adult survivors of childhood leukemia [who received chemotherapy and/or radiotherapy] is similar to the elderly rather than age-matched controls"[125]

Inflammation:

- Radiotherapy causes immediate inflammation[126]

Kidney Health:

- Radiotherapy causes kidney failure[127]

Liver Health:

- Radiotherapy causes liver disease[128]
- Radiotherapy causes liver failure[129]

Mental Health:

- Radiotherapy causes mental disorders, anxiety, depression and distress[131,132]
- Radiotherapy causes "significantly worse mental health before, during and 1 year after RT [radiotherapy] compared to the normal population."[133]

Muscle-Loss:

- Radiation-induced cachexia causes primates to lose as much as 50% of skeletal muscle[134]

Oral Health:

- Radiotherapy causes tooth decay[135]
- Radiotherapy causes jaw bone death (osteoradionecrosis)[136]

- Radiotherapy causes permanent salivary gland dysfunction[137]
- Radiotherapy causes restricted mouth opening (trismus)[130]
- Radiotherapy causes oral discomfort, oral mucositis, changes in taste, increased oral infections and difficulty swallowing (dysphagia)[138]

Post-Traumatic Stress:

- Radiotherapy causes post-traumatic stress disorder[139]

Quality of Life:

- Radiotherapy causes fatigue in up to 90% of patients[140]
- Radiotherapy causes intractable (untreatable) nausea, vomiting and headache[141]
- Radiotherapy causes unpredictable taste and smell changes in 48% of patients; some had a stronger sweet taste, some had a stronger salt taste and some a weaker sense of smell[142]
- Radio-chemotherapy causes 64% of patients to rely on tube feeding as their primary means of food intake[143]
- Radiotherapy considerably impairs overall quality of life[144,145]

Sexual Health:

- Radiotherapy causes "…increased incidence of numerical sex chromosomal abnormalities and high risk for reproductive and genetic diseases…"[146]
- Total-body irradiation causes an "extremely high rate of gonadal dysfunction"[147]
- Radiotherapy causes a high percentage of infertility in cervical and testicular cancer patients[148]
- Radiotherapy causes sexual dysfunction in 78% of women treated for cervical cancer[149]
- Radiotherapy causes testosterone deficiency[150]
- Radiotherapy causes erectile dysfunction in 93.9% of men after prostate irradiation[151]

Skin:

- Radiotherapy causes thickening and scarring of skin and connective tissues[152]
- Shoe-fitting fluoroscopes cause dermatitis with ulceration on foot[153]

Sleep:

- Radiotherapy causes sleep problems in nearly half of patients[154]
- Radiotherapy causes severe obstructive sleep apnea[155]

Speech:

- Radiotherapy causes degeneration of voice and speech[156]

Thyroid Health:

- Radiotherapy causes hypothyroidism in approximately 53% of patients[157]

Tumor Microenvironment:

- Radiotherapy increases free radicals[164]
- Radiotherapy increases cortisol[80]
- Radiotherapy increases adrenaline[165]
- Radiotherapy increases estrogen[62]
- Radiotherapy increases prolactin[166]
- Radiotherapy increases nitric oxide[81]
- Radiotherapy increases vascular endothelial growth factor[82]
- Radiotherapy increases epidermal growth factor[83]
- Radiotherapy increases tumor necrosis factor alpha[88]
- Radiotherapy increases interleukin-1 beta[88]
- Radiotherapy increases interleukin-4[84]
- Radiotherapy increases interleukin-6[88]
- Radiotherapy increases interleukin-8[85]
- Radiotherapy increases nuclear factor kappa b[86]
- Radiotherapy increases prostaglandins[87]
- Radiotherapy increases lactic acid[167]
- Radiotherapy increases stem cell production[89,90]
- Radiotherapy increases histamine[161]
- Radiotherapy increases serotonin[162]
- Radiotherapy increases high-mobility group box 1 protein[163]

Urinary Health:

- Radiotherapy causes involuntary urination in women[158] and men[159]
- Radiotherapy for rectal cancer causes long-term incontinence and major disturbances in bowel function[160]

TIMELESS QUOTES

"… I wouldn't have chemotherapy and radiation because I'm not interested in therapies that cripple the immune system, and, in my opinion, virtually ensure failure for the majority of cancer patients."
- Dr Julian Whitaker, M.D.

"I had a brain cancer specialist sit in my living room and tell me that he would never take radiation if he had a brain tumor. And I asked him, 'but, do you send people for radiation?' and he said, of course. 'I'd be drummed out of the hospital if I didn't."
- Dr. Ralph Moss

REFERENCES

1. Hall S, Rudrawar S, Zunk M, et al. Protection against Radiotherapy-Induced Toxicity. Antioxidants (Basel). 2016;5(3).

2. Nobel Lectures, *Physics 1901-1921*, Elsevier Publishing Company, Amsterdam, 1967. Available: http://www.nobelprize.org/nobel_prizes/physics/laureates/1901/rontgen-bio.html.(December 1, 2016).

3. Moss, Ralph W. The cancer industry: the classic exposé on the cancer establishment. Brooklyn, NY: Equinox Press, 1996. Page 64.

4. Inglis-Arkell, E. (2011). *When X-rays were Given in Shoe Stores.* Gizmodo [Online]. Available: http://io9.gizmodo.com/5843183/when-x-rays-were-given-in-shoe-stores [February 24, 2016].

5. Smullen MJ, Bertler DE. Basal cell carcinoma of the sole: possible association with the shoe-fitting fluoroscope. WMJ. 2007;106(5):275-8.

6. Gofman, J. Lecture. Stinson Beach, California. 1999. *Medical X-rays and Breast Cancer.* Available: https://www.youtube.com/watch?v=AzW0zIjKcmE [February 24, 2016].

7. Peat, R. Audio Interview. 2009. *Radiation 2.* Politics and Science. Available: https://www.youtube.com/watch?v=7NjCopysMzo [February 24, 2016].

8. Yablokov AV, Nesterenko VB, Nesterenko AV et al. Chernobyl, Consequences of the Catastrophe for People and the Environment. John Wiley & Sons; 2010.

9. Allison, W. (2009). *Public Trust in Nuclear Energy.* [Online]. Available: http://docplayer.net/21237548-Public-trust-in-nuclear-energy.html. [December 1, 2016].

10. Adair, FE. (1943). The Role of Surgery and Irradiation in Cancer of The Breast. *JAMA.* 1943;121(8):553-559.

11. Guttmann R. Radiotherapy in the treatment of primary operable carcinoma of the breast with proved lymph node metastases: approach and results. Am J Roentgenol Radium Ther Nucl Med. 1963;89:58-63.

12. Harrington SW. Results of surgical treatment of unilateral carcinoma of breast in women. J Am Med Assoc. 1952;148(12):1007-11.

13. Marshall SF, Hare HF. Carcinoma of the breast; results of combined treatment with surgery and roentgen rays. Ann Surg. 1947;125(6):688-702.

14. Watson TA. Carcinoma of the breast. Stage II--radiation range. Can survival be increased by postoperative irradiation following radical mastectomy?. JAMA. 1967;200(2):136-7.

15. Butcher HR, Seaman WB, Eckert C, Saltzstein S. An Assessment Of Radical Mastectomy and Postoperative Irradiation Therapy In The Treatment Of Mammary Cancer. Cancer. 1964;17:480-5.

16. Cantrel, S. T. and Buschke, F.: The Role of Roentgen Therapy in Carcinoma of the Breast. West. J. Surg. Obstet. Gynec. 54: 369, 1946.

17. Chu FC, Lucas JC, Farrow JH, Nickson JJ. Does prophylactic radiation therapy given for cancer of the breast predispose to metastasis?. Am J Roentgenol Radium Ther Nucl Med. 1967;99(4):987-94.

18. Easson, E. C.: Postoperative Radiotherapy in Breast Cancer in Symposium on Prognostic Factors in Breast Cancer. (Edinburgh: Livingston, 1968), pp. 118-127.

19. Haagensen, C. D. and Stout, A. P.: Carcinoma of the Breast. I. Results of Treatment. Ann. Surg., 116:801, 1942.

20. Elkins HB, Hickey RC, Kerr HD, Tidrick RT, Wieben EE. Cancer of the breast, 1661 patients. I. Considerations in future therapy. AMA Arch Surg. 1956;73(4):654-60.

21. Paterson, Ralston, and Marion H. Russell. "Clinical Trials in Malignant Disease." *Journal of the Faculty of Radiologists* 10.4 (1959): 175–180.

22. Robbins GF, Lucas JC, Fracchia AA, Farrow JH, Chu FC. An evaluation of postoperative prophylactic radiation therapy in breast cancer. Surg Gynecol Obstet. 1966;122(5):979-82.

23. Treves N, Holleb AI. A report of 549 cases of breast cancer in women 35 years of age or younger. Surg Gynecol Obstet. 1958;107(3):271-83.

24. Dao, T. L. and Kovaric, J.: Incidence of Pulmonary and Skin Metastases in Women with Breast Cancer Who Received Postoperative Irradiation. Surgery, 52:203, 1962.

25. DeCourmelles, F.: Action Atrophique Glandulaire Des Rayons X. C. R. Acad. Sci (Paris), 140:606, 1905.

26. Fisher B, Slack NH, Cavanaugh PJ, Gardner B, Ravdin RG. Postoperative radiotherapy in the treatment of breast cancer: results of the NSABP clinical trial. Ann Surg. 1970;172(4):711-32.

27. Stjernswärd J. Decreased survival related to irradiation postoperatively in early operable breast cancer. Lancet. 1974;2(7892):1285-6.

28. Effects of radiotherapy and surgery in early breast cancer. An overview of the randomized trials. Early Breast Cancer Trialists' Collaborative Group. N Engl J Med. 1995;333(22):1444-55.

29. Postoperative radiotherapy in non-small-cell lung cancer: systematic review and meta-analysis of individual patient data from nine randomised controlled trials. PORT Meta-analysis Trialists Group. Lancet. 1998;352(9124):257-63.

30. Burdett S, Stewart L. Postoperative radiotherapy in non-small-cell lung cancer: update of an individual patient data meta-analysis. Lung Cancer. 2005;47(1):81-3.

31. Brown BW, Brauner C, Minnotte MC. Noncancer deaths in white adult cancer patients. J Natl Cancer Inst. 1993;85(12):979-87.

32. Adjuvant radiotherapy for rectal cancer: a systematic overview of 8,507 patients from 22 randomised trials. Lancet. 2001;358(9290):1291-304.

33. Clarke M, Collins R, Darby S, et al. Effects of radiotherapy and of differences in the extent of surgery for early breast cancer on local recurrence and 15-year survival: an overview of the randomised trials. Lancet. 2005;366(9503):2087-106.

34. Karadağ O, Demiröz abakay C, Özkan L, Sağlam H, Demirkaya M. Evaluation of late effects of postoperative radiotherapy in patients with medulloblastoma. Turk J Pediatr. 2015;57(2):167-71.

35. Kreiker J, Kattan J. Second colon cancer following Hodgkin's disease. A case report. J Med Liban. 1996;44(2):107-8.

36. Boulaâmane L, Tazi el M, Glaoui M, et al. [Hodgkin's disease and secondary colon cancer: report of a case]. Pan Afr Med J. 2011;9:25.

37. Kleinerman RA. Cancer risks following diagnostic and therapeutic radiation exposure in children. Pediatr Radiol. 2006;36 Suppl 2:121-5.

38. Shore RE, Moseson M, Xue X, Tse Y, Harley N, Pasternack BS. Skin cancer after X-ray treatment for scalp ringworm. Radiat Res. 2002;157(4):410-8.

39. Karagas MR, Nelson HH, Zens MS, et al. Squamous cell and basal cell carcinoma of the skin in relation to radiation therapy and potential modification of risk by sun exposure. Epidemiology. 2007;18(6):776-84.

40. Schellong G, Riepenhausen M, Ehlert K, et al. Breast cancer in young women after treatment for Hodgkin's disease during childhood or adolescence--an observational study with up to 33-year follow-up. Dtsch Arztebl Int. 2014;111(1-2):3-9.

41. Van den belt-dusebout AW, Aleman BM, Besseling G, et al. Roles of radiation dose and chemotherapy in the etiology of stomach cancer as a second malignancy. Int J Radiat Oncol Biol Phys. 2009;75(5):1420-9.

42. Hancock SL, Tucker MA, Hoppe RT. Breast cancer after treatment of Hodgkin's disease. J Natl Cancer Inst. 1993;85(1):25-31.

43. Hauptmann M, Børge johannesen T, Gilbert ES, et al. Increased pancreatic cancer risk following radiotherapy for testicular cancer. Br J Cancer. 2016;115(7):901-8.

44. Hauptmann M, Fossa SD, Stovall M, et al. Increased stomach cancer risk following radiotherapy for testicular cancer. Br J Cancer. 2015;112(1):44-51.

45. Griem ML, Kleinerman RA, Boice JD, Stovall M, Shefner D, Lubin JH. Cancer following radiotherapy for peptic ulcer. J Natl Cancer Inst. 1994;86(11):842-9.

46. Lawrence TS, Ten Haken RK, Giaccia A. Principles of Radiation Oncology. In: DeVita VT Jr., Lawrence TS, Rosenberg SA, editors. *Cancer: Principles and Practice of Oncology*. 8th ed. Philadelphia: Lippincott Williams and Wilkins, 2008.

47. Nagasawa H, Little JB. Induction of sister chromatid exchanges by extremely low doses of alpha-particles. Cancer Res. 1992;52(22):6394-6.

48. Koturbash I, Kutanzi K, Hendrickson K, Rodriguez-juarez R, Kogosov D, Kovalchuk O. Radiation-induced bystander effects in vivo are sex specific. Mutat Res. 2008;642(1-2):28-36.

49. Mothersill C, Bucking C, Smith RW, et al. Communication of radiation-induced stress or bystander signals between fish in vivo. Environ Sci Technol. 2006;40(21):6859-64.

50. Khan MA, Van dyk J, Yeung IW, Hill RP. Partial volume rat lung irradiation; assessment of early DNA damage in different lung regions and effect of radical scavengers. Radiother Oncol. 2003;66(1):95-102.

51. Kovalchuk A, Mychasiuk R, Muhammad A, et al. Liver irradiation causes distal bystander effects in the rat brain and affects animal behaviour. Oncotarget. 2016;7(4):4385-98.

52. Koturbash I, Loree J, Kutanzi K, Koganow C, Pogribny I, Kovalchuk O. In vivo bystander effect: cranial X-irradiation leads to elevated DNA damage, altered cellular proliferation and apoptosis, and increased p53 levels in shielded spleen. Int J Radiat Oncol Biol Phys. 2008;70(2):554-62.

53. Whiteside JR, Mcmillan TJ. A bystander effect is induced in human cells treated with UVA radiation but not UVB radiation. Radiat Res. 2009;171(2):204-11.

54. Hujoel PP, Bollen AM, Noonan CJ, Del aguila MA. Antepartum dental radiography and infant low birth weight. JAMA. 2004;291(16):1987-93.

55. Li F, Liu P, Wang T, et al. The induction of bystander mutagenic effects in vivo by alpha-particle irradiation in whole Arabidopsis thaliana plants. Radiat Res. 2010;174(2):228-37.

56. Shao C, Folkard M, Prise KM. Role of TGF-beta1 and nitric oxide in the bystander response of irradiated glioma cells. Oncogene. 2008;27(4):434-40.

57. Yakovlev VA. Role of nitric oxide in the radiation-induced bystander effect. Redox Biol. 2015;6:396-400.

58. Han W, Wu L, Chen S, et al. Constitutive nitric oxide acting as a possible intercellular signaling molecule in the initiation of radiation-induced DNA double strand breaks in non-irradiated bystander cells. Oncogene. 2007;26(16):2330-9.

59. Xiao L, Liu W, Li J, et al. Irradiated U937 cells trigger inflammatory bystander responses in human umbilical vein endothelial cells through the p38 pathway. Radiat Res. 2014;182(1):111-21.

60. Peer G, Itzhakov E, Wollman Y, et al. Methylene blue, a nitric oxide inhibitor, prevents haemodialysis hypotension. Nephrol Dial Transplant. 2001;16(7):1436-41.

61. Sokolov MV, Smilenov LB, Hall EJ, Panyutin IG, Bonner WM, Sedelnikova OA. Ionizing radiation induces DNA double-strand breaks in bystander primary human fibroblasts. Oncogene. 2005;24(49):7257-65.

62. Shao C, Folkard M, Held KD, Prise KM. Estrogen enhanced cell-cell signalling in breast cancer cells exposed to targeted irradiation. BMC Cancer. 2008;8:184.

63. Boroujerdi, A. Estrogen Exposure Rapidly Elevates Nitric Oxide Production in Cerebral Vessels. [Online]. Available: http://www.urop.uci.edu/journal/journal03/01_AminBoroujerdi/boroujerdi.pdf [December 1, 2016].

64. García-durán M, De frutos T, Díaz-recasens J, et al. Estrogen stimulates neuronal nitric oxide synthase protein expression in human neutrophils. Circ Res. 1999;85(11):1020-6.

65. Han W, Wu L, Chen S, et al. Constitutive nitric oxide acting as a possible intercellular signaling molecule in the initiation of radiation-induced DNA double strand breaks in non-irradiated bystander cells. Oncogene. 2007;26(16):2330-9.

66. Sypniewska RK, Millenbaugh NJ, Kiel JL, et al. Protein changes in macrophages induced by plasma from rats exposed to 35 GHz millimeter waves. Bioelectromagnetics. 2010;31(8):656-63.

67. Pall ML. Electromagnetic fields act via activation of voltage-gated calcium channels to produce beneficial or adverse effects. J Cell Mol Med. 2013;17(8):958-65.

68. Myung SK, Ju W, Mcdonnell DD, et al. Mobile phone use and risk of tumors: a meta-analysis. J Clin Oncol. 2009;27(33):5565-72.

69. Hardell L, Carlberg M, Söderqvist F, Mild KH. Case-control study of the association between malignant brain tumours diagnosed between 2007 and 2009 and mobile and cordless phone use. Int J Oncol. 2013;43(6):1833-45.

70. Morgan LL, Miller AB, Sasco A, Davis DL. Mobile phone radiation causes brain tumors and should be classified as a probable human carcinogen (2A) (review). Int J Oncol. 2015;46(5):1865-71.

71. Crocetti E, Trama A, Stiller C, et al. Epidemiology of glial and non-glial brain tumours in Europe. Eur J Cancer. 2012;48(10):1532-42.

72. Coureau G, Bouvier G, Lebailly P, et al. Mobile phone use and brain tumours in the CERENAT case-control study. Occup Environ Med. 2014;71(7):514-22.

73. Benson VS, Pirie K, Schüz J, et al. Mobile phone use and risk of brain neoplasms and other cancers: prospective study. Int J Epidemiol. 2013;42(3):792-802.

74. Sadetzki S, Chetrit A, Jarus-hakak A, et al. Cellular phone use and risk of benign and malignant parotid gland tumors--a nationwide case-control study. Am J Epidemiol. 2008;167(4):457-67.

75. Karipidis KK, Benke G, Sim MR, et al. Occupational exposure to ionizing and non-ionizing radiation and risk of non-Hodgkin lymphoma. Int Arch Occup Environ Health. 2007;80(8):663-70.

76. West JG, Kapoor NS, Liao SY, Chen JW, Bailey L, Nagourney RA. Multifocal Breast Cancer in Young Women with Prolonged Contact between Their Breasts and Their Cellular Phones. Case Rep Med. 2013;2013:354682.

77. Stang A, Anastassiou G, Ahrens W, Bromen K, Bornfeld N, Jöckel KH. The possible role of radiofrequency radiation in the development of uveal melanoma. Epidemiology. 2001;12(1):7-12.

78. Lala PK, Chakraborty C. Role of nitric oxide in carcinogenesis and tumour progression. Lancet Oncol. 2001;2(3):149-56.

79. Engin AB. Dual function of nitric oxide in carcinogenesis, reappraisal. Curr Drug Metab. 2011;12(9):891-9.

80. Shimon I, Manisterski Y, Kanner AA. Acute cortisol release during stereotactic fractionated radiotherapy to an ACTH-secreting pituitary macroadenoma. Pituitary. 2012;15 Suppl 1:S41-5.

81. Sonveaux P, Brouet A, Havaux X, et al. Irradiation-induced angiogenesis through the up-regulation of the nitric oxide pathway: implications for tumor radiotherapy. Cancer Res. 2003;63(5):1012-9.

82. Hovinga KE, Stalpers LJ, Van bree C, et al. Radiation-enhanced vascular endothelial growth factor (VEGF) secretion in glioblastoma multiforme cell lines--a clue to radioresistance?. J Neurooncol. 2005;74(2):99-103.

83. Ozbilgin MK, Aktas C, Uluer ET, Buyukuysal MC, Gareveran MS, Kurtman C. Influence of Radiation Exposure During Radiotherapy. Evidence for the Increase of Versican and Heparin-Binding EGF-like Growth Factor Concentrations. Anal Quant Cytopathol Histpathol. 2016;38(2):126-32.

84. Kim ES, Choi YE, Hwang SJ, Han YH, Park MJ, Bae IH. IL-4, a direct target of miR-340/429, is involved in radiation-induced aggressive tumor behavior in human carcinoma cells. Oncotarget. 2016.

85. Tabatabaei P, Visse E, Bergström P, Brännström T, Siesjö P, Bergenheim AT. Radiotherapy induces an immediate inflammatory reaction in malignant glioma: a clinical microdialysis study. J Neurooncol. 2016.

86. Yeoh AS, Bowen JM, Gibson RJ, Keefe DM. Nuclear factor kappaB (NFkappaB) and cyclooxygenase-2 (Cox-2) expression in the irradiated colorectum is associated with subsequent histopathological changes. Int J Radiat Oncol Biol Phys. 2005;63(5):1295-303.

87. Ziboh VA, Mallia C, Morhart E, Taylor JR. Induced biosynthesis of cutaneous prostaglandins by ionizing irradiation. Proc Soc Exp Biol Med. 1982;169(3):386-91.

88. Ong ZY, Gibson RJ, Bowen JM, et al. Pro-inflammatory cytokines play a key role in the development of radiotherapy-induced gastrointestinal mucositis. Radiat Oncol. 2010;5:22.

89. Mccue JL, Sheffield JP, Phillips RK. Adjuvant radiotherapy and anastomosis in rectal cancer--disturbing evidence from animal studies. Dis Colon Rectum. 1995;38(2):152-8.

90. Printz C. Radiation treatment generates therapy-resistant cancer stem cells from less aggressive breast cancer cells. Cancer. 2012;118(13):3225.

91. Whitcroft, I. (2008). Why won't our doctors face up to the dangers of radiotherapy? [Online]. Available: http://www.dailymail.co.uk/health/article-1089091/Why-wont-doctors-face-dangers-radiotherapy.html [December 1, 2016].

92. Bogdanich, W. (2010). Radiation Offers New Cures, and Ways to Do Harm. New York Times. [Online]. Available: http://www.nytimes.com/2010/01/24/health/24radiation.html [February 24, 2016].

93. Macbeth FR, Wheldon TE, Girling DJ, et al. Radiation myelopathy: estimates of risk in 1048 patients in three randomized trials of palliative radiotherapy for non-small cell lung cancer. The Medical Research Council Lung Cancer Working Party. Clin Oncol (R Coll Radiol). 1996;8(3):176-81.

94. Keus RB, Rutgers EJ, Ho GH, Gortzak E, Albus-lutter CE, Hart AA. Limb-sparing therapy of extremity soft tissue sarcomas: treatment outcome and long-term functional results. Eur J Cancer. 1994;30A(10):1459-63.

95. Hutchinson ID, Olson J, Lindburg CA, et al. Total-body irradiation produces late degenerative joint damage in rats. Int J Radiat Biol. 2014;90(9):821-30.

96. Kahalley LS, Ris MD, Grosshans DR, et al. Comparing Intelligence Quotient Change After Treatment With Proton Versus Photon Radiation Therapy for Pediatric Brain Tumors. J Clin Oncol. 2016;34(10):1043-9.

97. Greene-schloesser D, Robbins ME, Peiffer AM, Shaw EG, Wheeler KT, Chan MD. Radiation-induced brain injury: A review. Front Oncol. 2012;2:73.

98.   Fernandez G, Pocinho R, Travancinha C, Netto E, Roldão M. Quality of life and radiotherapy in brain metastasis patients. Rep Pract Oncol Radiother. 2012;17(5):281-7.

99.   Dorresteijn LD, Kappelle AC, Boogerd W, et al. Increased risk of ischemic stroke after radiotherapy on the neck in patients younger than 60 years. J Clin Oncol. 2002;20(1):282-8.

100.   Uzun S, Toyran S, Akay F, Gundogan FC. Delayed visual loss due to radiation retinopathy. Pak J Med Sci. 2016;32(2):516-8.

101.   Zeng KL, Kuruvilla S, Sanatani M, Louie AV. Bilateral Blindness Following Chemoradiation for Locally Advanced Oropharyngeal Carcinoma. Cureus. 2015;7(10):e352.

102.   Metz JM, Smith D, Mick R, et al. A phase I study of topical Tempol for the prevention of alopecia induced by whole brain radiotherapy. Clin Cancer Res. 2004;10(19):6411-7.

103.   Kiang JG, Garrison BR, Burns TM, et al. Wound trauma alters ionizing radiation dose assessment. Cell Biosci. 2012;2(1):20.

104.   Wang Q, Dickson GR, Abram WP, Carr KE. Electron irradiation slows down wound repair in rat skin: a morphological investigation. Br J Dermatol. 1994;130(5):551-60.

105.   Tibbs MK. Wound healing following radiation therapy: a review. Radiother Oncol. 1997;42(2):99-106.

106.   Guimas V, Thariat J, Graff-cailleau P, et al. [Intensity modulated radiotherapy for head and neck cancer, dose constraint for normal tissue: Cochlea vestibular apparatus and brainstem]. Cancer Radiother. 2016;20(6-7):475-83.

107.   Upadhya I, Jariwala N, Datar J. Ototoxic effects of irradiation. Indian J Otolaryngol Head Neck Surg. 2011;63(2):151-4.

108.   Kirchmann M, Karnov K, Hansen S, Dethloff T, Stangerup SE, Caye-thomasen P. Ten-Year Follow-up on Tumor Growth and Hearing in Patients Observed With an Intracanalicular Vestibular Schwannoma. Neurosurgery. 2016.

109.   Bass JK, Hua CH, Huang J, et al. Hearing Loss in Patients Who Received Cranial Radiation Therapy for Childhood Cancer. J Clin Oncol. 2016;34(11):1248-55.

110.   Cuomo JR, Sharma GK, Conger PD, Weintraub NL. Novel concepts in radiation-induced cardiovascular disease. World J Cardiol. 2016;8(9):504-519.

111.   Boivin JF, Hutchison GB, Lubin JH, Mauch P. Coronary artery disease mortality in patients treated for Hodgkin's disease. Cancer. 1992;69(5):1241-7.

112.   Gyenes G, Rutqvist LE, Liedberg A, Fornander T. Long-term cardiac morbidity and mortality in a randomized trial of pre- and postoperative radiation therapy versus surgery alone in primary breast cancer. Radiother Oncol. 1998;48(2):185-90.

113.   Fontanelli A, Bernardi G, Morocutti G, Di chiara A. [A case of radiation-induced coronary occlusion treated with elective and emergency PTCA]. G Ital Cardiol. 1995;25(7):877-84.

114.   Roychoudhuri R, Robinson D, Putcha V, Cuzick J, Darby S, Møller H. Increased cardiovascular mortality more than fifteen years after radiotherapy for breast cancer: a population-based study. BMC Cancer. 2007;7:9.

115.   Darby SC, Mcgale P, Taylor CW, Peto R. Long-term mortality from heart disease and lung cancer after radiotherapy for early breast cancer: prospective cohort study of about 300,000 women in US SEER cancer registries. Lancet Oncol. 2005;6(8):557-65.

116.   Standish LJ, Torkelson C, Hamill FA, et al. Immune defects in breast cancer patients after radiotherapy. J Soc Integr Oncol. 2008;6(3):110-21.

117.   Girod DA, Mcculloch TM, Tsue TT, Weymuller EA. Risk factors for complications in clean-contaminated head and neck surgical procedures. Head Neck. 1995;17(1):7-13.

118. Thorgersen EB, Goscinski MA, Spasojevic M, et al. Deep Pelvic Surgical Site Infection After Radiotherapy and Surgery for Locally Advanced Rectal Cancer. Ann Surg Oncol. 2016.

119. Lalla RV, Latortue MC, Hong CH, et al. A systematic review of oral fungal infections in patients receiving cancer therapy. Support Care Cancer. 2010;18(8):985-92.

120. Cheung JP, Mak KC, Tsang HH, Luk KD. A Lethal Sequelae of Spinal Infection Complicating Surgery and Radiotherapy for Head and Neck Cancer. Asian Spine J. 2015;9(4):617-20.

121. Sbitany H, Wang F, Peled AW, et al. Immediate implant-based breast reconstruction following total skin-sparing mastectomy: defining the risk of preoperative and postoperative radiation therapy for surgical outcomes. Plast Reconstr Surg. 2014;134(3):396-404.

122. Low WK, Rangabashyam M, Wang F. Management of major post-cochlear implant wound infections. Eur Arch Otorhinolaryngol. 2014;271(9):2409-13.

123. De araujo TB, Jue xu M, Susarla SM, et al. Impact of Prior Unilateral Chest Wall Radiotherapy on Outcomes in Bilateral Breast Reconstruction. Plast Reconstr Surg. 2016;138(4):575-580.

124. Hughes MA, Parisi M, Grossman S, Kleinberg L. Primary brain tumors treated with steroids and radiotherapy: low CD4 counts and risk of infection. Int J Radiat Oncol Biol Phys. 2005;62(5):1423-6.

125. Azanan MS, Abdullah NK, Chua LL, et al. Immunity in young adult survivors of childhood leukemia is similar to the elderly rather than age-matched controls: Role of cytomegalovirus. Eur J Immunol. 2016;46(7):1715-26.

126. Tabatabaei P, Visse E, Bergström P, Brännström T, Siesjö P, Bergenheim AT. Radiotherapy induces an immediate inflammatory reaction in malignant glioma: a clinical microdialysis study. J Neurooncol. 2016.

127. Poskurica M, Petrović D, Poskurica M. [Acute renal failure in patients with tumour lysis sindrome]. Srp Arh Celok Lek. 2016;144(3-4):232-9.

128. Huang Y, Chen SW, Fan CC, Ting LL, Kuo CC, Chiou JF. Clinical parameters for predicting radiation-induced liver disease after intrahepatic reirradiation for hepatocellular carcinoma. Radiat Oncol. 2016;11(1):89.

129. Kitajima T, Fujimoto Y, Hatano E, et al. Salvage living-donor liver transplantation for liver failure following definitive radiation therapy for recurrent hepatocellular carcinoma: a case report. Transplant Proc. 2015;47(3):804-8.

130. Gebre-medhin M, Haghanegi M, Robért L, Kjellén E, Nilsson P. Dose-volume analysis of radiation-induced trismus in head and neck cancer patients. Acta Oncol. 2016;55(11):1313-1317.

131. Hernández blázquez M, Cruzado JA. A longitudinal study on anxiety, depressive and adjustment disorder, suicide ideation and symptoms of emotional distress in patients with cancer undergoing radiotherapy. J Psychosom Res. 2016;87:14-21.

132. Khalil A, Faheem M, Fahim A, et al. Prevalence of Depression and Anxiety amongst Cancer Patients in a Hospital Setting: A Cross-Sectional Study. Psychiatry J. 2016.

133. Sveistrup J, Mortensen OS, Bjørner JB, Engelholm SA, Munck af rosenschöld P, Petersen PM. Prospective assessment of the quality of life before, during and after image guided intensity modulated radiotherapy for prostate cancer. Radiat Oncol. 2016;11(1):117.

134. Cui W, Bennett AW, Zhang P, et al. A non-human primate model of radiation-induced cachexia. Sci Rep. 2016;6:23612.

135. Dobroś K, Hajto-bryk J, Wróblewska M, Zarzecka J. Radiation-induced caries as the late effect of radiation therapy in the head and neck region. Contemp Oncol (Pozn). 2016;20(4):287-90.

136. Maesschalck T, Dulguerov N, Caparrotti F, et al. Comparison of the incidence of osteoradionecrosis with conventional radiotherapy and intensity-modulated radiotherapy. Head Neck. 2016;38(11):1695-1702.

137. Ship JA, Eisbruch A, D'hondt E, Jones RE. Parotid sparing study in head and neck cancer patients receiving bilateral radiation therapy: one-year results. J Dent Res. 1997;76(3):807-13.

138. Grundmann O, Mitchell GC, Limesand KH. Sensitivity of salivary glands to radiation: from animal models to therapies. J Dent Res. 2009;88(10):894-903.

139. Kangas M, Milross C, Taylor A, Bryant RA. A pilot randomized controlled trial of a brief early intervention for reducing posttraumatic stress disorder, anxiety and depressive symptoms in newly diagnosed head and neck cancer patients. Psychooncology. 2013;22(7):1665-73.

140. Hofman M, Ryan JL, Figueroa-moseley CD, Jean-pierre P, Morrow GR. Cancer-related fatigue: the scale of the problem. Oncologist. 2007;12 Suppl 1:4-10.

141. Ahuja D, Bharati SJ, Gupta N, Kumar R, Bhatnagar S. Possible role of aprepitant for intractable nausea and vomiting following whole brain radiotherapy-a case report. Ann Palliat Med. 2016;5(4):315-318.

142. Spotten L, Corish C, Lorton C, et al. Subjective taste and smell changes in treatment-naive people with solid tumours. Support Care Cancer. 2016;24(7):3201-8.

143. Graner DE, Foote RL, Kasperbauer JL, et al. Swallow function in patients before and after intra-arterial chemoradiation. Laryngoscope. 2003;113(3):573-9.

144. Peters E, Mendoza schulz L, Reuss-borst M. Quality of life after cancer-How the extent of impairment is influenced by patient characteristics. BMC Cancer. 2016;16(1):787.

145. Oates JE, Clark JR, Read J, et al. Prospective evaluation of quality of life and nutrition before and after treatment for nasopharyngeal carcinoma. Arch Otolaryngol Head Neck Surg. 2007;133(6):533-40.

146. Le W, Huang S, Gui Y, et al. Assessment of numerical chromosomal abnormalities of the sperms before and after radiotherapy in seminoma patient. Int J Clin Exp Med. 2014;7(3):703-8.

147. Brignardello E, Felicetti F, Castiglione A, et al. Gonadal status in long-term male survivors of childhood cancer. J Cancer Res Clin Oncol. 2016;142(5):1127-32.

148. Apperley JF, Reddy N. Mechanism and management of treatment-related gonadal failure in recipients of high dose chemoradiotherapy. Blood Rev. 1995;9(2):93-116.

149. Zhou W, Yang X, Dai Y, Wu Q, He G, Yin G. Survey of cervical cancer survivors regarding quality of life and sexual function. J Cancer Res Ther. 2016;12(2):938-44.

150. Bandak M, Jørgensen N, Juul A, et al. Testosterone deficiency in testicular cancer survivors - a systematic review and meta-analysis. Andrology. 2016;4(3):382-8.

151. Resnick MJ, Koyama T, Fan KH, et al. Long-term functional outcomes after treatment for localized prostate cancer. N Engl J Med. 2013;368(5):436-45.

152. Hojan K, Milecki P. Opportunities for rehabilitation of patients with radiation fibrosis syndrome. Rep Pract Oncol Radiother. 2014;19(1):1-6.

153. Kopp H. Radiation damage caused by shoe-fitting fluoroscope. Br Med J. 1957;2(5057):1344-5.

154. Knobf MT, Sun Y. A longitudinal study of symptoms and self-care activities in women treated with primary radiotherapy for breast cancer. Cancer Nurs. 2005;28(3):210-8.

155. Piccin O, Sorrenti G, Milano F. Two Cases of Severe Obstructive Sleep Apnea Induced by Neck Radiotherapy Treated with an Oral Device. J Maxillofac Oral Surg. 2016;15(3):400-403.

156. Bergström L, Ward EC, Finizia C. Voice rehabilitation for laryngeal cancer patients: Functional outcomes and patient perceptions. Laryngoscope. 2016;126(9):2029-35.

157. Alba JR, Basterra J, Ferrer JC, Santonja F, Zapater E. Hypothyroidism in patients treated with radiotherapy for head and neck carcinoma: standardised long-term follow-up study. J Laryngol Otol. 2016;130(5):478-81.

158. Rayome RG, King C, King T. Patient with nocturnal enuresis and stress incontinence after previous hysterectomy and radiation therapy for cervical cancer. J Wound Ostomy Continence Nurs. 1995;22(1):64-7.

159. Faithfull S. 'Just grin and bear it and hope that it will go away': coping with urinary symptoms from pelvic radiotherapy. Eur J Cancer Care (Engl). 1995;4(4):158-65.

160. Kollmorgen CF, Meagher AP, Wolff BG, Pemberton JH, Martenson JA, Illstrup DM. The long-term effect of adjuvant postoperative chemoradiotherapy for rectal carcinoma on bowel function. Ann Surg. 1994;220(5):676-82.

161. Müller K, Meineke V. Radiation-induced mast cell mediators differentially modulate chemokine release from dermal fibroblasts. J Dermatol Sci. 2011;61(3):199-205.

162. Müller K, Gilbertz KP, Meineke V. Serotonin and ionizing radiation synergistically affect proliferation and adhesion molecule expression of malignant melanoma cells. J Dermatol Sci. 2012;68(2):89-98.

163. Sohun M, Shen H. The implication and potential applications of high-mobility group box 1 protein in breast cancer. Ann Transl Med. 2016;4(11):217.

164. Azzam EI, Jay-gerin JP, Pain D. Ionizing radiation-induced metabolic oxidative stress and prolonged cell injury. Cancer Lett. 2012;327(1-2):48-60.

165. Bravatà V, Minafra L, Russo G, et al. High-dose Ionizing Radiation Regulates Gene Expression Changes in the MCF7 Breast Cancer Cell Line. Anticancer Res. 2015;35(5):2577-91.

166. Constine LS, Rubin P, Woolf PD, Doane K, Lush CM. Hyperprolactinemia and hypothyroidism following cytotoxic therapy for central nervous system malignancies. J Clin Oncol. 1987;5(11):1841-51.

167. Judge JL, Owens KM, Pollock SJ, et al. Ionizing radiation induces myofibroblast differentiation via lactate dehydrogenase. Am J Physiol Lung Cell Mol Physiol. 2015;309(8):879-887.

CHAPTER 4

EARLY DETECTION, EARLY CURE?

LIKE ALL BUSINESSES, the cancer industry requires a steady flow of customers in order to generate revenue. The way it accomplishes this is by popularizing the idea that detecting and treating cancer in its early stages improves survival. 'Early detection saves lives' is a marketing strategy used to motivate people who have no signs or symptoms of cancer, to undergo regular screening for cancer.

The World Health Organization claims that "Cancer mortality can be reduced if cases are detected and treated early,"[1] and the American Cancer Society states, "Most doctors feel that early detection tests for breast cancer save thousands of lives each year. Many more lives probably could be saved if even more women and their health care providers took advantage of these tests."[2]

If early detection and treatment do in fact save lives, then this is indeed a righteous proposal, but the thing about 'early detection' is that - in order for it to be beneficial - the 'early treatment' that follows must be effective. And based on our investigations into orthodox cancer treatments in the preceding chapters, it seems incredibly unlikely that inflicting severe damage upon a sick person *at any stage* of their illness could improve their health. But rather than speculating, let's take a closer look at two of the most popular cancer screening tests and decide for ourselves if we think early detection saves lives.

THE PSA TEST - PROSTATE CANCER SCREENING

For a man, the road to being diagnosed with prostate cancer begins with a blood test called the prostate-specific antigen (PSA) test. A urologist might claim the PSA test is an accurate way to detect prostate cancer, but when we take a closer look, we come face-to-face with an uncomfortable reality: PSA cannot diagnose prostate cancer.[3] Dr. Richard Ablin - the man who discovered the prostate-specific antigen in 1970 - calls the widespread misuse of the PSA test "a public health disaster."

In his book *The Great Prostate Hoax*, Dr. Ablin reveals that prostate-specific antigen - a protein secreted by the prostate - is not cancer-specific. In other words, PSA is secreted by all prostates - both healthy and cancerous - and therefore, using it as a screening tool for prostate cancer is completely inappropriate.

If a man has his PSA levels tested and they end up being 4 or higher, the doctor will refer him to a urologist for a biopsy, which is the next step on the assembly line towards radiotherapy or surgical removal of the prostate (radical prostatectomy). But since PSA levels are increased by exercise, ejaculation and everyday stress, using them to determine whether or not a man is at risk for having cancer is no better than a coin toss. "You can biopsy according to whether a man has blue eyes or green eyes and get pretty much the same results as biopsying according to PSA," wrote Urologist Thomas Stamey, MD. "It is vital to understand that a man might have a PSA of 0.5 and have prostate cancer, yet another man whose number is an alarming 11 could be cancer free," Dr. Ablin explains.

Dr. Thomas Stamey and his colleagues at Stanford University studied prostate tissues collected over a 20-year period since the dawn of the PSA test in the early 1990's. Their 2004 study focused the scientific community's attention on what PSA-pioneer Dr. Richard Ablin had been saying for decades – the PSA test is virtually worthless in determining if men have prostate cancer; "the test indicates nothing more than the size of the prostate gland," Dr. Stamey declared, "The prostate specific antigen era in the united states is over."[4]

In 2011, the U.S. Preventive Services Task Force - an independent group of national experts in prevention and evidence-based medicine – reversed their previous position and recommended against the use of PSA screening with "moderate or high certainty that the service has no net benefit or that the harms outweigh the benefits."[5]

A CLOSER LOOK...

- Scientists from Rockville, Maryland conducted an updated review on PSA screening in 2011. Results showed that "After about 10 years, PSA-based screening results in the detection of more cases of prostate cancer, but small to no reduction in prostate cancer-specific mortality."[6]

- 76,685 men aged 55-74 years were examined for prostate mortality after undergoing the PSA test in *The Prostate, Lung, Colorectal, and Ovarian (PLCO) Cancer Screening Trial* of 2012. Published in the *Journal of the National Cancer Institute*, the study found "no evidence of a mortality benefit for organized annual [PSA] screening" after 13-years of follow-up. In fact, prostate cancer mortality was slightly *increased* in the screened group: 3.7 per 10,000 person-years, versus 3.4 for unscreened men.[7]

- A 2012 study published in *The New England Journal of Medicine* compared the efficacy of surgery versus no treatment in men diagnosed with prostate cancer by the PSA test. The study concluded that "radical prostatectomy [surgery] did not significantly reduce all-cause or prostate-cancer mortality, as compared with observation, through at least 12 years of follow-up."[8]

Despite clear evidence showing PSA screening fails to reduce mortality from prostate cancer[6-8] and the recommendation against the use of the PSA test by the Task Force, seductive celebrity-endorsed marketing campaigns pushing "prostate cancer awareness" continue luring men in to have their

PSA's tested to this day.[9] Once the money train begins to roll, it can be difficult to stop.

"The prostate gland is at the epicenter of a worldwide trillion-dollar industry and the PSA test is its kingpin... if the test were made irrelevant, an industry would crumble."
- Dr. Richard Ablin

OVERDIAGNOSIS AND OVERTREATMENT

Of the 3.7 million men diagnosed with prostate cancer in the US between 1986 and 2005, "our paper estimates about 1.3 million are attributable solely to the test... and would not have occurred without it," said Dr. H. Gilbert Welch about his 2009 study published in the *Journal of the National Cancer Institute.*[10]

If the PSA test was only finding cancers that were problematic, explains Dr. Welch, the number of new prostate cancer cases would have stayed the same in the early 1990's after the test was introduced. But instead, the number of diagnosed cancer cases skyrocketed, and the rate is still higher than it used to be. "It looks more like a stock market graph than a graph of cancer biology," says Welch. "These are the most erratic graphs in cancer anywhere."[11]

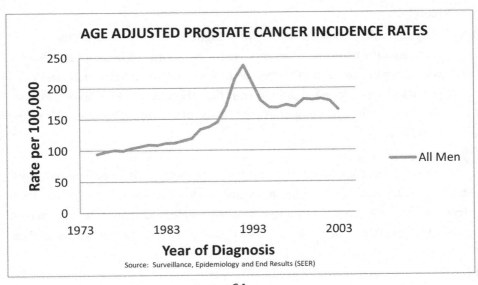

AGE ADJUSTED PROSTATE CANCER INCIDENCE RATES

Rate per 100,000

All Men

Year of Diagnosis

Source: Surveillance, Epidemiology and End Results (SEER)

As a consequence of using the PSA test to detect prostate cancer, as many as 85% of men diagnosed with the disease don't have anything that will ever kill or even harm them at all.[12,13] What they have shouldn't even be called cancer and tragically, many end up receiving unnecessary cancer treatments which often result in severe, life-changing side effects.

A BIG PRICE TO PAY

During a prostate biopsy, a urologist will stick an 18-gauge needle through a man's rectal wall into his prostate gland 6 to 12 times, punching out core tissues for examination. It's well-established that biopsies suppress the immune system and promote cancer metastasis,[14-17] but there are a number of other reasons why a man might want to avoid a prostate biopsy.

A biopsy of the prostate can cause residual pain, blood in the urine, rectal bleeding,[18] erectile dysfunction,[19] and life-threatening infections.[20,21] This is probably because the biopsy needle first enters the rectum before piercing through the rectal wall into the prostate, which drags bacteria and fecal matter along with it. "The risk of hospitalization within 30 days of prostate biopsy was significantly higher than in a control population."[22] But the damage caused by punching holes in the prostate is minor compared to irradiating or surgically removing the prostate.

The two most common complications associated with having the prostate gland irradiated or removed are involuntary urination (urinary incontinence) and erectile dysfunction. *The New England Journal of Medicine* published a study in 2013 reporting that erectile dysfunction was "nearly universal" in patients 15 years after treatment for prostate cancer; "87.0% of those in the prostatectomy group and 93.9% of those in the radiotherapy group reporting an inability to achieve an erection sufficient for intercourse." Furthermore, all men experienced a decline in urinary continence that worsened as time went on. Some men had to wear diapers to prevent urinary leakage for the full 15-year follow-up period and probably for the rest of their lives.[23]

Despite the fact that the PSA test cannot detect prostate cancer and the extraordinary risk of a man having his sexuality and dignity stolen as a consequence of the test, almost 66% of men who undergo the PSA test are not even aware they've had it done;[24] their doctors simply do it as part of their routine physical, without their consent and without telling them the potential implications.[25]

MAMMOGRAPHY - BREAST CANCER SCREENING

First introduced in the 1970's,[26] mammography is an x-ray procedure that captures a photograph of the human breast used to detect breast cancer. While those who are invested in expensive mammography machinery or who rely on breast cancer screening to earn a living will assure you that mammography reduces breast cancer death rates, a number of large-scale studies have demonstrated that mammography provides no mortality benefit.[27-29]

A CLOSER LOOK...

- The *Canadian National Breast Screening Study 1* involved 50,000 women aged 40 to 49 years and compared women who received 5 years of annual mammography screening and physical breast examinations with women who received only one physical breast examination. The study found that five annual mammograms and breast examinations in women aged 40 to 49 caused "no reduction in breast cancer mortality."[27]
- The *Canadian National Breast Screening Study 2* involved 40,000 women aged 50 to 59 years and compared women who received five years of physical breast exams and mammography screening with women who received physical examinations only. The study concluded that in women aged 50 to 59, "the addition of annual mammography screening to physical examination has no impact on breast cancer mortality."[28]
- The 25-year combined follow-up of the *Canadian National Breast Screening Study 1 and 2* was one of the largest and most meticulous studies ever conducted on mammography. Published in the *British Medical Journal* in 2014, results showed that "Annual mammography in women aged 40-59 does not reduce mortality from breast cancer beyond that of physical examination..."[29]

OVERDIAGNOSIS AND OVERTREATMENT

One of the major failures of mammography is how frequently it results in misdiagnosis of breast cancer. Over the course of 10 mammograms, women in the United States have between a 58-77% chance of being falsely diagnosed with breast cancer.[30] Another study found that for women with multiple breast cancer risk factors, like a strong family history, prolonged use of the contraceptive pill, etc. – the ones most strongly urged to have annual mammograms – the 10-year cumulative risk of being falsely diagnosed is "as high as 100 percent."[31] And of course, most will end up undergoing unnecessary treatments and suffering the horrendous side effects and mutilations associated with surgery and radiotherapy.

A 2012 study published in the *New England Journal of Medicine* concluded that one in three women (33%) diagnosed with breast cancer from a mammogram are misdiagnosed, and that a whopping 1.3 million women have been overdiagnosed by mammography in the past 30 years.[32]

A BIG PRICE TO PAY

Although the PSA test and mammography both fail to achieve their intended purpose of prolonging life, the PSA test involves only a blood sample while mammography exposes patients to damaging ionizing radiation and other harmful procedures.

First, the breast is tightly (and often painfully[33]) compressed between two imaging plates. If cancer is present in the breast during this compression it can result in metastasis.[34] Next, the x-ray image is taken and the patient receives a 10 mSv (millisievert) dose of ionizing radiation, approximately "1000 times greater than that from a chest x-ray," according to Dr. Samuel Epstein.[35]

THE DANGERS OF LOW-DOSE IONIZING RADIATION

The US government has long-held the position that low-doses of ionizing radiation are not hazardous to human health,[36] but since the early 1950's scientific research has indicated repeatedly that low-doses of radiation, like those administered to patients during x-ray imaging, do in fact cause increased rates of cancer.[37-53]

A CLOSER LOOK...

- Researchers from the University of California investigated the relationship between x-ray exposure early in life and childhood leukemia in 2010. "Exposure to post-natal diagnostic X-rays is associated with increased risk of childhood ALL [acute childhood leukemia], the study concluded."[53]

- A 1981 study published in *The Lancet* looked at cancer incidence in female factory workers who had been producing paint containing the radioactive element radium. The workers received radiation doses of 1-4mGy (milligray) per week and the study found, "Those in the group who were under 30 years of age when they started work show a significantly increased risk of dying from breast cancer."[46]

- In 1989, scientists from Atlanta, Georgia investigated 1,030 women with scoliosis who had received multiple x-rays during childhood. Published in *The Journal of the National Cancer Institute*, at an average follow-up of 26 years, the study found an 83% greater incidence of cancer in the women compared to the general population. Importantly, their rate of cancer actually increased with time; women assessed more than 30 years later had a 140% greater incidence of cancer than the general population.[43]

LOW DOSES WORSE THAN HIGHER DOSES

Groundbreaking research, mostly on atomic bomb survivors and nuclear workers, is beginning to uncover a startling detail – not only are low doses of ionizing radiation enough to cause cancer, but low doses can actually be *more harmful* than larger ones.[54-57] E.B. Burlakova, director of the Radiobiology Committee of the Russian Academy of Sciences, has published a number of studies showing that the true dose-response of ionizing radiation is *biphasic*, meaning the damage increases from zero dose and then falls and then increases again.[58]

A Closer Look...

- A 2008 study from Japan compared cancer prevalence in Hiroshima atomic bomb survivors with an unexposed population. The study found a significantly elevated risk of cancer in the exposed population, "Even at low and very low dose categories."[56]

- Italian researchers exposed a group of mice to 1 Gy (gray) of ionizing radiation and another group of mice to 0.1 Gy of ionizing radiation and compared the effects. Results were published in the *International Journal of Radiation Biology* in 2008 and found, "In mice exposed to 1 Gy genetic damage was initially high and decreased during the experimental-time, while in the 0.1 Gy group damage, at first low, persisted and slightly increased."[54]

- In 2016, researchers from Germany and Latvia questioned the validity of the current worldwide radiation risk model by investigating the genetic risks of exposure to low doses of radiation. The study found that, "Nearly all types of hereditary defects were found at doses as low as one to 10 mSv" and concluded that the current worldwide risk model for genetic effects of ionizing radiation is unsafe. Importantly, their work "supports a dose response relationship which is non-linear and is either biphasic or supralinear (hogs-back) and largely either saturates or falls above 10 mSv."[57]

How can a lower dose of ionizing radiation be *more* harmful than a larger dose? "Cancer arises when the DNA in cells is damaged, but the cells are not killed. Higher radiation doses are more likely to kill cells outright. So the lower doses are disproportionately carcinogenic," explains scientist Dr. Chris Busby.[59]

I asked Dr. Ray Peat the same question and he wrote, "The greatest effect per dose at low doses is sort of analogous to a car getting good gas mileage at low speeds with low wind resistance, compared to poor gas mileage at 80 to 100 mph, with considerable wind resistance. It isn't surprising if you think in terms of 'relatively mild electronic excitation,' producing chronic inflammatory signals, rather than all-or-nothing mutagenic events."

IS X-RAY IMAGING WORTH THE RISK?

A number of outspoken scientists have come to some startling conclusions regarding the use of medical imaging that the world needs to know about.

In 1971, Dr. Robert W. Gibson and his colleagues at the University of Buffalo conducted a study on the health effects of low-dose radiation from x-ray imaging. The researchers concluded that undergoing less than a dozen routine medical x-rays to the same part of the body increases the risk of leukemia by *at least* 60%.[60]

Dr. Irwin Bross headed the Tri-State Leukemia Study in the 1970's to determine what had been causing the alarming increases in leukemia at the time. The experiment included 16 million people from New York, Maryland, and Minnesota, and after exploring wide-ranging factors - including health history, occupational history, residential history, family background, cause of death for parents and grandparents, exposure to farm animals, pet ownership, whether or not the pets had ever been sick - Dr. Bross concluded that medical radiation in the form of diagnostic medical x-rays was *the main cause* of the rising rates of leukemia.[61]

Dr. John Gofman, medical physicist from the University of California, became a spokesman for the United States Atomic Energy Commission in the 1940's and spent almost 30 years travelling around glorifying the use of x-rays and other forms of radiation while denying that ionizing radiation had any harmful effects. Then, right in the middle of one of his speeches in the late 1960's, he realized that what he had been saying for three decades was insane:

"The big moment in my life happened while I was giving a health lecture to nuclear engineers. In the middle of my talk it hit me! What the hell am I saying? If you don't know whether low doses are safe or not, going ahead is exactly wrong. At that moment, I changed my position entirely."

Dr. Gofman suddenly went from being a government and nuclear industry 'talking head' to one of their biggest threats and soon found himself campaigning against the use of nuclear and medical x-ray technologies as well as writing a number of groundbreaking books.

The most significant conclusion made by Dr. Gofman after a lifetime of investigation into the biological effects of low-dose x-ray radiation was that accumulated radiation exposure from medical diagnostics is *the main cause* of over 50% of cancer deaths, 60% of heart disease deaths and over 80% of breast cancer deaths in the United States. While Dr. Gofman acknowledged other causes of cancer such as smoking, poor food quality and environmental toxins, he maintained that more than half the deaths from cancer and heart disease would not have occurred if it weren't for medical x-rays.[62]

Of course, none of the evidence above can be officially acknowledged or it would mean the death of the entire nuclear industry: power, weapons and medical imaging.

CANCER SCREENING: A PUBLIC HEALTH DISASTER

If mammography reveals an abnormality that the doctor suspects might be cancer, a biopsy will be performed. And if the biopsy reveals what the doctor interprets to be cancer, the woman suddenly becomes a breast cancer patient and will receive the whole works - surgery, chemotherapy and radiotherapy.

Despite evidence showing that surgical removal of one or both breasts (mastectomy) results in increased tumor recurrences and higher mortality,[63] or at best provides no additional benefit,[64] mastectomies have been on the rise in recent years.[65]

A CLOSER LOOK...

- A 1995 study published in the *New England Journal of Medicine* followed up with breast cancer patients 10-years after receiving a mastectomy (surgical removal of one or both breasts) or a simple lumpectomy (surgical removal of only the tumor and some surrounding tissue) followed by whole-breast irradiation. Patients who received the mastectomy had more tumor recurrences and higher mortality 10-years following treatment than those who received the less invasive lumpectomy.[63]

This trend has a lot to do with the dramatic increase in biased media coverage of celebrity mastectomies since 2004, wrote scientists from the University of Michigan. "The surgical treatment was significantly more likely to be mentioned [in the media] when a celebrity had bilateral mastectomies than unilateral mastectomy or breast conservation," their study concluded.[66]

One of the side effects a surgeon will probably fail to mention before performing a mastectomy is the subsequent almost-universal decline in self-esteem that women experience following the procedure.[67,68] "Patients who had had a mastectomy felt less attractive, less sexually desirable, and more ashamed of their breasts. They also experienced less enjoyment in their sexual relationships than they had before treatment."[69] To combat this hopelessness, many women return to their surgeons for breast implants, which unfortunately, only make a bad situation worse; as breast implants following mastectomy have been associated with a 3-fold increase in the risk of suicide.[70]

Now we return to our original question from the beginning of this chapter: does early detection and treatment of cancer save lives?

We've examined a number of studies showing that neither the PSA test nor mammography provide any mortality benefit whatsoever to the men and women who undergo them. Rather than saving lives, the widespread implementation of prostate and breast cancer screening has only enhanced the amount of men and women diagnosed and treated for cancer.

While this is obviously a lucrative and rewarding situation for the cancer industry, the mass overdiagnosis and overtreatment that sustains the booming cancer business comes at a considerable price; it means patients are frequently told they have cancer when they don't, and are frequently treated aggressively for diseases they don't have.

Maybe this is why Dr. Dean Burk once said of the American Cancer Society, "They lie like scoundrels," or why Dr. James Watson, the man who discovered DNA, declared before the California Assembly Committee of Health in 1976, "The American public is being sold a nasty bill of goods about cancer... Today, the press releases coming out of the National Cancer Institute have all the honesty of the Pentagon's."

TIMELESS QUOTES

"It is utter nonsense to claim that catching cancer symptoms early enough will increase the patient's chances of survival: not one scientist or study has proven that in any way."
- Dr. Hardin B. Jones

"There is simply no evidence that early detection of prostate cancer improves the health of patients."
- Dr. Steven H. Woolf, science advisor for US Preventive Services Task Force

"We're going to look back at this century and we're going to laugh eventually, but we'll cry first. This is one of the most barbaric periods. It's going to be called the Dark Ages of Medicine."
- Dr. Richard Shulze

REFERENCES

1. World Health Organization. (2017). Cancer Fact Sheet. Available: http://www.who.int/mediacentre/factsheets/fs297/en. [February 3rd, 2017].

2. American Cancer Society. Breast Cancer Early Detection and Diagnosis. Available: https://www.cancer.org/cancer/breast-cancer/screening-tests-and-early-detection.html. [January 15th, 2017].

3. Kuriyama M, Wang MC, Lee CL, et al. Multiple marker evaluation in human prostate cancer with the use of tissue-specific antigens. J Natl Cancer Inst. 1982;68(1):99-105.

4. Stamey TA, Caldwell M, Mcneal JE, Nolley R, Hemenez M, Downs J. The prostate specific antigen era in the United States is over for prostate cancer: what happened in the last 20 years?. J Urol. 2004;172(4 Pt 1):1297-301.

5. Volk RJ, Wolf AM. Grading the new US Preventive Services Task Force prostate cancer screening recommendation. JAMA. 2011;306(24):2715-6.

6. Lin K, Croswell JM, Koenig H, Lam C, Maltz A. Prostate-Specific Antigen-Based Screening for Prostate Cancer: An Evidence Update for the U.S. Preventive Services Task Force. 2011; report no. 12-05160-EF-1.

7. Andriole GL, Crawford ED, Grubb RL, et al. Prostate cancer screening in the randomized Prostate, Lung, Colorectal, and Ovarian Cancer Screening Trial: mortality results after 13 years of follow-up. J Natl Cancer Inst. 2012;104(2):125-32.

8. Wilt TJ, Brawer MK, Jones KM, et al. Radical prostatectomy versus observation for localized prostate cancer. N Engl J Med. 2012;367(3):203-13.

9. Ablin J.R. 2010. The Great Prostate Mistake. *The New York Times.* Available: http://www.nytimes.com/2010/03/10/opinion/10Ablin.html. [February 3, 2017].

10. Welch HG, Albertsen PC. Prostate cancer diagnosis and treatment after the introduction of prostate-specific antigen screening: 1986-2005. J Natl Cancer Inst. 2009;101(19):1325-9.

11. Langreth, R. 2009. The Dark Side of Prostate Cancer Screening. *Forbes.* Available: http://www.forbes.com/2009/08/31/prostate-cancer-screening-business-healthcare-prostate.html. [February 3, 2017].

12. Aizer AA, Gu X, Chen MH, et al. Cost implications and complications of overtreatment of low-risk prostate cancer in the United States. J Natl Compr Canc Netw. 2015;13(1):61-8.

13. Seu K, Casciotti D, Bravo BFD, Chen M, Jury NJ. 2016. Are annual prostate cancer screenings necessary? Should early stage prostate cancer be treated? *National Center for Health Research.* Available: http://center4research.org/child-teen-health/general-health-and-mental-health/are-annual-prostate-cancer-screenings-necessary-should-early-stage-prostate-cancer-be-treated. [February 3, 2017].

14. Hansen NM, Ye X, Grube BJ, Giuliano AE. Manipulation of the primary breast tumor and the incidence of sentinel node metastases from invasive breast cancer. Arch Surg. 2004;139(6):634-9.

15. Hoover HC, Ketcham AS. Techniques for inhibiting tumor metastases. Cancer. 1975;35(1):5-14.

16. Mathenge EG, Dean CA, Clements D, et al. Core needle biopsy of breast cancer tumors increases distant metastases in a mouse model. Neoplasia. 2014;16(11):950-60.

17. Hobson J, Gummadidala P, Silverstrim B, et al. Acute inflammation induced by the biopsy of mouse mammary tumors promotes the development of metastasis. Breast Cancer Res Treat. 2013;139(2):391-401.

18. Rosario DJ, Lane JA, Metcalfe C, et al. Short term outcomes of prostate biopsy in men tested for cancer by prostate specific antigen: prospective evaluation within ProtecT study. BMJ. 2012;344:d7894.

19. Helfand BT, Glaser AP, Rimar K, et al. Prostate cancer diagnosis is associated with an increased risk of erectile dysfunction after prostate biopsy. BJU Int. 2013;111(1):38-43.

20. Hwang EC, Yu HS, Jung SI, Park HJ. Infectious Complications after Prostate Biopsy: A Prospective Multicenter Prostate Biopsy Study. Urogenit Tract Infect 2016;11(1):17-24.

21. Gallina A, Suardi N, Montorsi F, et al. Mortality at 120 days after prostatic biopsy: a population-based study of 22,175 men. Int J Cancer. 2008;123(3):647-52.

22. Loeb S, Carter HB, Berndt SI, Ricker W, Schaeffer EM. Complications after prostate biopsy: data from SEER-Medicare. J Urol. 2011;186(5):1830-4.

23. Resnick MJ, Koyama T, Fan KH, Albertsen PC, Goodman M, Hamilton AS, Hoffman RM, Potosky AL, Stanford JL, Stroup AM, Van Horn RL, Penson DF. Long-term functional outcomes after treatment for localized prostate cancer. N Engl J Med 2013;368(5):436-45. doi: 10.1056/NEJMoa1209978. Urol Oncol. 2013;32(4):513-4.

24. Lamplugh M, Gilmore P, Quinlan T, Cornford P. PSA testing: are patients aware of what lies ahead?. Ann R Coll Surg Engl. 2006;88(3):284-8.

25. Justman S. Uninformed consent: mass screening for prostate cancer. Bioethics. 2012;26(3):143-8.

26. Retsky M, Demicheli R, Hrushesky W, Baum M, Gukas I. Surgery triggers outgrowth of latent distant disease in breast cancer: an inconvenient truth?. Cancers (Basel). 2010;2(2):305-37.

27. Miller AB, To T, Baines CJ, Wall C. The Canadian National Breast Screening Study-1: breast cancer mortality after 11 to 16 years of follow-up. A randomized screening trial of mammography in women age 40 to 49 years. Ann Intern Med. 2002;137(5 Part 1):305-12.

28. Miller AB, To T, Baines CJ, Wall C. Canadian National Breast Screening Study-2: 13-year results of a randomized trial in women aged 50-59 years. J Natl Cancer Inst. 2000;92(18):1490-9.

29. Miller AB, Wall C, Baines CJ, Sun P, To T, Narod SA. Twenty five year follow-up for breast cancer incidence and mortality of the Canadian National Breast Screening Study: randomised screening trial. BMJ. 2014;348:g366.

30. Von euler-chelpin M, Kuchiki M, Vejborg I. Increased risk of breast cancer in women with false-positive test: the role of misclassification. Cancer Epidemiol. 2014;38(5):619-22.

31. Christiansen CL, Wang F, Barton MB, et al. Predicting the cumulative risk of false-positive mammograms. J Natl Cancer Inst. 2000;92(20):1657-66.

32. Bleyer A, Welch HG. Effect of three decades of screening mammography on breast-cancer incidence. N Engl J Med. 2012;367(21):1998-2005.

33. Kornguth PJ, Keefe FJ, Conaway MR. Pain during mammography: characteristics and relationship to demographic and medical variables. Pain. 1996;66(2-3):187-94.

34. Van netten JP, Cann SA, Hall JG. Mammography controversies: time for informed consent?. J Natl Cancer Inst. 1997;89(15):1164-5.

35. Epstein SE. 2002. Mammography Doesn't Come Without Risk. Los Angeles Times. Available: http://articles.latimes.com/2002/feb/25/opinion/oe-epstein25 [February 3, 2017].

36. Eon3. Sept 29, 2015. Pt. 1 – Medical X-rays and Breast Cancer – Dr. John Gofman. Available: https://www.youtube.com/watch?v=AzW0zIjKcmE [February 3, 2017].

37. Modan B, Ron E, Werner A. Thyroid cancer following scalp irradiation. Radiology. 1977;123(3):741-4.

38. Boice JD, Preston D, Davis FG, Monson RR. Frequent chest X-ray fluoroscopy and breast cancer incidence among tuberculosis patients in Massachusetts. Radiat Res. 1991;125(2):214-22.

39. Baverstock KF, Vennart J. A note on radium body content and breast cancer in U.K. radium luminisers. Health Phys. 1983;44 Suppl 1:575-7.

40.   Boice JD, Monson RR. Breast cancer in women after repeated fluoroscopic examinations of the chest. J Natl Cancer Inst. 1977;59(3):823-32.

41.   Boice JD, Rosenstein M, Trout ED. Estimation of breast doses and breast cancer risk associated with repeated fluoroscopic chest examinations of women with tuberculosis. Radiat Res. 1978;73(2):373-90.

42.   Harvey EB, Boice JD, Honeyman M, Flannery JT. Prenatal x-ray exposure and childhood cancer in twins. N Engl J Med. 1985;312(9):541-5.

43.   Hoffman DA, Lonstein JE, Morin MM, Visscher W, Harris BS, Boice JD. Breast cancer in women with scoliosis exposed to multiple diagnostic x rays. J Natl Cancer Inst. 1989;81(17):1307-12.

44.   Miller AB, Howe GR, Sherman GJ, et al. Mortality from breast cancer after irradiation during fluoroscopic examinations in patients being treated for tuberculosis. N Engl J Med. 1989;321(19):1285-9.

45.   Modan B, Chetrit A, Alfandary E, Katz L. Increased risk of breast cancer after low-dose irradiation. Lancet. 1989;1(8639):629-31.

46.   Baverstock KF, Papworth D, Vennart J. Risks of radiation at low dose rates. Lancet. 1981;1(8217):430-3.

47.   Myrden JA, Hiltz JE. Breast cancer following multiple fluoroscopies during artificial pneumothorax treatment of pulmonary tuberculosis. Can Med Assoc J. 1969;100(22):1032-4.

48.   Giles D, Hewitt D, Stewart A, Webb J. Malignant disease in childhood and diagnostic irradiation in utero. Lancet. 1956;271(6940):447.

49.   Stewart A, Webb J, Hewitt D. A survey of childhood malignancies. Br Med J. 1958;1(5086):1495-508.

50.   Stewart A, Kneale GW. Radiation dose effects in relation to obstetric x-rays and childhood cancers. Lancet. 1970;1(7658):1185-8.

51.   Andrieu N, Easton DF, Chang-claude J, et al. Effect of chest X-rays on the risk of breast cancer among BRCA1/2 mutation carriers in the international BRCA1/2 carrier cohort study: a report from the EMBRACE, GENEPSO, GEO-HEBON, and IBCCS Collaborators' Group. J Clin Oncol. 2006;24(21):3361-6.

52.   Giles D, Hewitt D, Stewart A, Webb J. Malignant disease in childhood and diagnostic irradiation in utero. Lancet. 1956;271(6940):447.

53.   Bartley K, Metayer C, Selvin S, Ducore J, Buffler P. Diagnostic X-rays and risk of childhood leukaemia. Int J Epidemiol. 2010;39(6):1628-37.

54.   Giovanetti A, Deshpande T, Basso E. Persistence of genetic damage in mice exposed to low dose of X rays. Int J Radiat Biol. 2008;84(3):227-35.

55.   Goto H, Watanabe T, Miyao M, Fukuda H, Sato Y, Oshida Y. Cancer mortality among atomic bomb survivors exposed as children. Environ Health Prev Med. 2012;17(3):228-34.

56.   Watanabe T, Miyao M, Honda R, Yamada Y. Hiroshima survivors exposed to very low doses of A-bomb primary radiation showed a high risk for cancers. Environ Health Prev Med. 2008;13(5):264-70.

57.   Schmitz-feuerhake I, Busby C, Pflugbeil S. Genetic radiation risks: a neglected topic in the low dose debate. Environ Health Toxicol. 2016;31:e2016001.

58.   Burlakova, E.B. 2000. *Low Doses of Radiation: Are They Dangerous?* Nova Science Pub Inc. 378 pps.

59.   Busby, C. (2016). The 'Genetics' letter, the Euratom suicide clause, and the death of the nuclear industry. *The   Ecologist.*   Available: http://www.theecologist.org/campaigning/2988466/the_genetics_letter_the_euratom_suicide_clause_and_t he_death_of_the_nuclear_industry.html. [February 3, 2017].

60.   R.W. Gibson, M.D., National Enquirer, December 5, 1971, 11) as reported in the book Indicted!: The People Vs the Medical & Drug Cartel by James Henderson. (2009).

61.   Leslie Freeman, ed., Nuclear Witnesses: Insiders Speak Out, New York: Norton, 1982, p.27.

62.   Peat, R. (2011). Radiation and growth: Incoherent imprinting from inappropriate irradiation. Available: http://raypeat.com/pdf/Radiation-and-Growth-January-2011.pdf. [February 3, 2017].

63. Jacobson JA, Danforth DN, Cowan KH, et al. Ten-year results of a comparison of conservation with mastectomy in the treatment of stage I and II breast cancer. N Engl J Med. 1995;332(14):907-11.

64. Vila J, Gandini S, Gentilini O. Overall survival according to type of surgery in young (≤40 years) early breast cancer patients: A systematic meta-analysis comparing breast-conserving surgery versus mastectomy. Breast. 2015;24(3):175-81.

65. Kummerow KL, Du L, Penson DF, Shyr Y, Hooks MA. Nationwide trends in mastectomy for early-stage breast cancer. JAMA Surg. 2015;150(1):9-16.

66. Sabel MS, Dal cin S. Trends in Media Reports of Celebrities' Breast Cancer Treatment Decisions. Ann Surg Oncol. 2016;23(9):2795-801.

67. Polivy J. Psychological effects of mastectomy on a woman's feminine self-concept. J Nerv Ment Dis. 1977;164(2):77-87.

68. José Manuel García Arroyo and María Luisa Domínguez López, "Psychological Problems Derived from Mastectomy: A Qualitative Study," International Journal of Surgical Oncology, vol. 2011, Article ID 132461, 8 pages, 2011.

69. Margolis G, Goodman RL, Rubin A. Psychological effects of breast-conserving cancer treatment and mastectomy. Psychosomatics. 1990;31(1):33-9.

70. Le GM, O'malley CD, Glaser SL, et al. Breast implants following mastectomy in women with early-stage breast cancer: prevalence and impact on survival. Breast Cancer Res. 2005;7(2):184-193.

CHAPTER 5

THE BATTLE FOR TRUTH

A MONUMENTAL RULING was made in US federal court in 2006 when a judge declared cigarette manufacturers *guilty* of conspiracy, fraud and racketeering. "They knew that cigarettes caused cancer, and they lied about it. They knew that nicotine was addictive, and they lied about that, too. They manipulated the levels of nicotine in cigarettes to sustain a smoker's addiction. And they denied that, knowing that that was incorrect. They lied about marketing to youth," said Dr. David Kessler, the government's lead witness in the case.[1]

By now, it shouldn't come as a surprise to most people that the tobacco industry engaged in conspiracy to sell their harmful products - but what might be surprising is that despite 100 million cigarette-induced deaths in the 20th century,[2] the judge imposed only minor penalties against the companies with "no hard hits on their wallets," reported the *Los Angeles Times*.[3]

THE PSYCHOLOGY OF THE RICH

For most of us, the idea of murdering over 100 million people for the sake of profit is incomprehensible. Scientists analyzing this bewildering psychology for a number of decades have come to the conclusion that higher social class "predicts increased unethical behavior."[4-6] A 2012 review on the subject noted that upper-class individuals were more likely to break the law, steal, lie, endorse unethical behavior and cheat to increase their chances of winning a prize.

With a $35 billion dollar annual 'prize' at stake for the tobacco industry,[7] perhaps now we can begin to understand the motivation behind their dreadful conduct, and also why the cancer industry - with its $125 billion dollar annual 'prize' - might be guilty of similar crimes.

THE CANCER INDUSTRY'S BAG OF TRICKS

There are a number of simple schemes used by the cancer industry to increase profits and a number that have taken greater effort to orchestrate. Starting simple, a 2015 study found that between the years 1995 to 2013, the average launch price of new cancer drugs increased by an average of $8,500 (10%) per year.[8] Some of the newest cancer drugs can cost patients over $150,000 USD for one year of treatment.[9]

Have the production costs of these new drugs increased? No.
Are they more effective? No.
Pharmaceutical companies charge more for cancer drugs merely because they can.

Another trick used to boost chemotherapy drug earnings was exposed in a 2016 study titled *Overspending driven by oversized single dose vials of cancer drugs*.[10] Simply by selling one-size-fits-all vials of chemotherapy containing far more than what most patients need, an additional $3 billion is generated every year pushing product that ends up not being used.

SUPPRESSED CANCER CURES?

Most people I've talked to suspect the cancer industry has been involved in suppressing cancer cures from the public. From armed raids on the *Burzynski cancer clinic* in Texas to the political extinguishing of Renee Caisse's cancer clinic in Canada to the incredible story of Krebiozen – the active suppression of medicines that have threatened the profits of the cancer establishment have not been uncommon. One of the most fascinating accounts comes to us from Dr. Stan Monteith, who recently unlocked a story through the freedom of information act that had been hidden from the public for over 50 years.

In the 1950's, a man named Charles Tobey Jr. was diagnosed with cancer and told he had less than two years to live. But instead of submitting to the toxic orthodox cancer treatments that were recommended to him by his doctors, Tobey Jr. discovered an alternative approach that he opted for instead. The treatment was known as *The Lincoln Treatment*.

Developed by physician Dr. Robert Lincoln of Medford, Massachusetts, the Lincoln treatment consisted of taking viral and bacterial samples from patients, culturing them and then administering them back to patients through a nebulizer. Dr. Lincoln never charged more than $5 for the treatment and according to Tobey Jr. it had cured many people. "I saw hundreds of people who were getting well; I saw hundreds of husbands and wives who felt that they had new hope, and felt they were going to some one who was honestly trying to help them." Tobey Jr. underwent the Lincoln treatment, experienced a full recovery from cancer and credits the treatment for saving his life.[11]

After hearing that his son was cancer free and watching U.S. health authorities refuse to investigate the Lincoln treatment, his father – the prominent U.S. Senator Charles Toby - launched an official investigation into the cancer establishment. For the position, Toby appointed investigator Benedict Fitzgerald of the US Interstate Commerce Commission. His findings, titled *The Fitzgerald Report*, were presented to the U.S. senate in 1953, but the senate took no action and the inquest was never made public.[12] Here are some conclusions from his investigation, finally made public in 2007:

"My investigation to date should convince this committee that a conspiracy does exist to stop the free flow and use of drugs in interstate commerce which allegedly has solid therapeutic value. Public and private funds have been thrown around like confetti at a country fair to close up and destroy clinics, hospitals, and scientific research laboratories which do not conform to the viewpoint of medical associations.

There is reason to believe that the AMA [American Medical Association] has been hasty, capricious, arbitrary, and outright dishonest...in an interstate conspiracy of alarming proportions. Behind and over all this is the weirdest conglomeration of corrupt motives, intrigue, selfishness, jealousy, obstruction and conspiracy that I have ever seen."
- Benedict F. Fitzgerald, Jr.

FRAUDULENT CANCER RESEARCH?

One of the schemes used by the tobacco industry to mislead the American public about the safety of cigarettes was they paid scientists to fabricate evidence declaring cigarettes weren't harmful.[13] Is it possible that the cancer industry too has been involved in fabricating scientific evidence to misrepresent the safety and efficacy of its cancer screening tools or treatments?

One study cited repeatedly by the industry in recent years as 'the perfect example' of the benefits of mammography was conducted in Denmark and published in 2005. Looking at the effects of mammography screening on women from Copenhagen for the first 10 years after it had been introduced in 1991, the study reported that mammography decreased mortality by 25%.[14]

However, in 2010, scientists from the Nordic Cochrane Centre in Denmark re-analyzed this group's findings and came to some startling conclusions. By expanding the scope of the study to include breast cancer mortality data from 10 years before screening was introduced and 10 years after screening was in practice in areas that weren't using screening, they discovered significant flaws in the original work. Published in the *British*

Medical Journal, the study concluded that breast cancer actually slightly *increased* as a result of mammography screening.[15]

With an estimated 48 million mammograms performed in the United States every year,[17] at prices ranging from $43 to $1,989 for the test,[18] mammography represents between $2 billion and $91 billion dollars in annual revenue for the cancer industry, let alone the treatments that follow.

I contacted the Nordic Cochrane Centre and asked them if they knew of any industry funding behind this original work. They replied, "No industry funding of the BMJ-study you refer to. The problem is intellectual bias, which is sometimes a problem of similar magnitude."

What the cancer industry did do in this case was exploit flawed research to sell a service that often causes unnecessary mutilation and increased death – which is no less immoral. There are a number of other studies that may have been funded by the industry to deliberately confuse the issue of mammography's safety and effectiveness. I'll present them and we can let the judge decide.

One of the most damning studies ever conducted on cancer screening and treatment was published in the journal *Medical Hypotheses* in 1996.[16] For the study, scientists re-examined 7 randomized mammography screening trials commonly cited as having produced evidence for reduced breast cancer mortality in order to resolve opposing claims about whether or not lives are saved through early detection. Their conclusions were as follows:

Early detection:
"No correlation was found between reduced breast cancer mortality and earlier surgical intervention. In fact, the trial with the most earlier surgical intervention had the smallest reduction in mortality; and that with the least earlier surgical intervention had the largest reduction in mortality. This demonstrates that the earlier-diagnosis hypothesis is invalid."

Cancer surgery:
"The conclusion from the previous analysis, that surgery has not been shown to reduce mortality for any form of cancer, is therefore still valid."

Radiotherapy:
"Some correlation was established between reduced mortality and reduced use of radiotherapy…"

While inspecting the 7 mammography screening trials, researchers identified up to five factors that were variable in each trial, confounding the results. The reduction in deaths attributed to mammographic screening in the 7 trials resulted from the use of flawed statistical data that had reclassified a number of breast cancer deaths "as deaths from other causes following ischaemic heart damage caused by radiotherapy." In other words, people who were killed by radiotherapy treatment following early detection with mammography were labeled dead for reasons other than breast cancer, creating the false appearance of reduced breast cancer deaths and thus, the false appearance of a mortality benefit from both treatment and screening. Sound familiar?

You'll recall from the radiotherapy chapter, as first exposed by Dr. Ralph Moss, that official cancer mortality statistics have been altered to make it appear that cancer treatments are more effective than they actually are.[19-22]

By setting up a system where cancer mortality statistics are generated using death certificates, the stage was set so that even unbiased scientists would draw favorable conclusions for the ineffectual cancer screening programs and orthodox treatments; concealing the truth about their dangers and temporarily circumventing the cancer industry's inevitable collapse.

THE BATTLE FOR TRUTH

The unceasing battle being waged before us is one between individuals seeking empirical truth and those seeking monetary gain. The way people and organizations respond to criticisms of cancer screening tools and treatments reveals which side they are on.

When the U.S. Preventive Services Task Force publically recommended against PSA screening in 2011 "with moderate to high certainty" that its harms outweigh its benefits, the urology community - who rely on the steady influx of mostly-misdiagnosed prostate cancer patients provided by the PSA test to stay in business - fought back.

But instead of searching for flaws in the evidence used by the Task Force to make their recommendation, the urology community responded emotionally, calling their decision "cynical," "wreckless," and "unconscionable."[23] Skip Lockwood, CEO of the non-profit prostate cancer organization ZERO even went as far as saying their decision would amount to a death sentence for thousands of men each year. "The decision of no confidence on the PSA test by the U.S. government condemns tens of thousands of men to die this year and every year going forward..."[24]

Dr. Peter Gotzsche, leading Danish professor, statistician and head of the Nordic Cochrane Center, has been studying mammography for over two decades. Not only do mammograms do little to reduce death from breast cancer, but because women haven't been told the truth about the risks of mammography, he explains, some endure painful disfigurement and completely unnecessary treatment that may have shortened their lives.[25]

In 2000, Dr. Gotzsche and his colleague conducted a meta-analysis of eight randomized trials on mammography screening.[26] All six trials that had reported a mortality benefit from screening were found to have imbalances or inconsistencies in the way they were randomized, and of the two remaining trials that had been randomized adequately, neither reported a mortality benefit, prompting researchers to conclude, "Screening for breast cancer with mammography is unjustified." The study was published in *The Lancet* and its results generated a furious response.

In typical fashion of an industry fighting for its existence, the profiteers of mammography and breast cancer treatment didn't challenge the validity of Dr. Gotzsche's findings, but instead chose to attack him personally. "Often the attacks didn't even challenge my research - they were simply personal. I was said to be ignorant, careless and on a crusade against screening," said Gotzsche. Industry 'experts' urged women to ignore the report, government 'authorities' claimed there was no evidence behind it and Laszlo Tabar – author of one of the trials analyzed in the study – branded Gotzsche a 'woman hater.'[25]

The backlash against scientists reporting the ineffectiveness and dangers of cancer screening and treatments represents a desperate struggle by those who profit from cancer screening and treatment to prevent the public from realizing their greatest fear: *we are better off without them.*

MANY 'CANCERS' NOT EVEN HARMFUL

In a 2016 study published in the *Journal of the American Medical Association,* an international panel of doctors declared that a type of thyroid cancer, called Encapsulated Follicular Variant of Papillary Thyroid Carcinoma, is no longer cancer.[27] Although these tumors have been diagnosed as cancer and treated for decades, they have been found to never actually produce symptoms or any problems at all for patients when left untreated.

The push for reclassification began after Dr. Yuri E. Nikiforov from the University of Pittsburgh was asked his opinion about a small thyroid tumor in a 19-year-old woman. "I told the surgeon, who was a good friend, 'This is a very low grade tumor. You do not have to do anything else.'" But the surgeon replied that guidelines mandate she must remove the woman's entire thyroid gland and treat her with radioactive iodine. "I said, 'That's enough. Someone has to take responsibility and stop this madness."

As a result of Dr. Nikiforov's successful initiative, "…thousands of patients will be spared removal of their thyroid, treatment with radioactive iodine and regular checkups for the rest of their lives…" reported the *New York Times.*[28] But this particular type of thyroid tumor is not the only type of cancer that is harmless and in need of reclassification.

PROSTATE CANCER

The most astounding thing about the worldwide trillion-dollar[29] prostate cancer industry is that, even without treatment, almost no men diagnosed with prostate cancer will die from the disease.

In 1992, researchers followed up with untreated prostate cancer patients 10 years after they were diagnosed to determine their rate of survival. Results showed that only 8.5% of patients had died of prostate cancer. Some of the patients died of other causes but the overall survival rate of untreated prostate cancer patients at 10 years was almost 90%.[30] **But there's a catch:** some of the patients were given the hormone estrogen as treatment, which was probably rationalized by the mistaken belief that prostate cancer is caused by testosterone.[31,74-77] Since estrogen is officially classified a carcinogen, the 10-year survival rate of untreated prostate cancer patients - who are not given estrogen - is likely even greater. I searched for more studies on long-term survival rates of untreated prostate cancer patients and found the following.

In 2010, Swedish researchers published a study in the *Journal of the National Cancer Institute* that looked at how many men with untreated prostate cancer actually died from it. 10-years after being diagnosed with early-stage prostate cancer, results showed that only 2.4% of men died from the disease.[32]

"Of all the men diagnosed each year with prostate cancer, their lifetime risk of death from the disease is only 3 percent, which means, of course, that a man has 97% chance of surviving a diagnosis of prostate cancer..." explains Dr. Richard Ablin.

Because of the misuse of a simple test, millions of men have been shelling out $20,000-$50,000 or more[33] for treatments that have left them impotent and having to wear diapers - sometimes for the rest of their lives - all to treat a 'cancer' that was never even a threat.

BREAST CANCER

More than 60,000 women in the United States are diagnosed every year with a type of early-stage breast cancer called ductal carcinoma in situ (DCIS). [34] Between the years 1983 and 2003 there was a 500% increase in the number of women diagnosed with DCIS,[35] most of whom underwent damaging and unnecessary surgical procedures.[36] And in similar fashion to prostate cancer, virtually no women diagnosed with DCIS will die if their 'cancer' is left untreated.[27,39]

A study published in the *Journal of the American Medical Association* in 2015 investigated the 20-year mortality rates of more than 108,196 women diagnosed with ductal carcinoma in situ. Results showed that 20-years after diagnosis, treated or not, only 3.3% of the women died of breast cancer.[37]

The results of this study prompted Laura Esserman, M.D., and her colleague Christina Yau, Ph.D., from the University of California to write an editorial, in which they stated, "Given the low breast cancer mortality risk, we should stop telling women that DCIS is an emergency and that they should schedule definitive surgery within 2 weeks of diagnosis."[38] While women diagnosed with DCIS are routinely frightened into quickly undergoing treatment, this study suggests the best treatment for these patients is no treatment.

MANY OTHER CANCERS

One of Dr. Peter Gotzsche's critical messages is that many of the occult tumors detected during breast[39] and prostate cancer screening[40] may never become advanced enough to harm patients. As a result, thousands of people who would have remained perfectly healthy – because their cancers would have never caused a problem – become cancer patients.

"It is a biological fact of life that we cannot avoid getting cancer as we get older," says Dr. Gotzsche. "It's so common nearly all middle-aged people will have some sign of it and most of them will die without having had any symptoms as a result."[25]

For years, many cancer experts have been calling for the reclassification of small cancers of the breast and prostate, lung, brain, thyroid, skin and kidney.[27] A growing body of experiments conducted by forward-thinking scientists are showing that when we avoid harming the body with destructive treatments, many cancers may ultimately undergo spontaneous regression.

SPONTANEOUS REGRESSION OF CANCER

Spontaneous regression, or the complete disappearance of cancer in the absence of treatment, was first documented in the medical literature in 1742.[41] Since then, spontaneous regression has been documented in virtually every type of cancer; including breast,[42] prostate,[43] sarcoma,[44] seminoma,[45] melanoma,[46] basal cell carcinoma,[46] leukemia,[47] stomach,[48] kidney,[47] colon,[49] cervical,[50] liver,[51] lung[51] and brain.[52]

In the early to mid-1900's, the frequency of spontaneous regression of cancer was believed to be 1 in 80,000-100,000 patients,[61] but modern research is showing that spontaneous regression is vastly more common. "One of the reasons that spontaneous regression of tumors seems so rare is undoubtedly that most tumors are quickly cut out by surgeons," wrote Dr. Ray Peat.

When patients aren't scared-to-death and rushed into treatment by their doctors, rates of spontaneous regression can be seen as high as 7% in renal carcinoma patients,[62] up to 15% in melanoma patients[63] and up to 20% in patients with low-grade lymphoma.[64] Some studies have recorded even higher rates of spontaneous regression.[65-68]

A CLOSER LOOK...

- A 1984 study from the *New England Journal of Medicine* examined survival rates of 83 untreated cancer patients with advanced non-Hodgkin's lymphoma. Results showed that 83% of patients were alive at 5-years and 73% were still alive at 10-years and remarkably, "Spontaneous regressions occurred in 19 untreated patients (23 percent)."[65]

- A 2008 American study examined the prevalence of invasive breast cancer in 100,000 women who received either mammography screening or no screening. The first group was screened every two years (receiving six more mammograms per woman on average) and the control group underwent a single screening at the end of their six-year observation period to assess for cancer. At the end of the six-years, the study found that 22% more women in the screening group had invasive breast cancer than the control group - suggesting that 22% of cancers detected by repeated mammographic screening had spontaneously regressed in the absence of screening. In other words, by simply avoiding the repeated doses of ionizing radiation administered during mammography, the body is given a chance to heal on its own; and often it does.[66]

- In 1997, scientists from the Royal Prince Alfred Hospital in Australia looked at the prevalence of spontaneous regression in skin tumors. Published in *The Australasian Journal of Dermatology*, the study found that 25% of melanomas and 50% of basal cell carcinomas spontaneously regressed on their own. Additionally, in two other types of skin tumors called keratoacanthoma and epithelioma, "nearly all the tumours regress completely."[67]

A number of studies have suggested that spontaneous regression is mediated by the body's immune system;[53-60] "Analysis of the regressing tumors revealed heavy infiltration by T lymphocytes as compared to non-regressing tumors," concluded scientists from Kuwait University in 2005.[60]

Given that only about 2 percent of patients survive 5-years following chemotherapy, simply by rejecting harmful orthodox cancer treatments, survival rates can be increased by 5-times, 10-times, even 25-times. Now, imagine the prospect of survival if the rejection of orthodox cancer treatments is accompanied by the use of medicines that are both safe and effective.

THE CANCER INDUSTRY'S BIGGEST SECRET

There's a reason why women and men are never fully-informed about the dangers and potential implications of mammography screening, PSA screening, surgery, chemotherapy or radiotherapy - because if they were, nobody would ever agree to undergo them.

Doctors see first hand that surgery, chemotherapy and radiotherapy commonly increase the rate of cancer metastasis 100-fold,[78] and that's why almost 90% of doctors have said they would refuse these treatments for themselves if they were terminally ill and dying.[79]

In the previous chapter, three large mammography screening trials, all of which reported no mortality benefits from mammography screening were presented. A closer look at the data from two of those studies reveals that mortality was actually *increased* in women who underwent mammography screening.[69,70]

A CLOSER LOOK...

- At the 7-year follow-up for the *Canadian National Breast Screening Study 1,* researchers discovered a 36% *increased* mortality among women in the mammography screening group; "38 women in the mammography group and 28 women in the usual care group had died of breast cancer."[69]

- At the 25-year follow-up of the *Canadian National Breast Screening Study* 1 and 2, researchers found that 180 women died of breast cancer in the mammography screening group and only 171 women in the control group.[70]

Another large-scale mammography study was The Malmö Mammographic Screening Trial of 1988. The Malmö study included over 40,000 women to determine whether repeated mammographic screening reduces mortality from breast cancer. At an average follow-up of 9 years, results showed that in women under the age of 55 who underwent mammography screening, breast cancer deaths *increased* by 29%.[71]

THE UNTREATED LIVE LONGER

In 1979, American Biologist Dr. Maurice Fox published an article in the *Journal of the American Medical Association* comparing survival rates of breast cancer patients treated using orthodox methods with those who were left untreated. After reviewing data from studies conducted at the Harvard School of Public Health, Dr. Fox concluded, "Those who refused medical procedures had a lower mortality rate than those who submitted."[72]

Dr. Hardin B. Jones, professor of medical physics at the University of California, Berkeley and leading US cancer statistician for over 30 years, sent shockwaves through a 1969 seminar for the American Cancer Society when he announced the results of his 25-year study[73] comparing survival rates of treated cancer patients with untreated cancer patients:

"My studies have proved conclusively that untreated cancer victims live up to four times longer than treated individuals. If one has cancer and opts to do nothing at all, he will live longer and feel better than if he undergoes radiation, chemotherapy or surgery, other than when used in immediate life-threatening situations."

In 1975, twice as many women were diagnosed with breast cancer than in 1935 and twice as many women died,[72] evidencing what appears to be the most vile, appalling and despicable truth those in the cancer industry have worked so diligently to conceal: Cancer deaths have increased in parallel to the number of people treated.

TIMELESS QUOTES

"We have a multi-billion dollar industry that is killing people, right and left, just for financial gain."
- Dr. Glen Warner

"If I contracted cancer, I would never go to a standard cancer treatment centre. Cancer victims who live far from such centers have a chance."
- Professor Charles Mathe

"You see, it is not the cancer that kills the victim. It's the breakdown of the defense mechanism that eventually brings death. With every cancer patient who keeps in excellent physical shape and boosts his health to build up his natural resistance, there's a high chance that the body will find its own defense against cancer. He may have many good years left in good health. He shouldn't squander them by being made into a hopeless invalid through radical intervention which has zero chance of extending his life."
- Dr. Hardin B. Jones, Ph.D.,quoted at Midnight, September 1, 1975.

"It is better not to apply any treatment in cases of occult cancer; for if treated, the patients die quickly; but if not treated, they hold out for a long time."
- Hippocrates (460-370 BC)

"It is from nature that the disease comes, and from nature comes the cure, not from physicians."
- Paracelsus (1493-1541)

REFERENCES

1. Brown, J. (2006). *Judge Finds Big Tobacco Guilty of Racketeering, Conspiracy.* [Online]. Available: http://www.pbs.org/newshour/bb/law-july-dec06-smoking_08-18. [February 3, 2017].

2. Proctor RN. The history of the discovery of the cigarette-lung cancer link: evidentiary traditions, corporate denial, global toll. Tob Control. 2012;21(2):87-91.

3. Levin M. (2006). *Big Tobacco is Guilty of Conspiracy.* Los Angeles Times. [Online]. Available: http://articles.latimes.com/2006/aug/18/nation/na-smoke18.[February 5, 2017].

4. Piff PK, Stancato DM, Côté S, Mendoza-denton R, Keltner D. Higher social class predicts increased unethical behavior. Proc Natl Acad Sci USA. 2012;109(11):4086-91.

5. Côté S, Piff PK, Willer R. For whom do the ends justify the means? Social class and utilitarian moral judgment. J Pers Soc Psychol. 2013;104(3):490-503.

6. Dubois D, Rucker DD, Galinsky AD. Social class, power, and selfishness: when and why upper and lower class individuals behave unethically. J Pers Soc Psychol. 2015;108(3):436-49.

7. Bowers, S. (2012). *Global profits for tobacco trade total $35bn as smoking deaths top 6 million.* The Guardian. [Online]. Available: https://www.theguardian.com/business/2012/mar/22/tobacco-profits-deaths-6-million.[February 5, 2017].

8. Howard DH, Bach PB, Berndt ER, Conti RM. Pricing in the Market for Anticancer Drugs. J Econ Perspec. 2015; 29(1):139-162.

9. (2016). *These New Cancer Drugs Are Helping Patients Live Years Longer.* Fortune. [Online]. Available: http://fortune.com/2016/05/19/cancer-drugs-keytruda-opdivo.[February 5, 2017].

10. Bach PB, Conti RM, Muller RJ, Schnorr GC, Saltz LB. Overspending driven by oversized single dose vials of cancer drugs. BMJ. 2016;352:i788.

11. Tobey Jr, C. *Charles Tobey Jr. Reports On Cancer and The Venal Medical Conspiracy.* Whale.to. [Online]. Available: http://www.whale.to/p/tobey.html. [February 5, 2017].

12. Hon. William Langer, US Congressional Record, August 3, 1953, p. A 5352. Available: http://www.newmediaexplorer.org/chris/Fitzgerald%20Report%201953.pdf.[February 5, 2017].

13. Drope J, Chapman S. Tobacco industry efforts at discrediting scientific knowledge of environmental tobacco smoke: a review of internal industry documents. J Epidemiol Community Health. 2001;55(8):588-94.

14. Olsen AH, Njor SH, Vejborg I, et al. Breast cancer mortality in Copenhagen after introduction of mammography screening: cohort study. BMJ. 2005;330(7485):220.

15. Jørgensen KJ, Zahl PH, Gøtzsche PC. Breast cancer mortality in organised mammography screening in Denmark: comparative study. BMJ. 2010;340:c1241.

16. Benjamin DJ. The efficacy of surgical treatment of breast cancer. Med Hypotheses. 1996;47(5):389-97.

17. Castillo, M. (2012). *Bra aims to detect breast cancer before mammogram.* CBS News. [Online]. Available: http://www.cbsnews.com/news/bra-aims-to-detect-breast-cancer-before-mammogram/.[February 5, 2017].

18. Fowler, E. (2015). *New Study Finds Huge Price Differences For Mammograms & Other Critical Women's Health Procedures in the 30 Largest U.S. Cities.* Castlight Health. [Online]. Available: http://www.castlighthealth.com/press-releases/new-study-finds-huge-price-differences-for-mammograms-other-critical-womens-health-procedures-in-the-30-largest-u-s-cities.[February 5, 2017].

19. Effects of radiotherapy and surgery in early breast cancer. An overview of the randomized trials. Early Breast Cancer Trialists' Collaborative Group. N Engl J Med. 1995;333(22):1444-55.

20. Adjuvant radiotherapy for rectal cancer: a systematic overview of 8,507 patients from 22 randomised trials. Lancet. 2001;358(9290):1291-304.

21. Clarke M, Collins R, Darby S, et al. Effects of radiotherapy and of differences in the extent of surgery for early breast cancer on local recurrence and 15-year survival: an overview of the randomised trials. Lancet. 2005;366(9503):2087-106.

22. Brown BW, Brauner C, Minnotte MC. Noncancer deaths in white adult cancer patients. J Natl Cancer Inst. 1993;85(12):979-87.

23. (2012). *U.S. Preventive Servies Task Force Ruling on PSA Testing a Major Blow to Men's Health.* [Online]. Available: http://pintsforprostates.org/u-s-preventive-services-task-force-ruling-on-psa-testing-a-major-blow-to-mens-health/.[February 5, 2017].

24. Public and Professional Reactions to U.S. Preventive Services Task Force Recommendations on PSA Screening. Dr. Catalona. [Online]. Available: http://www.drcatalona.com/quest/Winter2011/article2.html.[February 5, 2017].

25. Burne, J. (2012). *The expert branded a woman hater for saying breast cancer screening ruins lives.* [Online].Available: http://www.dailymail.co.uk/health/article-2120750/The-expert-branded-woman-hater-saying-breast-cancer-screening-ruins-lives.html#ixzz1qOQwifwi.[February 5, 2017].

26. Gøtzsche PC, Olsen O. Is screening for breast cancer with mammography justifiable?. Lancet. 2000;355(9198):129-34.

27. Nikiforov YE, Seethala RR, Tallini G, et al. Nomenclature Revision for Encapsulated Follicular Variant of Papillary Thyroid Carcinoma: A Paradigm Shift to Reduce Overtreatment of Indolent Tumors. JAMA Oncol. 2016;2(8):1023-9.

28. Kolata, G. (2016). *It's Not Cancer: Doctors Reclassify a Thyroid Tumor.* [Online]. Available: https://www.nytimes.com/2016/04/15/health/thyroid-tumor-cancer-reclassification.html?_r=2.[February 5, 2017].

29. Ablin, R.J. and Piana R. 2014. The Great Prostate Hoax: How Big Medicine Hijacked the PSA Test and Caused a Public Health Disaster. St. Martin's Press., New York, NY.

30. Johansson JE, Adami HO, Andersson SO, Bergström R, Holmberg L, Krusemo UB. High 10-year survival rate in patients with early, untreated prostatic cancer. JAMA. 1992;267(16):2191-6.

31. Schweizer MT, Antonarakis ES, Wang H, et al. Effect of bipolar androgen therapy for asymptomatic men with castration-resistant prostate cancer: results from a pilot clinical study. Sci Transl Med. 2015;7(269).

32. Stattin P, Holmberg E, Johansson JE, et al. Outcomes in localized prostate cancer: National Prostate Cancer Register of Sweden follow-up study. J Natl Cancer Inst. 2010;102(13):950-8.

33. Cooperberg MR, Ramakrishna NR, Duff SB, et al. Primary treatments for clinically localised prostate cancer: a comprehensive lifetime cost-utility analysis. BJU Int. 2013;111(3):437-50.

34. American Cancer Society. (2015). *Breast Carcinoma in Situ Cancer Facts & Figures.* [Online]. Available: https://www.cancer.org/content/dam/cancer-org/research/cancer-facts-and-statistics/annual-cancer-facts-and-figures/2015/special-section-breast-carcinoma-in-situ-cancer-facts-and-figures-2015.pdf.[February 5, 2017].

35. Kerlikowske K. Epidemiology of ductal carcinoma in situ. J Natl Cancer Inst Monographs. 2010;2010(41):139-41.

36. Demicheli R, Retsky MW, Hrushesky WJ, Baum M, Gukas ID. The effects of surgery on tumor growth: a century of investigations. Ann Oncol. 2008;19(11):1821-8.

37. Narod SA, Iqbal J, Giannakeas V, Sopik V, Sun P. Breast Cancer Mortality After a Diagnosis of Ductal Carcinoma In Situ. JAMA Oncol. 2015;1(7):888-96.

38. Esserman L, Yau C. Rethinking the Standard for Ductal Carcinoma In Situ Treatment. JAMA Oncol. 2015;1(7):881-3.

39. Drew PJ, Turnbull LW, Kerin MJ, Carleton PJ, Fox JN. Multicentricity and recurrence of breast cancer. Lancet. 1997;349(9046):208-9.

40. Penson DF, Albertsen PC. *The Natural History of Prostate Cancer*. Springer Netherlands. 2007. Available: http://link.springer.com/chapter/10.1007/978-1-4020-5847-9_2 [February 5, 2017].

41. Le Dran HF. Traite des operations de chirurgie. Paris: C. Osmont; 1742.

42. Larsen SU, Rose C. [Spontaneous remission of breast cancer. A literature review]. Ugeskr Laeg. 1999;161(26):4001-4.

43. Monzen Y, Nakahara M, Nishisaka T. Spontaneous regression of primary malignant lymphoma of the prostate. Case Rep Urol. 2013;2013:363072.

44. Banihani MN, Al manasra AR. Spontaneous regression in alveolar soft part sarcoma: case report and literature review. World J Surg Oncol. 2009;7:53.

45. Tanaka K, Hamada T, Takasaki H, Yokoyama S. Spontaneous regression of mediastinal seminoma. OAI. 1989.

46. Printz C. Spontaneous Regression of Melanoma May Offer Insight Into Cancer Immunology. J Nat Can Inst. 2001; 93 (14): 1047-1048.

47. Papac RJ. Spontaneous regression of cancer: possible mechanisms. In Vivo. 1998;12(6):571-8.

48. Ogawa D, Uemura N, Sasaki N, et al. Spontaneous regression of malignant lymphoma of the stomach. J Med. 1998;29(5-6):381-93.

49. Bir AS, Fora AA, Levea C, Fakih MG. Spontaneous regression of colorectal cancer metastatic to retroperitoneal lymph nodes. Anticancer Res. 2009;29(2):465-8.

50. Stefani C, Liverani CA, Bianco V, et al. Spontaneous regression of low-grade cervical intraepithelial lesions is positively improved by topical bovine colostrum preparations (GINEDIE®). A multicentre, observational, italian pilot study. Eur Rev Med Pharmacol Sci. 2014;18(5):728-33.

51. Iwanaga T. [Studies on cases of spontaneous regression of cancer in Japan in 2011, and of hepatic carcinoma, lung cancer and pulmonary metastases in the world between 2006 and 2011]. Gan To Kagaku Ryoho. 2013;40(11):1475-87.

52. Davis T, Doyle H, Tobias V, Ellison DW, Ziegler DS. Case Report of Spontaneous Resolution of a Congenital Glioblastoma. Pediatrics. 2016;137(4).

53. Isobe Y, Aritaka N, Sasaki M, Oshimi K, Sugimoto K. Spontaneous regression of natural killer cell lymphoma. J Clin Pathol. 2009;62(7):647-50.

54. Crisci A, Corsale I, Abrami F, et al. [Spontaneous regression of lung metastases from renal cell carcinoma: the importance of immunogenetic factors and a review of the literature]. Minerva Urol Nefrol. 2008;60(2):123-35.

55. Bir AS, Fora AA, Levea C, Fakih MG. Spontaneous regression of colorectal cancer metastatic to retroperitoneal lymph nodes. Anticancer Res. 2009;29(2):465-8.

56. Paredes BE. [Regression in malignant melanoma. Definition, etiopathogenesis, morphology and differential diagnosis]. Pathologe. 2007;28(6):453-63.

57. Khar A, Muralikrishna K, Varalakshmi C. High intratumoural level of cytokines mediates efficient regression of a rat histiocytoma. Clin Exp Immunol. 1997;110(1):127-31.

58. Wong DA, Bishop GA, Lowes MA, Cooke B, Barnetson RS, Halliday GM. Cytokine profiles in spontaneously regressing basal cell carcinomas. Br J Dermatol. 2000;143(1):91-8.

59. Mueller N. Overview of the epidemiology of malignancy in immune deficiency. J Acquir Immune Defic Syndr. 1999;21 Suppl 1:S5-10.

60. Saleh F, Renno W, Klepacek I, et al. Direct evidence on the immune-mediated spontaneous regression of human cancer: an incentive for pharmaceutical companies to develop a novel anti-cancer vaccine. Curr Pharm Des. 2005;11(27):3531-43.

61. Schilder H, de Vries MJ, Goodkin K, Antoni M. Psychological Changes Preceding Spontaneous Remission of Cancer. Clinical Case Studies. 2004; 3(4):288-312.

62. Oliver RT, Nethersell AB, Bottomley JM. Unexplained spontaneous regression and alpha-interferon as treatment for metastatic renal carcinoma. Br J Urol. 1989;63(2):128-31.

63. Sroujieh AS. Spontaneous regression of intestinal malignant melanoma from an occult primary site. Cancer. 1988;62(6):1247-50.

64. Drobyski WR, Qazi R. Spontaneous regression in non-Hodgkin's lymphoma: clinical and pathogenetic considerations. Am J Hematol. 1989;31(2):138-41.

65. Horning SJ, Rosenberg SA. The natural history of initially untreated low-grade non-Hodgkin's lymphomas. N Engl J Med. 1984;311(23):1471-5.

66. Zahl PH, Maehlen J, Welch HG. The natural history of invasive breast cancers detected by screening mammography. Arch Intern Med. 2008;168(21):2311-6.

67. Barnetson RS, Halliday GM. Regression in skin tumours: a common phenomenon. Australas J Dermatol. 1997;38 Suppl 1:S63-5.

68. Zahl PH, Gøtzsche PC, Mæhlen J. Natural history of breast cancers detected in the Swedish mammography screening programme: a cohort study. Lancet Oncol. 2011;12(12):1118-24.

69. Miller AB, To T, Baines CJ, Wall C. The Canadian National Breast Screening Study-1: breast cancer mortality after 11 to 16 years of follow-up. A randomized screening trial of mammography in women age 40 to 49 years. Ann Intern Med. 2002;137(5 Part 1):305-12.

70. Miller AB, Wall C, Baines CJ, Sun P, To T, Narod SA. Twenty five year follow-up for breast cancer incidence and mortality of the Canadian National Breast Screening Study: randomised screening trial. BMJ. 2014;348.

71. Andersson I, Aspegren K, Janzon L, et al. Mammographic screening and mortality from breast cancer: the Malmö mammographic screening trial. BMJ. 1988;297(6654):943-8.

72. Fox MS. On the Diagnosis and Treatment of Breast Cancer. *JAMA.* 1979;241(5):489-494.

73. Jones HB. Demographic consideration of the cancer problem. Trans N Y Acad Sci. 1956;18(4):298-333.

74. Rubinow DR, Roca CA, Schmidt PJ, et al. Testosterone suppression of CRH-stimulated cortisol in men. Neuropsychopharmacology. 2005;30(10):1906-12.

75. Buchanan KL, Evans MR, Goldsmith AR, Bryant DM, Rowe LV. Testosterone influences basal metabolic rate in male house sparrows: a new cost of dominance signalling?. Proc Biol Sci. 2001;268(1474):1337-44.

76. Hofling M, Hirschberg AL, Skoog L, Tani E, Hägerström T, Von schoultz B. Testosterone inhibits estrogen/progestogen-induced breast cell proliferation in postmenopausal women. Menopause. 2007;14(2):183-90.

77. Dicker A, Rydén M, Näslund E, et al. Effect of testosterone on lipolysis in human pre-adipocytes from different fat depots. Diabetologia. 2004;47(3):420-8.

78. Hanin L, Zaider M. Effects of Surgery and Chemotherapy on Metastatic Progression of Prostate Cancer: Evidence from the Natural History of the Disease Reconstructed through Mathematical Modeling. Cancers (Basel). 2011;3(3):3632-60.

79. Periyakoil VS, Neri E, Fong A, Kraemer H. Do unto others: doctors' personal end-of-life resuscitation preferences and their attitudes toward advance directives. PLoS ONE. 2014;9(5).

CONCLUSION

WHEN A HUMAN BEING is sick with cancer, they deserve the absolute safest and most effective medicines known to man. Period.

Yet in this world, cancer patients are routinely rushed into oncology centers where doctors sentence them to death using treatments that make industrial animal slaughterhouses look humane.

When somebody survives the total onslaught of surgery, chemotherapy and radiotherapy, they have not survived because these war weapons have somehow healed them; they have survived *despite* these so-called treatments because they are extraordinarily strong and have an unrelenting will to survive.

In writing this book I have come to the realization that what I had long suspected about my mother's death was in fact true: My mother didn't die of cancer. She was murdered-for-profit by an industry that cares more about making money than saving lives.

What else are we to expect from an enterprise claiming that butchering sick people with knives, poisoning them with mustard gas and burning them with ionizing radiation will improve their health?

The monstrous $126 billion dollar cancer industry, hell-bent on preserving its profits at any cost, continues its murderous rampage to this day. The mind of the beast wells up with excitement at the thought of 50% of all human beings alive being one day diagnosed with cancer. Only an informed population of people, willing to stand up for themselves and make their own health decisions, can put an end to the cancer industry's reign of terror.

With this raging bull charging directly at humanity the question remains: Are we going to continue letting the cancer industry annihilate us and everyone we love until there's no one left - or stand up for ourselves and watch this beast plummet into the eternal, fiery depths of hell?

THE CANCER INDUSTRY CRUMBLES

If our goal as a society is to reduce the suffering in this world and create better future for all human beings, then it's clear the present screening tests and treatments offered by the cancer industry no longer have a place here.

If you've decided you will never submit to the cancer industry's diagnostic tests or its so-called treatments, then make that decision clear to yourself and to the people around you. Be vocal about it and speak the truth.

Never be afraid to assert yourself and say '*no*' to your doctor or anybody trying to sell you a product or service. Remember, it's your body and your choice.

This is literally all it will take in order for us to forever eliminate the insane practice of using weapons of war on the sickest among us. As with all products and services that go unpurchased, they will quickly cease being produced.

HEALING THE WORLD AND ENDING CANCER

We know that our chances of survival from cancer are greatly increased simply by saying '*no*' to useless cancer screening tests and mainstream cancer treatments like surgery, chemotherapy and radiotherapy. Now imagine our prognosis if we couple the elimination of these damaging treatments with healing protocols that actually enhance both the speed and quality of healing without side effects.

This is the next step in our investigation into cancer. Equally critical as understanding that the cancer industry is doing more harm than good is knowing what to replace that void with.

The goal of the next book in this *Curing Cancer Series* will be to finally solve some of the greatest mysteries of cancer, some of which have escaped scientists for centuries, including:

- What is cancer?

- What causes cancer?

- What is a tumor?

- What are the safest and most effective ways to prevent and reverse cancer?

Thank you for reading this book. I hope it empowers you to make your own rational and informed health decisions and live a long, healthy and cancer-free   life.

BOOK 2

CANCER: THE METABOLIC DISEASE

CHAPTER 6

TARGETING THE TUMOR MICROENVIRONMENT

The tumor microenvironment is one of the most important areas of cancer research. Understanding what the tumor microenvironment is and how it works is critical for understanding the disease of cancer. Despite this, the concept has never been announced publically and most people are entirely unaware of it.

The tumor microenvironment is the area surrounding a tumor, which contains a network of different signaling molecules, hormones and other factors which are in constant interaction with tumor cells.[55] Depending on which substances are present within the tumor microenvironment, a tumor will either be signaled to grow and spread to other areas of the body or to shrink and resolve itself. Put simply, the substances present within the tumor microenvironment are the ultimate mediators of the fate of a tumor.

The following tumor microenvironmental factors, first presented in book 1 of this series titled *The Cancer Industry*, seem to exist together and promote cancer growth and spread within the body.

Nitric Oxide - Anytime a tissue has been injured, nitric oxide and other growth factors are released to signal cells to grow and divide to replace lost cells.[56] In a person with cancer, tumor cells caught in the crossfire of nitric oxide signaling will also be signaled to grow, which is why nitric oxide is a well-known promoter of angiogenesis and tumor progression.[57-60]

Nitric Oxide - Nitric oxide has also been demonstrated to trigger the adhesion of circulating tumor cells (like the ones released during cancer surgery) onto body tissues, which is the first step in new tumor formation.[61]

Vascular Endothelial Growth Factor – Similar to nitric oxide, VEGF is a protein that signals growth to help repair injured tissues.[90] Elevated blood levels of VEGF have been associated with the growth and progression of cancer.[91]

Epidermal Growth Factor – EGF, like nitric oxide and VEGF, enhances the growth, invasion and metastasis of tumors.[92] High levels of EGF are associated with poor prognosis in cancer patients.[93]

Free Radicals – Free radicals are highly-reactive molecules that are balanced by the body's antioxidant system. In excess, the oxidative damage caused by free radicals results in aging, cardiovascular disease, cancer and other chronic diseases.[112]

Adrenaline – The stress hormone adrenaline is one of the primary triggers of the breakdown of fat for energy (lipolysis).[89] Anytime unsaturated fatty acids enter the bloodstream, prostaglandins are formed,[62] which are carcinogenic.[63]

106

CANCER CURED

Cortisol - People with cancer have higher cortisol levels than people without cancer,[64] and a number of studies have shown that cancer patients with the highest levels of cortisol have the greatest risk of dying from the disease.[65,66]

Estrogen - The presence of cortisol in the bloodstream leads to increased production of the hormone estrogen.[67-69] The famous 1990's Women's Health Initiative study tested the effects of supplemental estrogen on women, but was forced to stop early after participants began developing cardiovascular disease, stroke, dementia and cancer.[70]

Serotonin - Since cortisol's basic action is to catabolize muscle tissue and muscle meat contains high levels of the amino acid tryptophan (a precursor for serotonin), stress increases serotonin production.[71] While most people think of serotonin as a 'happy hormone,' this cultural belief appears misguided, since serotonin is not a hormone and lowering it can alleviate depression.[87] Serotonin is part of the body's stress response and has been shown in numerous studies to promote tumor growth.[71-75]

Histamine - Histamine is an inflammatory mediator commonly known for its role in allergic reactions.[76,77] Substances that inhibit histamine prevent cancer growth and progression.[78-80]

Lactic Acid - Lactic acid is produced by cells that aren't getting what they need to produce energy efficiently. Lactic acid suppresses the immune system,[81] promotes cancer growth and metastasis[82] and also triggers the release of cortisol,[83] perpetuating the cycle of stress.

Prolactin - Elevated blood concentrations of the hormone prolactin trigger inflammation by amplifying the production of inflammatory cytokines,[84] and promote the formation and progression of numerous types of cancer.[85,86,88]

Tumor Necrosis Factor alpha – TNFalpha is an inflammatory cytokine released by macrophages in response to toxins or other stressors.[95] Due to its extreme toxicity, TNFalpha has been shown to kill cancer cells,[96] but the rest of the body is severely damaged in the process.[97-99] TNFalpha promotes

107

inflammation, is involved in cancer growth and metastasis, and its presence in the body increases with age,[100] like cancer's.[101]

Nuclear Factor Kappa b – TNFalpha triggers the production of NFKB,[102] which is a protein that signals inflammation[103] and plays a key role in tumor formation, growth and spread.[104,105] Many ancient natural medicines found to be effective against cancer inhibit NFKB.[106]

Interleukin 6 – IL-6 is a highly-toxic pro-inflammatory cytokine[107-108] that plays a key role in the formation of numerous types of cancer, including colorectal,[94] pancreatic,[110] liver[111] and prostate.[114]

High-Mobility Group Box 1 Protein – HMGB1 is a pro-inflammatory protein that signals immune system activation in response to injury.[113] Overexpression of HMGB1 promotes inflammation, carcinogenesis, angiogenesis and metastasis. "Our studies and those of our colleagues suggest that HMGB1 is central to cancer."[109]

Interestingly, in *The Cancer Industry* it was established using existing scientific research that surgery, chemotherapy and radiotherapy – whether administered individually or in combination - significantly elevate all of the aforementioned substances within the body (See figure 1 on next page).

Figure 1.	Surgery	Chemotherapy	Radiotherapy
Free Radicals	✓	✓	✓
TNF-alpha	✓	✓	✓
Interleukin-1beta	✓	✓	✓
Interleukin-4	✓	No evidence found	✓
Interleukin-6	✓	✓	✓
Interleukin-8	✓	✓	✓
NFKb	✓	✓	✓
Cortisol	✓	✓	✓
Adrenaline	✓	✓	✓
Prolactin	✓	✓	✓
High mobility group box 1 protein	✓	✓	✓
VEGF	✓	✓	✓
EGF	✓	✓	✓
Nitric oxide	✓	✓	✓
Lactic acid	✓	✓	✓
Estrogen	✓	✓	✓
Prostaglandins	✓	✓	✓
Serotonin	✓	✓	✓
Histamine	✓	✓	✓

These are the precise biochemical mechanisms which explain why mainstream cancer treatments ultimately make the health of cancer patients far worse. These findings further substantiate the conclusions of many reknowned doctors and scientists over the preceding decades: The absolute last thing a cancer patient needs are treatments involving knives, poisons and ionizing radiation.

As it turns out, these cancer-promoting factors reside not just in the tumor microenvironment but in all areas of the body of a cancer patient. Although they appear to be particularly concentrated within the tumor microenvironment, studies on untreated cancer patients have found high levels of these cancer-promoting substances throughout their bodies.

THE TUMOR MICROENVIRONMENT OF UNTREATED CANCER PATIENTS

- Elevated free radicals[1-3]
- Elevated tumor necrosis factor-alpha[4,5]
- Elevated interleukin-1[5,6]
- Elevated interleukin-4[48]
- Elevated interleukin-6[5,6]
- Elevated interleukin-8[5,6]
- Elevated nuclear factor-kappa b[7]
- Elevated cortisol[8-10]
- Elevated adrenaline[47]
- Elevated prolactin[11-13]
- Elevated high mobility group box 1 protein[49]
- Elevated vascular endothelial growth factor[50]
- Elevated epidermal growth factor[51]
- Elevated nitric oxide[14,15]
- Elevated lactic acid[16-18]
- Elevated estrogen[10,19]
- Elevated prostaglandins[20,21]
- Elevated serotonin[24,25]
- Elevated histamine[22,23]

These key hormonal and pro-inflammatory substances are what trigger the formation of cancer in the body. They also cause existing cancers to progress.

The questions that must be asked and answered now include:

- Is there anything we can do to safely reduce these substances in cancer patients?

- And if so, what happens to the health of a cancer patient once they are reduced?

- Is reducing these substances the most efficient way to restore health in a cancer patient?

DOWNREGULATING THE TUMOR PROMOTING FACTORS IN CANCER PATIENTS

We all eat food everyday, our lives depend on it. Once consumed, the food we eat is digested and used by our bodies as base materials to maintain and regenerate its structure and to power the energy-producing 'engines' within each of our cells, called mitochondria. Based on this, it's clear that the most fundamental way to affect human health either positively or negatively is to alter their intake of food.

If a person is ingesting everything they need to be healthy (water, air, protein, carbohydrates, fat, vitamins and minerals) and avoiding things they don't need (chemical poisons), they will be in good health. If they're not, the process of disease and degeneration will begin to occur.

Since food is our primary source of nourishment, let's explore which foods might act medicinally to downregulate the tumor-promoting factors within the body and tumor microenvironment.

One of the dietary recommendations Dr. Raymond Peat has been making for years is that people eat more oranges. After reading a number of studies on oranges, it became clear that this fruit indeed contains a number of powerful medicinal ingredients that might make it a good candidate to alter the tumor microenvironment. I explored the scientific literature to determine the impact of oranges on the tumor microenvironment and here are my findings.

ORANGES AND THE TUMOR MICROENVIRONMENT:

- Oranges reduce free radicals[26,27]
- Oranges reduce tumor necrosis factor-alpha[27,28]
- Oranges reduce interleukin-1[27,29]
- Oranges reduce interleukin-4[30]

- Oranges reduce interleukin-5[30]
- Oranges reduce interleukin-6[28]
- Oranges reduce interleukin-8[31]
- Oranges reduce interleukin-13[30]
- Oranges reduce nuclear factor kappa-b[31]
- Oranges reduce cortisol[32]
- Oranges reduce adrenaline[46]
- Oranges reduce prolactin[33,34]
- Oranges reduce high mobility group box 1 protein[52]
- Oranges reduce vascular endothelial growth factor[53]
- Oranges reduce epidermal growth factor[54]
- Oranges reduce nitric oxide[34-36]
- Oranges reduce lactic acid[37,38]
- Oranges reduce estrogen[34,39-41]
- Oranges reduce prostaglandins[26,35,36]
- Oranges reduce serotonin[44,45]
- Oranges reduce histamine[42,43]

As you can see, there is abundant scientific evidence suggesting that oranges can diminish not just one, but *all* of the cancer-promoting substances in the human body and tumor microenvironment. Before doing this work I had suspected that oranges would reduce at least a few of these substances, but to my surprise it seems to be able to downregulate every single of them. We are off to a great start.

Next we will conduct a thorough scientific investigation into oranges to find out what they can do in animal and human experiments of cancer. Following this, similar investigations will be conducted on two other medicines and then we will return to synthesize the information and unravel the mysteries of cancer in our final chapter.

REFERENCES

1. Suhail N, Bilal N, Khan HY, et al. Effect of vitamins C and E on antioxidant status of breast-cancer patients undergoing chemotherapy. J Clin Pharm Ther. 2012;37(1):22-6.

2. Yuvaraj S, Premkumar VG, Vijayasarathy K, Gangadaran SG, Sachdanandam P. Augmented antioxidant status in Tamoxifen treated postmenopausal women with breast cancer on co-administration with Coenzyme Q10, Niacin and Riboflavin. Cancer Chemother Pharmacol. 2008;61(6):933-41.

3. De cavanagh EM, Honegger AE, Hofer E, et al. Higher oxidation and lower antioxidant levels in peripheral blood plasma and bone marrow plasma from advanced cancer patients. Cancer. 2002;94(12):3247-51.

4. Sheen-chen SM, Chen WJ, Eng HL, Chou FF. Serum concentration of tumor necrosis factor in patients with breast cancer. Breast Cancer Res Treat. 1997;43(3):211-5.

5. Kaminska J, Kowalska M, Kotowicz B, et al. Pretreatment serum levels of cytokines and cytokine receptors in patients with non-small cell lung cancer, and correlations with clinicopathological features and prognosis. M-CSF - an independent prognostic factor. Oncology. 2006;70(2):115-25.

6. Kaminska J, Nowacki MP, Kowalska M, et al. Clinical significance of serum cytokine measurements in untreated colorectal cancer patients: soluble tumor necrosis factor receptor type I-- an independent prognostic factor. Tumour Biol. 2005;26(4):186-94.

7. Ismail S, Mayah W, Battia HE, et al. Plasma nuclear factor kappa B and serum peroxiredoxin 3 in early diagnosis of hepatocellular carcinoma. Asian Pac J Cancer Prev. 2015;16(4):1657-63.

8. Sharma P, Mathur K, Sharma R, et al. Serum Cortisol Level in Lung Cancer Patients at Various Stages of Diagnosis. International Journal of Basic & Applied Physiology. 2014. Available: http://ijbap.weebly.com/uploads/1/3/1/4/13145127/10.pdf . [January 1, 2016].

9. Zeitzer JM, Nouriani B, Rissling MB, et al. Aberrant nocturnal cortisol and disease progression in women with breast cancer. Breast Cancer Res Treat. 2016;158(1):43-50.

10. Fabre B, Grosman H, Gonzalez D, et al. Prostate Cancer, High Cortisol Levels and Complex Hormonal Interaction. Asian Pac J Cancer Prev. 2016;17(7):3167-71.

11. Tworoger SS, Eliassen AH, Sluss P, Hankinson SE. A prospective study of plasma prolactin concentrations and risk of premenopausal and postmenopausal breast cancer. J Clin Oncol. 2007;25(12):1482-8.

12. Bhatavdekar JM, Patel DD, Shah NG, et al. Prolactin as a local growth promoter in patients with breast cancer: GCRI experience. Eur J Surg Oncol. 2000;26(6):540-7.

13. Fernandez I, Touraine P, Goffin V. Prolactin and human tumourogenesis. J Neuroendocrinol. 2010;22(7):771-7.

14. Ratajczak-wrona W, Jablonska E, Antonowicz B, Dziemianczyk D, Grabowska SZ. Levels of biological markers of nitric oxide in serum of patients with squamous cell carcinoma of the oral cavity. Int J Oral Sci. 2013;5(3):141-5.

15. H. Higashino, M. Tabuchi, S. Yamagata, T. Kurita, H. Miya, H. Mukai and Y. Miya, 2010. Serum Nitric Oxide Metabolite Levels in Groups of Patients with Various Diseases in Comparison of Healthy Control Subjects. Journal of Medical Sciences, 10: 1-11.

16. John AP. Dysfunctional mitochondria, not oxygen insufficiency, cause cancer cells to produce inordinate amounts of lactic acid: the impact of this on the treatment of cancer. Med Hypotheses. 2001;57(4):429-31.

17. Fischer K, Hoffmann P, Voelkl S, et al. Inhibitory effect of tumor cell-derived lactic acid on human T cells. Blood. 2007;109(9):3812-9.

18. San-millán I, Brooks GA. Reexamining cancer metabolism: lactate production for carcinogenesis could be the purpose and explanation of the Warburg Effect. Carcinogenesis. 2016.

19. Wang WS, Liu C, Li WJ, Zhu P, Li JN, Sun K. Involvement of CRH and hCG in the induction of aromatase by cortisol in human placental syncytiotrophoblasts. Placenta. 2014;35(1):30-6.

20. Pugh S, Thomas GA. Patients with adenomatous polyps and carcinomas have increased colonic mucosal prostaglandin E2. Gut. 1994;35(5):675-8.

21. Bennett A, Charlier EM, Mcdonald AM, Simpson JS, Stamford IF, Zebro T. Prostaglandins and breast cancer. Lancet. 1977;2(8039):624-6.

22. Medina VA, Brenzoni PG, Lamas DJ, et al. Role of histamine H4 receptor in breast cancer cell proliferation. Front Biosci (Elite Ed). 2011;3:1042-60.

23. Kennedy L, Hodges K, Meng F, Alpini G, Francis H. Histamine and histamine receptor regulation of gastrointestinal cancers. Transl Gastrointest Cancer. 2012;1(3):215-227.

24. Mccall CM, Shi C, Klein AP, et al. Serotonin expression in pancreatic neuroendocrine tumors correlates with a trabecular histologic pattern and large duct involvement. Hum Pathol. 2012;43(8):1169-76.

25. Nilsson O, Ahlman H, Ericson LE, Skolnik G, Dahlström A. Release of serotonin from human carcinoid tumor cells in vitro and grown in the anterior eye chamber of the rat. Cancer. 1986;58(3):676-84.

26. Rangel-huerta OD, Aguilera CM, Martin MV, et al. Normal or High Polyphenol Concentration in Orange Juice Affects Antioxidant Activity, Blood Pressure, and Body Weight in Obese or Overweight Adults. J Nutr. 2015;145(8):1808-16.

27. Kwatra M, Jangra A, Mishra M, et al. Naringin and Sertraline Ameliorate Doxorubicin-Induced Behavioral Deficits Through Modulation of Serotonin Level and Mitochondrial Complexes Protection Pathway in Rat Hippocampus. Neurochem Res. 2016;41(9):2352-66.

28. Buscemi S, Rosafio G, Arcoleo G, et al. Effects of red orange juice intake on endothelial function and inflammatory markers in adult subjects with increased cardiovascular risk. Am J Clin Nutr. 2012;95(5):1089-95.

29. Hirata M, Matsumoto C, Takita M, Miyaura C, Masaki I. Naringin Suppresses Osteoclast Formation and Enhances Bone Mass in Mice. Journal of Health Sciences. 2009. Vol. 55.

30. Jiao HY, Su WW, Li PB, et al. Therapeutic effects of naringin in a guinea pig model of ovalbumin-induced cough-variant asthma. Pulm Pharmacol Ther. 2015;33:59-65.

31. Liu Y, Su WW, Wang S, Li PB. Naringin inhibits chemokine production in an LPS-induced RAW 264.7 macrophage cell line. Mol Med Rep. 2012;6(6):1343-50.

32. Peters EM, Anderson R, Theron AJ. Attenuation of increase in circulating cortisol and enhancement of the acute phase protein response in vitamin C-supplemented ultramarathoners. Int J Sports Med. 2001;22(2):120-6.

33. Casanueva E, Ripoll C, Meza-camacho C, Coutiño B, Ramírez-peredo J, Parra A. Possible interplay between vitamin C deficiency and prolactin in pregnant women with premature rupture of membranes: facts and hypothesis. Med Hypotheses. 2005;64(2):241-7.

34. Arivazhagan L, Sorimuthu pillai S. Tangeretin, a citrus pentamethoxyflavone, exerts cytostatic effect via p53/p21 up-regulation and suppresses metastasis in 7,12-dimethylbenz(α)anthracene-induced rat mammary carcinoma. J Nutr Biochem. 2014;25(11):1140-53.

35. Chao CL, Weng CS, Chang NC, Lin JS, Kao ST, Ho FM. Naringenin more effectively inhibits inducible nitric oxide synthase and cyclooxygenase-2 expression in macrophages than in microglia. Nutr Res. 2010;30(12):858-64.

36. Raso GM, Meli R, Di carlo G, Pacilio M, Di carlo R. Inhibition of inducible nitric oxide synthase and cyclooxygenase-2 expression by flavonoids in macrophage J774A.1. Life Sci. 2001;68(8):921-31.

37. Moran L, Giraldez FJ, Bodas R, Benavides J, Prieto N, Andres S. Metabolic acidosis corrected by including antioxidants in diets of fattening lambs. Small Ruminant Research.2013. Volume 109, Issues 2-3, Pages 133–135.

38. Murunga AN, Miruka DO, Driver C, Nkomo FS, Cobongela SZ, Owira PM. Grapefruit Derived Flavonoid Naringin Improves Ketoacidosis and Lipid Peroxidation in Type 1 Diabetes Rat Model. PLoS ONE. 2016;11(4):e0153241.

39. Huang Z, Fasco MJ, Kaminsky LS. Inhibition of estrone sulfatase in human liver microsomes by quercetin and other flavonoids. J Steroid Biochem Mol Biol. 1997;63(1-3):9-15.

40. Bulzomi P, Bolli A, Galluzzo P, Leone S, Acconcia F, Marino M. Naringenin and 17beta-estradiol coadministration prevents hormone-induced human cancer cell growth. IUBMB Life. 2010;62(1):51-60.

41. Sanderson JT, Hordijk J, Denison MS, Springsteel MF, Nantz MH, Van den berg M. Induction and inhibition of aromatase (CYP19) activity by natural and synthetic flavonoid compounds in H295R human adrenocortical carcinoma cells. Toxicol Sci. 2004;82(1):70-9.

42. Kawai M, Hirano T, Higa S, et al. Flavonoids and related compounds as anti-allergic substances. Allergol Int. 2007;56(2):113-23.

43. Park HH, Lee S, Son HY, et al. Flavonoids inhibit histamine release and expression of proinflammatory cytokines in mast cells. Arch Pharm Res. 2008;31(10):1303-11.

44. Rahman MS, Thomas P. Interactive effects of hypoxia with estradiol-17β on tryptophan hydroxylase activity and serotonin levels in the Atlantic croaker hypothalamus. Gen Comp Endocrinol. 2013;192:71-6.

45. Hiroi R, Mcdevitt RA, Neumaier JF. Estrogen selectively increases tryptophan hydroxylase-2 mRNA expression in distinct subregions of rat midbrain raphe nucleus: association between gene expression and anxiety behavior in the open field. Biol Psychiatry. 2006;60(3):288-95.

46. Peters EM, Anderson R, Nieman DC, Fickl H, Jogessar V. Vitamin C supplementation attenuates the increases in circulating cortisol, adrenaline and anti-inflammatory polypeptides following ultramarathon running. Int J Sports Med. 2001;22(7):537-43.

47. Vistelle R, Grulet H, Gibold C, et al. High permanent plasma adrenaline levels: a marker of adrenal medullary disease in medullary thyroid carcinoma. Clin Endocrinol (Oxf). 1991;34(2):133-8.

48. Mojtahedi Z, Khademi B, Yehya A, Talebi A, Fattahi MJ, Ghaderi A. Serum levels of interleukins 4 and 10 in head and neck squamous cell carcinoma. J Laryngol Otol. 2012;126(2):175-9.

49. Tang D, Kang R, Zeh HJ, Lotze MT. High-mobility group box 1 and cancer. Biochim Biophys Acta. 2010;1799(1-2):131-40.

50. Liu Y, Tamimi RM, Collins LC, et al. The association between vascular endothelial growth factor expression in invasive breast cancer and survival varies with intrinsic subtypes and use of adjuvant systemic therapy: results from the Nurses' Health Study. Breast Cancer Res Treat. 2011;129(1):175-84.

51. Pfeiffer P, Clausen PP, Andersen K, Rose C. Lack of prognostic significance of epidermal growth factor receptor and the oncoprotein p185HER-2 in patients with systemically untreated non-small-cell lung cancer: an immunohistochemical study on cryosections. Br J Cancer. 1996;74(1):86-91.

52. Gil M, Kim YK, Hong SB, Lee KJ. Naringin Decreases TNF-α and HMGB1 Release from LPS-Stimulated Macrophages and Improves Survival in a CLP-Induced Sepsis Mice. PLoS ONE. 2016;11(10):e0164186.

53. Luo H, Jiang BH, King SM, Chen YC. Inhibition of cell growth and VEGF expression in ovarian cancer cells by flavonoids. Nutr Cancer. 2008;60(6):800-9.

54. Wenzel U, Kuntz S, Daniel H. Flavonoids with epidermal growth factor-receptor tyrosine kinase inhibitory activity stimulate PEPT1-mediated cefixime uptake into human intestinal epithelial cells. J Pharmacol Exp Ther. 2001;299(1):351-7.

55. Catalano V, Turdo A, Di franco S, Dieli F, Todaro M, Stassi G. Tumor and its microenvironment: a synergistic interplay. Semin Cancer Biol. 2013;23(6 Pt B):522-32.

56. Morbidelli L, Donnini S, Ziche M. Role of nitric oxide in the modulation of angiogenesis. Curr Pharm Des. 2003;9(7):521-30.

57. Morbidelli L, Donnini S, Ziche M. Role of nitric oxide in tumor angiogenesis. Cancer Treat Res. 2004;117:155-67.

58. Ziche M, Morbidelli L. Nitric oxide and angiogenesis. J Neurooncol. 2000;50(1-2):139-48.

59. Morbidelli L, Donnini S, Ziche M. Role of nitric oxide in tumor angiogenesis. Cancer Treat Res. 2004;117:155-67.

60. Gallo O, Masini E, Morbidelli L, et al. Role of nitric oxide in angiogenesis and tumor progression in head and neck cancer. J Natl Cancer Inst. 1998;90(8):587-96.

61. Vidal MJ, Zocchi MR, Poggi A, Pellegatta F, Chierchia SL. Involvement of nitric oxide in tumor cell adhesion to cytokine-activated endothelial cells. J Cardiovasc Pharmacol. 1992;20 Suppl 12:S155-9.

62. Shavit Y, Weidenfeld J, Dekeyser FG, et al. Effects of surgical stress on brain prostaglandin E2 production and on the pituitary-adrenal axis: attenuation by preemptive analgesia and by central amygdala lesion. Brain Res. 2005;1047(1):10-7.

63. Wolfle D. Enhancement of carcinogen-induced malignant cell transformation by prostaglandin F2a. 2003; Volume 188, Issues 2-3, pages 139-147.

64. Fabre B, Grosman H, Gonzalez D, et al. Prostate Cancer, High Cortisol Levels and Complex Hormonal Interaction. Asian Pac J Cancer Prev. 2016;17(7):3167-71.

65. Kim HM, Ha KS, Hwang IC, Ahn HY, Youn CH. Random Serum Cortisol as a Predictor for Survival of Terminally Ill Patients With Cancer: A Preliminary Study. Am J Hosp Palliat Care. 2016;33(3):281-5.

66. Cohen L, Cole SW, Sood AK, et al. Depressive symptoms and cortisol rhythmicity predict survival in patients with renal cell carcinoma: role of inflammatory signaling. PLoS ONE. 2012;7(8):e42324.

67. Schmidt M, Löffler G. Induction of aromatase in stromal vascular cells from human breast adipose tissue depends on cortisol and growth factors. FEBS Lett. 1994;341(2-3):177-81.

68. Wang WS, Liu C, Li WJ, Zhu P, Li JN, Sun K. Involvement of CRH and hCG in the induction of aromatase by cortisol in human placental syncytiotrophoblasts. Placenta. 2014;35(1):30-6.

69. Wang W, Li J, Ge Y, et al. Cortisol induces aromatase expression in human placental syncytiotrophoblasts through the cAMP/Sp1 pathway. Endocrinology. 2012;153(4):2012-22.

70. Women's Health Initiative. Available: https://www.nhlbi.nih.gov/whi/estro_alone.htm. [December 1, 2016].

71. Soll C, Jang JH, Riener MO, et al. Serotonin promotes tumor growth in human hepatocellular cancer. Hepatology. 2010;51(4):1244-54.

72. Gurbuz N, Ashour AA, Alpay SN, Ozpolat B. Down-regulation of 5-HT1B and 5-HT1D receptors inhibits proliferation, clonogenicity and invasion of human pancreatic cancer cells. PLoS ONE. 2014;9(8):e105245.

73. Pai VP, Marshall AM, Hernandez LL, Buckley AR, Horseman ND. Altered serotonin physiology in human breast cancers favors paradoxical growth and cell survival. Breast Cancer Res. 2009;11(6):R81.

74. Siddiqui EJ, Shabbir MA, Mikhailidis DP, Mumtaz FH, Thompson CS. The effect of serotonin and serotonin antagonists on bladder cancer cell proliferation. BJU Int. 2006;97(3):634-9.

75. Sui H, Xu H, Ji Q, et al. 5-hydroxytryptamine receptor (5-HT1DR) promotes colorectal cancer metastasis by regulating Axin1/β-catenin/MMP-7 signaling pathway. Oncotarget. 2015;6(28):25975-87.

76. Koh KJ, Pearce AL, Marshman G, Finlay-jones JJ, Hart PH. Tea tree oil reduces histamine-induced skin inflammation. Br J Dermatol. 2002;147(6):1212-7.

77. Adlesic M, Verdrengh M, Bokarewa M, Dahlberg L, Foster SJ, Tarkowski A. Histamine in rheumatoid arthritis. Scand J Immunol. 2007;65(6):530-7.

78. Lefranc F, Yeaton P, Brotchi J, Kiss R. Cimetidine, an unexpected anti-tumor agent, and its potential for the treatment of glioblastoma (review). Int J Oncol. 2006;28(5):1021-30.

79. Hsieh HY, Shen CH, Lin RI, et al. Cyproheptadine exhibits antitumor activity in urothelial carcinoma cells by targeting GSK3β to suppress mTOR and β-catenin signaling pathways. Cancer Lett. 2016;370(1):56-65.

80. Harris AL, Smith IE. Regression of carcinoid tumour with cyproheptadine. Br Med J (Clin Res Ed). 1982;285(6340):475.

81. Choi SY, Collins CC, Gout PW, Wang Y. Cancer-generated lactic acid: a regulatory, immunosuppressive metabolite?. J Pathol. 2013;230(4):350-5.

82. Dhup S, Dadhich RK, Porporato PE, Sonveaux P. Multiple biological activities of lactic acid in cancer: influences on tumor growth, angiogenesis and metastasis. Curr Pharm Des. 2012;18(10):1319-30.

83. Wahl P, Zinner C, Achtzehn S, Bloch W, Mester J. Effect of high- and low-intensity exercise and metabolic acidosis on levels of GH, IGF-I, IGFBP-3 and cortisol. Growth Horm IGF Res. 2010;20(5):380-5.

84. Brand JM, Frohn C, Cziupka K, Brockmann C, Kirchner H, Luhm J. Prolactin triggers pro-inflammatory immune responses in peripheral immune cells. Eur Cytokine Netw. 2004;15(2):99-104.

85. Tworoger SS, Eliassen AH, Zhang X, et al. A 20-year prospective study of plasma prolactin as a risk marker of breast cancer development. Cancer Res. 2013;73(15):4810-9.

86. Clevenger, C.V. Role of Prolactin/Prolactin Receptor Signaling in Human Breast Cancer. Breast Disease. 18(1):75.

87. Recchione C, Galante E, Secreto G, Cavalleri A, Dati V. Abnormal serum hormone levels in lung cancer. Tumori. 1983;69(4):293-8.

88. Capuron L, Ravaud A, Neveu PJ, Miller AH, Maes M, Dantzer R. Association between decreased serum tryptophan concentrations and depressive symptoms in cancer patients undergoing cytokine therapy. Mol Psychiatry. 2002;7(5):468-73.

89. Coppack SW, Jensen MD, Miles JM. In vivo regulation of lipolysis in humans. J Lipid Res. 1994;35(2):177-93.

90. Lee CG, Link H, Baluk P, et al. Vascular endothelial growth factor (VEGF) induces remodeling and enhances TH2-mediated sensitization and inflammation in the lung. Nat Med. 2004;10(10):1095-103.

91. Manzoor H, Qadir MI, Abbas K, et al. Vascular endothelial growth factor (VEGF) in cancer. African journal of pharmacy and pharmacology. 2014;8(37):917-923.

92. Sasaki T, Hiroki K, Yamashita Y. The role of epidermal growth factor receptor in cancer metastasis and microenvironment. Biomed Res Int. 2013;2013:546318.

93. Koenders PG, Beex LV, Kienhuis CB, Kloppenborg PW, Benraad TJ. Epidermal growth factor receptor and prognosis in human breast cancer: a prospective study. Breast Cancer Res Treat. 1993;25(1):21-7.

94. Waldner MJ, Foersch S, Neurath MF. Interleukin-6--a key regulator of colorectal cancer development. Int J Biol Sci. 2012;8(9):1248-53.

95. Lentz EK, Cherla RP, Jaspers V, Weeks BR, Tesh VL. Role of tumor necrosis factor alpha in disease using a mouse model of Shiga toxin-mediated renal damage. Infect Immun. 2010;78(9):3689-99.

96. Mocellin S, Rossi CR, Pilati P, Nitti D. Tumor necrosis factor, cancer and anticancer therapy. Cytokine Growth Factor Rev. 2005;16(1):35-53.

97. Ulich TR, Del castillo J, Ni RX, Bikhazi N, Calvin L. Mechanisms of tumor necrosis factor alpha-induced lymphopenia, neutropenia, and biphasic neutrophilia: a study of lymphocyte recirculation and hematologic interactions of TNF alpha with endogenous mediators of leukocyte trafficking. J Leukoc Biol. 1989;45(2):155-67.

98. Clark GC, Taylor MJ. Tumor necrosis factor involvement in the toxicity of TCDD: the role of endotoxin in the response. Exp Clin Immunogenet. 1994;11(2-3):136-41.

99. Degasperi GR, Romanatto T, Denis RG, et al. UCP2 protects hypothalamic cells from TNF-alpha-induced damage. FEBS Lett. 2008;582(20):3103-10.

100. Han D, Hosokawa T, Aoike A, Kawai K. Age-related enhancement of tumor necrosis factor (TNF) production in mice. Mech Ageing Dev. 1995;84(1):39-54.

101. Schmidlin K, Spoerri A, Egger M, et al. Cancer, a disease of aging (part 1) - trends in older adult cancer mortality in Switzerland 1991-2008. Swiss Med Wkly. 2012;142:w13637.

102. Pinna F, Sahle S, Beuke K, et al. A Systems Biology Study on NFκB Signaling in Primary Mouse Hepatocytes. Front Physiol. 2012;3:466.

103. Wang S, Liu Z, Wang L, Zhang X. NF-kappaB signaling pathway, inflammation and colorectal cancer. Cell Mol Immunol. 2009;6(5):327-34.

104. Sakamoto K, Maeda S, Hikiba Y, et al. Constitutive NF-kappaB activation in colorectal carcinoma plays a key role in angiogenesis, promoting tumor growth. Clin Cancer Res. 2009;15(7):2248-58.

105. Bharti AC, Aggarwal BB. Nuclear factor-kappa B and cancer: its role in prevention and therapy. Biochem Pharmacol. 2002;64(5-6):883-8.

106. Olivier S, Robe P, Bours V. Can NF-kappaB be a target for novel and efficient anti-cancer agents?. Biochem Pharmacol. 2006;72(9):1054-68.

107. Weber J, Yang JC, Topalian SL, et al. Phase I trial of subcutaneous interleukin-6 in patients with advanced malignancies. J Clin Oncol. 1993;11(3):499-506.

108. Weiss GR, Margolin KA, Sznol M, et al. A phase II study of the continuous intravenous infusion of interleukin-6 for metastatic renal cell carcinoma. J Immunother Emphasis Tumor Immunol. 1995;18(1):52-6.

109. Tang D, Kang R, Zeh HJ, Lotze MT. High-mobility group box 1 and cancer. Biochim Biophys Acta. 2010;1799(1-2):131-40.

110. Okada S, Okusaka T, Ishii H, et al. Elevated serum interleukin-6 levels in patients with pancreatic cancer. Jpn J Clin Oncol. 1998;28(1):12-5.

111. Tian G, Mi J, Wei X, et al. Circulating interleukin-6 and cancer: A meta-analysis using Mendelian randomization. Sci Rep. 2015;5:11394.

112. Lobo V, Patil A, Phatak A, Chandra N. Free radicals, antioxidants and functional foods: Impact on human health. Pharmacogn Rev. 2010;4(8):118-26.

113. Chen Q, Guan X, Zuo X, Wang J, Yin W. The role of high mobility group box 1 (HMGB1) in the pathogenesis of kidney diseases. Acta Pharm Sin B. 2016;6(3):183-8.

114. Nguyen DP, Li J, Tewari AK. Inflammation and prostate cancer: the role of interleukin 6 (IL-6). BJU Int. 2014;113(6):986-92.

CHAPTER 7

ORANGES

SWEET, POWERFULLY REFRESHING and bursting with flavor; it's no surprise that oranges are one of the most popular fruits in the world. Most people are aware that oranges are a potent source of vitamin C, but there are a number of other nutrients within an orange that boost its medicinal value considerably.

In this chapter, we will investigate the therapeutic potential of citrus flavonoids, modified citrus pectin, vitamin C and orange juice on cancer and overall health.

CITRUS FLAVONOIDS

Flavonoids are naturally occurring substances found in fruits, vegetables, teas and wines that are responsible for the diversity of colors produced by plants.[1] Epidemiological studies have shown that dietary consumption of flavonoids can reduce the risk of cardiovascular disease,[3] asthma, type 2 diabetes, heart disease, prostate cancer and lung cancer.[4]

More than 60 flavonoids have been identified in citrus fruit, making them one of the most concentrated and readily available sources of flavonoids.[366] A 2003 study from the UK found that a Sicilian variety of orange called *Tarocco* had higher concentrations of citrus flavonoids than 6 other orange varieties tested.[5] Interestingly, flavonoids are found more abundantly in the peel than in the pulp of citrus fruit.[2]

Some examples of citrus flavonoids include naringin, naringenin, diosmin, hesperetin, hesperidin, quercetin, tangeretin, nobiletin. In this section we will investigate three of them.

CITRUS FLAVONOIDS VS. CANCER

One of the methods used by scientists to test the therapeutic value of nutrients or drugs against cancer is to add them to a test tube containing cancer cells and observe the effects. Testing cancer cells outside of living organisms in this way is called *in vitro*. Sometimes effects observed in vitro are not the same as inside living organisms, or *in vivo*, but many times they are, as you will see.

NARINGIN

In vitro studies have confirmed naringin can inhibit the **growth** of stomach,[9] cervical,[12] breast,[14] and colon cancer cells,[11] the **spread** of brain[7,8] and bone cancer cells,[10] and trigger cancer cell death (**apoptosis**) in colon,[11,17] pancreatic,[17] stomach,[17] cervical,[12,13,17] liver[17] and breast cancer cells.[14,17]

Another popular method used by scientists to determine the value of nutrients or drugs against cancer is by inducing cancer in animals - usually by injecting carcinogenic chemicals into them - and then administering the treatment and observing the outcome.

In vivo studies have confirmed naringin can inhibit the **growth** of colon,[18] oral,[19] lung[20] and connective tissue tumors,[16,17] the **spread** of skin tumors[20] and trigger **apoptosis** in colon tumors.[18]

A Closer Look...

___

- In 2012, scientists from Sao Paulo, Brazil, investigated the effects of naringin on rats bearing connective tissue cancer. Results showed that a 25mg/kg dose of naringin administered daily for 50 days inhibited tumor growth by 75%. Naringin also increased survival and notably, "two rats presented complete tumor regression."[16]

One of the most exciting experiments on naringin was conducted in 2016 by Chinese researchers, who added naringin to skin cancer cells to determine its impact on cellular energy metabolism. One of the key changes in the metabolism of cancer cells is increased production of lactic acid, and not only did naringin inhibit lactic acid production in the skin cancer cells, but it also completely reversed them back into normal cells. "In summary, we demonstrated that naringin inhibits the malignant phenotype of A375 cells." they concluded.[15]

Perhaps best of all, the beneficial effects of naringin can be obtained "without adverse side effects."[59]

Normally, once a 'drug' has proven itself in vitro and in vivo, it would move on to human testing in clinical trials, but since the average cost of phase 1 clinical trial in the United States ranges from $1.4 million to $6.6 million dollars;[198] and since natural substances found in foods can't be patented or sold by drug companies, this type of research doesn't often receive funding and is thus rarely performed. Many times, the only reason in vitro and in vivo studies on food nutrients are funded is so drug companies can find medicines that work and then attempt to replicate similar chemicals to patent and sell.

NARINGENIN

A 2015 study identified naringenin as one of 10 therapeutic agents "that may warrant further investigation to target the tumor microenvironment" for preventing and treating cancer."[64]

In vitro experiments have established naringenin can inhibit the **growth** of breast,[65,73] stomach,[71] colon,[66,73] skin,[68,76] leukemia[75] and liver cancer cells,[67,77] the **spread** of breast,[65] liver,[67] skin,[68] bladder,[69] pancreatic,[70] and stomach cancer cells,[71] and trigger **apoptosis** in liver,[67,77] stomach,[71] colon,[72,73] breast,[73,74] leukemia[75] and skin cancer cells.[76]

Animal experiments have verified naringenin can inhibit the **growth** of oral,[19] stomach,[78] lung[81] and brain tumors,[80] prevent the **spread** of breast tumors[79] and trigger **apoptosis** in brain tumors.[82]

Synergistic enhancement of the anti-cancer effects of naringenin can be obtained by combining it with either curcumin[83] or vitamin E,[84] and one study reports that nano-encapsulated naringenin exhibits "significantly higher" antioxidant and anticancer properties than naringenin in free form.[86]

Naringenin has a "promising safety profile"[133] and remarkably, it maintains its cancer-killing effects even in the presence of the environmental toxin bisphenol A.[85]

HESPERIDIN

In vitro, hesperidin can inhibit the **growth** of breast,[134,135] immune,[138] leukemia,[140,141] and lung cancer cells,[143] the **spread** of skin cancer cells,[136] and trigger **apoptosis** in breast,[135,144] immune,[138] colon,[139] leukemia,[140,141] liver[137,142] and lung cancer cells.[143]

Animal studies have confirmed hesperidin can inhibit the **growth** of colon,[145] lung,[146] bladder,[147] oral,[148,149] throat[150] and stomach tumors,[151] and trigger **apoptosis** in stomach[151] and colon tumors.[152]

One study compared the medicinal potencies of a number of citrus flavonoids and found that hesperidin exerted a more powerful anti-cancer effect than neohesperidin, naringin and naringenin.[137] With that in mind, Tunisian researchers reported in 2016 that concentrations of hesperidin were greater in organically-grown oranges than in oranges grown conventionally.[6]

A safety study from 1990 fed rats dietary concentrations of 0%, 1.25% or 5% methyl hesperidin for two years and concluded that the substance "lacked any carcinogenicity" in rats.[193]

ADDITIONAL HEALTH EFFECTS

Antibacterial:

- Naringin exerts a "robust antibacterial effect"[21]

- Hesperidin inhibits growth of bifidobacteria[153]

Antioxidant:

- Naringin neutralizes the toxic effects of herbicide paraquat[22]
- Naringin prevents kidney and liver damage from acetaminophen[23] and sodium arsenite[24]
- Naringin prevents chemotherapy-induced kidney[25] and lung damage[26]
- Naringin reverses side effects of HIV medication[29,30]
- Naringenin prevents damage from lead[108] and endotoxin[87]
- Hesperidin prevents chemically-induced kidney damage[155-158]
- Hesperidin prevents chemotherapy-induced liver damage[161]

Antiviral:

- Naringin[28] and naringenin[93] inhibit infection by sindbis virus[28]
- Naringenin reduces hepatitis C virus secretions from infected cells by 80%[92]
- Hesperidin prevents replication of influenza A virus[162]
- Hesperidin inhibits infection by canine distemper virus[163] and rotavirus[164]
- Hesperidin inhibits combined viral-bacterial infections[165]

Arthritis:

- Naringin prevents inflammation associated with arthritis[31-34]
- Naringenin prevents inflammatory pain in mice[94,95]
- Hesperidin prevents chemically-induced arthritis[154,166,167]

Asthma:

- Naringin significantly reduces coughing (associated with a type of asthma that causes chronic coughing)[63]

Bone Health:

- Naringin prevents the destruction of cartilage[38]
- Naringin,[35,36] naringenin[96-99] and hesperidin[168-170] prevent bone loss and accelerate bone formation

Brain Health:

- Naringin improves brain function in mice with Alzheimer's disease[42,43]
- Naringin prevents brain degeneration in rats with Parkinson's disease[44-46]
- Naringin reverses chemically-induced memory deficits[39-41,47]
- Naringin prevents chemically-induced seizures[48]
- Naringenin reduces anxiety caused by lead poisoning[89]
- Naringenin prevents brain damage caused by neurotoxins[90] and iron[102]
- Naringenin prevents Alzheimer's disease[100]
- Naringenin improves learning and memory in rats with Alzheimer's disease[101]
- Naringenin prevents cognitive decline in rats with Parkinson's disease[103]
- Hesperidin prevents brain damage from pesticides,[171] heavy metals,[172] and other poisons[174]
- Hesperidin prevents cognitive impairment in mice with Alzheimer's disease[173]

Cooking:

- Naringenin prevents toxic acrylamides from forming in food during high-heat cooking[132]

Dental Health:

- Naringin remineralizes root caries (cavities) in teeth[37]

Depression:

- Naringenin produces antidepressant-like behavior in rats[106,107]
- Naringenin[105] and hesperidin[175-177] exert potent antidepressant effects

Detoxification:

- Naringenin chelates lead from the body[108]

Diabetes:

- Naringin prevents scarring of the heart caused by diabetes[49]
- Naringenin prevents kidney damage caused by diabetes[52,109]
- Naringenin improves glucose metabolism[110,111]

- Naringin improves insulin sensitivity[50,51]
- Hesperidin reduces diabetes and its complications[178]

Digestive Health:

- Naringenin an effective treatment for inflammatory bowel disease[120,121]
- Naringenin prevents defects of the intestinal barrier[122]

Exercise:

- Naringin in combination with treadmill exercise is more effective at increasing bone strength and density than either therapy alone[53]
- Hesperidin synergistically enhances the health benefits of exercise[179]

Eye Health:

- Naringenin eye drops prevent chemically-induced retinal damage[91]
- Hesperidin prevents eye damage caused by chemotherapy[159]

Food Production:

- Naringin and Hesperidin fed to chickens elevates antioxidant levels in chicken meat; are "important additives for both the consumer and the industry."[27]

Headaches:

- Drynaria quercifolia (a plant containing naringin) alleviates painful inflammatory conditions, like headache[54]
- Hesperidin may be useful for treating migraines[180]

Healing:

- Naringin[55] and hesperidin[191] accelerate wound healing

Heart Health:

- Naringin[56] and naringenin[113] prevent arterial plaque formation
- Naringinen reduces arterial stiffness[112]
- Naringenin prevents thickening of the heart muscle[114]

Immune System:

- Naringenin boosts the immune system[115,116]
- Naringenin significantly enhances anti-cancer immunity[117-119]
- Hesperidin enhances immune systems of mice[181] and irradiated mice[189]
- Hesperidin enhances immune systems of broiler chickens[182]

Obesity:

- Naringin significantly decreases fat mass[57,59]
- Naringin prevents formation of new fat tissue[58]
- Naringenin reduces body fat and suppresses weight gain[123-125]
- Hesperidin improves lipid metabolism in humans[183,184]

Radiation protective:

- Naringin protects skin from ultraviolet B radiation[61]
- Naringin[60] and naringenin[126] prevent genetic damage caused by ionizing radiation
- Naringenin prevents skin aging and wrinkle formation caused by ultraviolet B radiation[127-129]
- Naringenin added to conventional sunscreen reduces its toxicity[130]
- Hesperidin reduces damage caused by whole-body gamma ray irradiation[185]
- Hesperidin prevents ultraviolet B radiation damage[186,187]
- Hesperidin prevents brain damage caused by ionizing radiation[188]

Sexual Health:

- Naringenin aids the process of conception[104]
- Naringenin prevents testicle damage caused by insecticides[88]
- Hesperidin prevents testicle and sperm damage caused by chemotherapy[160]

Skin Health:

- Naringin[62] and hesperidin[192] promote the production of skin-protective melanin

- Naringenin "should be introduced into cosmetic products as natural tanning agents."[131]

Other:

- A mixture of citrus flavonoids Hesperidin, Troxerutin, and Diosmin applied to hemmorhoids reduces pain, bleeding and swelling in humans[190]

MODIFIED CITRUS PECTIN

Pectin is a complex of sugar molecules (polysaccharide) heavily concentrated in the pulp and peel of citrus fruit. Because of its gelling properties, pectin is a traditional ingredient used for making marmalades and jams.

Pectin's long-branched chains of polysaccharides make it virtually indigestible by humans, but researchers have discovered ways to *modify* pectin so it can be easily absorbed into the blood stream. Once in the bloodstream, modified citrus pectin (MCP) has proven useful for treating a number of conditions, including cancer.[317] Although heat treatment and pH modifications are commonly used to create modified citrus pectin,[315] high-intensity ultrasound is also effective and is said to be more 'environmentally friendly.'[316]

"The more we learn about MCP, the more impressive it becomes," said Dr. Isaac Eliaz. "With its ability to control aggressive cancers, reduce inflammation, enhance immunity, chelate heavy metals and work synergistically with a variety of chemotherapeutic agents, it has earned an important role within anti-cancer and chronic disease protocols."[367]

MODIFIED CITRUS PECTIN VS. CANCER

Scientists have observed modified citrus pectin prevent the **growth** of prostate cancer cells[320,322] and trigger **apoptosis** in lung,[321] liver,[321] prostate[322] and eight other types of cancer cells.[323]

Co-administration of modified citrus pectin with two herbal products have revealed synergistic inhibitory effects on the spread of breast and prostate cancer in vitro.[324] Modified citrus pectin can also eliminate chemotherapy resistance[325] and increase the apoptosis-inducing effects of chemotherapy in cell cultures.[326]

Modified citrus pectin can prevent the **growth** of skin[327] and sarcoma tumors in mice; including a 51% reduction in tumor size and increased survival compared to control mice.[323] Another study reported a 70% reduction in colon tumor size in mice after 20 days of MCP treatment.[332] Also in animals, the **spread** of breast,[328] prostate,[329] skin[330] and colon tumors can be inhibited by as much as 90% using modified citrus pectin.[331]

Scientists from the Harry S. Truman Memorial Veteran's Hospital in Missouri discovered that MCP prevents cancer metastasis by inhibiting circulating tumor cells from adhering and establishing themselves onto distal body tissues.[318] Another mechanism behind MCP's therapeutic effects is the inhibition of a substance called Galectin-3, which is involved in inflammation, fibrosis, heart disease, stroke and cancer.[319]

Studies report modified citrus pectin has no adverse side effects,[339] including one study in which 15 grams MCP was administered daily to humans for 12 consecutive months.[340]

ADDITIONAL HEALTH EFFECTS

Antioxidant:
- MCP prevents liver fibrosis[334]
- MCP prevents kidney injury[335]
- MCP prevents damage caused by endotoxin[336]

Arthritis:
- MCP is "a therapeutic approach for the treatment of inflammatory arthritis"[337]

Detoxification:
- MCP dramatically increases urinary excretion of arsenic, cadmium and lead in humans[338]
- MCP safely and dramatically detoxifies lead from children[339]

- MCP reduces toxic heavy metal burden in humans by an average of 74%[340]

Heart Health:

- MCP "may represent a new promising therapeutic option in heart failure"[341]
- MCP decreases cardiovascular fibrosis and inflammation[342,343,344]
- Galectin-3 inhibition "causes decreased atherosclerosis"[345]

Immune System:

- MCP enhances anti-cancer immunity[346]

Inflammation:

- MCP reduces inflammation and pain after spinal nerve injury[333]

Obesity:

- MCP prevents production of new fat tissue[347]

VITAMIN C

Although vitamin C (aka ascorbic acid or ascorbate) wasn't officially discovered until 1928 by Hungarian biochemist Albert Szent-Gyorgyi,[194] the manifestations of its deficiency, known as scurvy,[195] were first documented by the physician Hippocrates in ancient Greece (460BC-370BC).[368] In 1945, scientists from the University of Wisconsin found that when they deprived monkeys of vitamin C for just a few weeks, various dental issues including bleeding gums, loosening of the teeth and the formation of heavy tartar deposits were induced.[196]

The effects of supplemental vitamin C are highly-dependent on the dose administered. In low doses, vitamin C behaves as an anti-oxidant, helping the body neutralize toxins and eliminate waste products. And in high doses, vitamin C acts as a pro-oxidant that can selectively target unhealthy and even cancerous cells.[197] High-doses of intravenous vitamin C have been used to treat cancer since the 1970s.[200]

VITAMIN C VS. CANCER

One thing cancer patients all have in common is significantly depleted levels of vitamin C.[222] Remarkably, some researchers have said that vitamin C might be the most important nutritional factor needed by the body to resist cancer; "There is increasing recognition that resistance to cancer depends, to a certain extent, upon the availability of certain nutritional factors, of which ascorbic acid appears to be the most important," wrote scientist Ewan Cameron in 1982.[201]

An epidemiological study of people in Northern Italy reported that vitamin C intake has "possible protective activity" against skin cancer[202] and greater consumption of antioxidants was associated with less aggressive prostate cancer in the United States.[203] A 2014 systematic review by Chinese researchers concluded that low doses of vitamins, specifically vitamins A, C and E, can significantly reduce the risk of stomach cancer.[204]

In vitro studies have confirmed vitamin C can trigger **apoptosis** in colon,[206,207,214] breast,[207] skin,[208] blood,[209] bone marrow,[209] Ehrlich acites carcinoma,[205] melanoma[220] and four types of malignant mesothelioma cancer cells.[213] Co-administration of vitamin C and vitamin B2 can synergistically enhance apoptosis in multiple types of cancer cells.[210] Vitamin C loaded into tiny bubbles of fat (lipid nanoparticles) was shown to enter into cells more efficiently than free vitamin C[219] and vitamin C affixed to nano-sized polymer carriers has been shown to trigger apoptosis in brain cancer cells.[218]

In animals, vitamin C can prevent the **growth** of lung,[211] skin,[211] ovarian,[212] pancreatic,[212] brain,[212] malignant mesothelioma,[213] colon[214] and sarcoma tumors,[215] and can trigger **apoptosis** in liver tumors.[216] A nutrient mixture containing lysine, vitamin C, proline, green tea extract and other micronutrients fed to tumor-bearing mice "demonstrated a potent inhibition of [cervical] tumor growth."[217]

A CLOSER LOOK...

- An American group of scientists from Kansas administered 500mg/kg/day sodium ascorbate to liver tumor-bearing guinea pigs in 2006. Results showed that "Subcutaneous injections of ascorbate (500 mg/kg/day) inhibited tumor growth by as much as sixty-five percent, with oral supplementation reducing it by roughly fifty percent." [216]

In 1994, researchers from the Oregon Institute of Science and Medicine induced tumors in mice and treated them with high-doses of vitamin C along with variations in diet. Results showed that survival could be increased by up to 20-times simply by adjusting the animal's nutritional intake. [221]

Two-time Nobel Prize winner Linus Pauling and surgeon Ewan Cameron administered 10 grams/day of vitamin C to terminal cancer patients in 1976 and found that survival was increased "more than 4.2 times" compared to patients who weren't given vitamin C. [222] Other studies have confirmed vitamin C can increase survival and significantly improve the quality of life of terminal cancer patients. [223-225]

How does vitamin C exert its beneficial effects? When blood levels of vitamin C are maintained at a consistently high level, it is absorbed into cancerous tissue where it produces hydrogen peroxide that kills cancer cells. [199]

SAFETY

Thanks to the work of Dr. Frederick R. Klenner, it has been known for over 70 years that vitamin C doses as high as 300,000mg (300 grams) per day in humans are safe and modern research has confirmed this finding. [205,209,212,224,225,235,260]

A Korean study from 2007 acknowledged that vitamin C "is considered a safe and effective therapy" [225] and a 2008 study from the National Institutes of Health found that high-doses of vitamin C displayed "cytotoxicity toward a variety of cancer cells in vitro without adversely affecting normal cells." [212]

One thing to be aware of is that vitamin C can increase the absorption of iron, [307-309] which in small amounts is essential, but like all heavy metals, becomes toxic in excess [311] and can diminish the effectiveness of vitamin C treatment. [310] For these reasons, oral supplementation of vitamin C is probably best without food and to lower existing iron levels in the body, iron-chelating substances such as tetracycline, doxycycline, minocycline [312] or curcumin [369] can be used.

ORAL VS. INTRAVENOUS

There is some controversy surrounding the efficacy of various vitamin C administration methods. While Dr. Mark Levine of the NIH claims that "...only injected ascorbate might deliver the concentrations needed to see an anti-tumor effect,"[313] Dr. Steve Hickey has said, "it is not clear that intravenous vitamin C necessarily provides an advantage over oral supplements in the treatment of cancer."[314]

When the body is given a high enough dose of vitamin C intravenously, much of it goes unused and is excreted in the urine, according to Dr. Hickey. Furthermore, he makes the case that high-doses of orally administered vitamin C might even be *more* effective.[314]

While Dr. Levine claims that maximum blood levels of vitamin C are 200μM/L, Dr. Hickey maintains he has been able to generate blood levels of around 250μM/L with a single 5 gram oral dose of vitamin C and blood levels above 400μM/L with a single oral dose of liposomal vitamin C.[314]

DOSE

For many people, a single oral dose of 2 grams of vitamin C will cause a laxative effect and anything more will be eliminated from the body. Interestingly, bowel tolerance is said to increase dramatically when a person is ill.[314] In other words, a person who would normally be able to tolerate only 2 grams might be able to tolerate 100-times that amount when sick.

Maximum blood levels of orally-ingested vitamin C can be achieved by consuming about 3 grams every four hours. Since vitamin C is only active in the body for a few hours, frequent doses are critical to maintain consistently high blood levels.

SUCCESS STORIES

Dr. Victor Marcial, radiation oncologist:

"We studied patients with advanced cancer (stage 4). 40 patients received 40,000-75,000 mg intravenously several times a week. These are patients that have not responded to other treatments. The initial tumor response rate was achieved in 75% of patients, defined as a 50% reduction or more in tumor size... Once you start using IV vitamin C, the effect is so dramatic that it is difficult to go back to not using it."

Dr. Linus Pauling, 2x Nobel Prize Laureate:

"I became interested in vitamin C and cancer in 1971 and began working with Ewan Cameron, M.B., Ch.B., chief surgeon at Vale of Leven Hospital in Scotland. Cameron gave 10 grams of vitamin C a day to patients with untreatable, terminal cancer. These patients were then compared by Cameron and me to patients with the same kind of cancer at the same terminal stage who were being treated in the same hospital but by other doctors-doctors who didn't give vitamin C, but instead just gave conventional treatments. Cameron's terminal cancer patients lived far longer compared to the ones who didn't get 10 grams a day of vitamin C. The other patients lived an average of six months after they were pronounced terminal, while Cameron's patients lived an average of about six years."

Dr. Irwin Stone, American biochemist, chemical engineer:

"In one case where complete remission was achieved in myelogenous leukemia... the patient took 24-42 gms vitamin c per day... it is inconceivable that no-one appears to have followed this up... without the scurvy, leukemia may be a relatively benign, non-fatal condition. I wrote a paper... in an attempt to have the therapy clinically tested... I sent it to 3 cancer journals and 3 blood journals... it was refused by all... Two without even reading it."

ADDITIONAL HEALTH EFFECTS

Antioxidant:

- Vitamin C an antidote for snake venom[228]
- Vitamin C a cure for carbon monoxide poisoning[233]
- Vitamin C a cure for mushroom poisoning[229]
- Vitamin C prevents damage caused by agricultural fungicides[230] and insecticides[231]

- Vitamin C prevents liver damage caused by dexmedetomidine[236]
- Vitamin C prevents damage caused by monosodium glutamate[237]
- Vitamin C prevents damage caused by methylmercury,[238] formaldehyde[239] and endotoxin[241,242,245,246,248]
- Vitamin C prevents chemically-induced ulcer formation in rats[240]
- Vitamin C prevents septic organ injury in mice[243]
- Vitamin C prevents alcohol-induced liver fibrosis in mice[244]
- Vitamin C prevents the formation of nitric oxide[247]
- Vitamin C prevents kidney[249] and liver damage[250,251] caused by chemotherapy

Antiviral:

- Vitamin C "kills influenza virus"[252]
- Vitamin C shortens duration of the common cold, pneumonia, malaria and diarrhea infections[253]
- Vitamin C suppresses HIV replication by infected cells[254]
- Vitamin C successfully treats hepatitis, mononucleosis and pneumonia[255]
- Vitamin C successfully treats polio, diphtheria, herpes zoster, herpes simplex, chicken pox, influenza, measles, mumps and viral pneumonia[256]
- Vitamin C successfully treats Epstein-Barr virus[257]
- Vitamin C resolves all symptoms of Chikungunya fever in two days[260]

Arthritis:

- Elevated free radicals and oxidative stress found in patients with Rheumatoid Arthritis[227]

Bone Health:

- Vitamin C prevents bone loss[261]
- Vitamin C improves bone mineral density in postmenopausal women[262-264]
- Vitamin C is "a skeletal anabolic agent"[265]
- Vitamin A, C and E decrease risk of hip fracture[266]

Brain Health:

- Vitamin C prevents brain damage caused by methamphetamine,[267] insecticides[268,269] and glutamate[270]
- Vitamin C deficiency increases risk of seizures[271]
- Vitamin C (and zinc) deficiencies impair the physical and mental growth of children[287]
- Vitamin C levels in patients with severe Parkinson's disease were "significantly lower"[272]

Depression:

- Vitamin C reduces anxiety levels in highschool students after 14 days of supplementing 500mg[276]

Detoxification:

- Vitamin C chelates lead from the bloodstream[277]
- Vitamin C reduces blood levels of chemical pollutants[232]

Diabetes:

- Vitamin C reduces fasting blood sugar in diabetics[278,280]
- Vitamin C significantly lowers needed insulin dose for blood sugar control[279]

Exercise:

- Vitamin C and low-intensity exercise prevent seizures[281]
- Vitamin C has anti-seizure effects in rats performing endurance swimming[282]
- Vitamin C improves blood flow and oxygen use in muscles[283]

Food Production:

- Vitamin C improves growth performance and enhances stress resistance in fish[303]

Headaches:

- Vitamin C and Pinus Radiata bark extract ingested for 12 months reduces headache severity and frequency by 50%[284]

Healing:

- Vitamin C accelerates healing[235,301]
- Vitamin C enhances cell survival and DNA repair in human fibroblasts exposed to x-rays[299]

Heart Health:

- Vitamin C decreases length of hospital stay in patients following cardiac surgery[304]

Immune System:

- Vitamin C enhances anti-cancer immunity[285,289-292]
- Vitamin C significantly enhances immunity[286-288]

Inflammation:

- Vitamin C reduces inflammation[226]

Lifespan:

- Antioxidant-rich diet extends survival of mice exposed to endotoxin[234]
- Vitamin C extends lifespan of tetanus patients[258,259]

Obesity:

- Vitamin C intake reduces obesity in women[293]

Radiation protective:

- Vitamin C prevents damage caused by ionizing radiation[294,297,298]
- Vitamin C and vitamin E synergistically prevent damage caused by ionizing radiation[295]
- Vitamin C and melatonin synergistically prevent damage caused by ionizing radiation[296]

Sexual Health:

- Vitamin C "significantly improves sperm concentration and mobility" [274]
- Vitamin C prevents infertility in rats subjected to forced swimming stress[275]
- Vitamin C promotes a healthy pregnancy[273]

Sleep:

- Vitamin C prevents spatial memory impairment in rats following sleep deprivation[300]

Other:

- Vitamin C resolves symptoms of burning mouth syndrome in humans[302]
- Vitamin C diminishes microparticle elevations caused by SCUBA diving[305]
- Vitamin C prevents complex regional pain syndrome in humans[306]

ORANGE JUICE

If an orange contains all the medicines we've investigated above, then one would expect orange juice to have substantial therapeutic value as well.

ORANGE JUICE VS CANCER

Although studies are limited, scientists have investigated the therapeutic effects of orange juice on cancer cell cultures and in animals. In vitro studies have confirmed orange juice can trigger **apoptosis** in two types of blood cancer cells.[348]

In vivo, researchers have experimentally induced tumors in rats and then replaced their water with orange juice to determine its effects. Results show that orange juice can inhibit the **growth** of breast,[349] colon,[350-352] tongue[352] and lung tumors,[352] and can trigger **apoptosis** in colon tumors.[350]

A CLOSER LOOK...

- In 2015, Brazilian researchers incubated two types of blood cancer cells with orange juice – one with the juice of a red-fleshed sweet orange and the other with juice from a blond orange - for 24-hours and observed the results. At the end of the study, both varieties of orange juice were found to induce apoptosis in the blood cancer cells.[348]
- Mandarin orange juice was tested on rats induced with three types of cancers in a 2012 Japanese study from the *Journal of Biomedicine & Biotechnology*. Citrus juices from the satsuma mandarin orange were

found to inhibit the formation of chemically-induced colon, tongue and lung tumors in rats.[352]

- Canadian scientists from Western University in London, Ontario, chemically-induced breast tumors in rats and fed them orange juice to determine if it could prevent cancer formation. Published in the journal *Nutrition and Cancer* in 1996, results showed that rats given orange juice "had a smaller tumor burden than controls." [349]

ADDITIONAL HEALTH EFFECTS

Antibacterial:

- Tangerine juice concentrate is effective for "controlling unwanted microbial growth" [353]

Antioxidant:

- Orange juice consumption results in a "marked antioxidant effect"[355,356]

Bone Health:

- Orange juice increases bone strength in rats[358]
- Orange juice increases bone mineral density in children and adults[357]

Exercise:

- Orange juice prevents exercise-induced hypoxia[359]
- Orange juice improves physical performance in overweight women[360]

Heart Health:

- Fermented orange juice reduces cardiovascular risk factors[361]

Immune System:

- Orange juice enhances the immune system[362]

Inflammation:

- Orange juice reduces inflammation[354]

Obesity:

- Orange juice associated with healthier body composition in adults[363]
- Orange juice decreases risk of obesity[364]
- Orange juice prevents fatty liver disease[365]

REFERENCES

1. Patel K, Singh GK, Patel DK. A review on pharmacological and analytical aspects of naringenin. Chin J Integr Med. 2014.

2. Nakajima VM, Madeira JV, Macedo GA, Macedo JA. Biotransformation effects on anti lipogenic activity of citrus extracts. Food Chem. 2016;197 Pt B:1046-53.

3. Chanet A, Milenkovic D, Manach C, Mazur A, Morand C. Citrus flavanones: what is their role in cardiovascular protection?. J Agric Food Chem. 2012;60(36):8809-22.

4. Knekt P, Kumpulainen J, Järvinen R, et al. Flavonoid intake and risk of chronic diseases. Am J Clin Nutr. 2002;76(3):560-8.

5. Proteggente AR, Saija A, De pasquale A, Rice-evans CA. The compositional characterisation and antioxidant activity of fresh juices from sicilian sweet orange (Citrus sinensis L. Osbeck) varieties. Free Radic Res. 2003;37(6):681-7.

6. Letaief H, Zemni H, Mliki A, Chebil S. Composition of Citrus sinensis (L.) Osbeck cv «Maltaise demi-sanguine» juice. A comparison between organic and conventional farming. Food Chem. 2016;194:290-5.

7. Aroui S, Aouey B, Chtourou Y, Meunier AC, Fetoui H, Kenani A. Naringin suppresses cell metastasis and the expression of matrix metalloproteinases (MMP-2 and MMP-9) via the inhibition of ERK-P38-JNK signaling pathway in human glioblastoma. Chem Biol Interact. 2016;244:195-203.

8. Aroui S, Najlaoui F, Chtourou Y, et al. Naringin inhibits the invasion and migration of human glioblastoma cell via downregulation of MMP-2 and MMP-9 expression and inactivation of p38 signaling pathway. Tumour Biol. 2016;37(3):3831-9.

9. Raha S, Yumnam S, Hong GE, et al. Naringin induces autophagy-mediated growth inhibition by downregulating the PI3K/Akt/mTOR cascade via activation of MAPK pathways in AGS cancer cells. Int J Oncol. 2015;47(3):1061-9.

10. Tan TW, Chou YE, Yang WH, Hsu CJ, Fong YC, Tang CH. Naringin suppress chondrosarcoma migration through inhibition vascular adhesion molecule-1 expression by modulating miR-126. Int Immunopharmacol. 2014;22(1):107-14.

11. Vadde R, Radhakrishnan S, Reddivari L, Vanamala JK. Triphala Extract Suppresses Proliferation and Induces Apoptosis in Human Colon Cancer Stem Cells via Suppressing c-Myc/Cyclin D1 and Elevation of Bax/Bcl-2 Ratio. Biomed Res Int. 2015;2015:649263.

12. Zeng L, Zhen Y, Chen Y, et al. Naringin inhibits growth and induces apoptosis by a mechanism dependent on reduced activation of NF-κB/COX-2-caspase-1 pathway in HeLa cervical cancer cells. Int J Oncol. 2014;45(5):1929-36.

13. Ramesh E, Alshatwi AA. Naringin induces death receptor and mitochondria-mediated apoptosis in human cervical cancer (SiHa) cells. Food Chem Toxicol. 2013;51:97-105.

14. Li H, Yang B, Huang J, et al. Naringin inhibits growth potential of human triple-negative breast cancer cells by targeting β-catenin signaling pathway. Toxicol Lett. 2013;220(3):219-28.

15. Guo B, Zhang Y, Hui Q, Wang H, Tao K. Naringin suppresses the metabolism of A375 cells by inhibiting the phosphorylation of c-Src. Tumour Biol. 2016;37(3):3841-50.

16. Camargo CA, Gomes-marcondes MC, Wutzki NC, Aoyama H. Naringin inhibits tumor growth and reduces interleukin-6 and tumor necrosis factor α levels in rats with Walker 256 carcinosarcoma. Anticancer Res. 2012;32(1):129-33.

17. Kanno S, Tomizawa A, Hiura T, et al. Inhibitory effects of naringenin on tumor growth in human cancer cell lines and sarcoma S-180-implanted mice. Biol Pharm Bull. 2005;28(3):527-30.

18. Zhang YS, Li Y, Wang Y, et al. Naringin, a natural dietary compound, prevents intestinal tumorigenesis in Apc (Min/+) mouse model. J Cancer Res Clin Oncol. 2016;142(5):913-25.

19. Miller EG, Peacock JJ, Bourland TC, et al. Inhibition of oral carcinogenesis by citrus flavonoids. Nutr Cancer. 2008;60(1):69-74.

20. Menon LG, Kuttan R, Kuttan G. Inhibition of lung metastasis in mice induced by B16F10 melanoma cells by polyphenolic compounds. Cancer Lett. 1995;95(1-2):221-5.

21. Ozçelik B, Kartal M, Orhan I. Cytotoxicity, antiviral and antimicrobial activities of alkaloids, flavonoids, and phenolic acids. Pharm Biol. 2011;49(4):396-402.

22. Blanco-ayala T, Andérica-romero AC, Pedraza-chaverri J. New insights into antioxidant strategies against paraquat toxicity. Free Radic Res. 2014;48(6):623-40.

23. Adil M, Kandhare AD, Ghosh P, Venkata S, Raygude KS, Bodhankar SL. Ameliorative effect of naringin in acetaminophen-induced hepatic and renal toxicity in laboratory rats: role of FXR and KIM-1. Ren Fail. 2016;:1-14.

24. Adil M, Kandhare AD, Visnagri A, Bodhankar SL. Naringin ameliorates sodium arsenite-induced renal and hepatic toxicity in rats: decisive role of KIM-1, Caspase-3, TGF-β, and TNF-α. Ren Fail. 2015;37(8):1396-407.

25. Chtourou Y, Aouey B, Aroui S, Kebieche M, Fetoui H. Anti-apoptotic and anti-inflammatory effects of naringin on cisplatin-induced renal injury in the rat. Chem Biol Interact. 2016;243:1-9.

26. Turgut NH, Kara H, Elagoz S, Deveci K, Gungor H, Arslanbas E. The Protective Effect of Naringin against Bleomycin-Induced Pulmonary Fibrosis in Wistar Rats. Pulm Med. 2016;2016:7601393.

27. Goliomytis M, Kartsonas N, Charismiadou MA, Symeon GK, Simitzis PE, Deligeorgis SG. The Influence of Naringin or Hesperidin Dietary Supplementation on Broiler Meat Quality and Oxidative Stability. PLoS ONE. 2015;10(10):e0141652.

28. Paredes A, Alzuru M, Mendez J, Rodríguez-ortega M. Anti-Sindbis activity of flavanones hesperetin and naringenin. Biol Pharm Bull. 2003;26(1):108-9.

29. Adebiyi OO, Adebiyi OA, Owira PM. Naringin Reverses Hepatocyte Apoptosis and Oxidative Stress Associated with HIV-1 Nucleotide Reverse Transcriptase Inhibitors-Induced Metabolic Complications. Nutrients. 2015;7(12):10352-68.

30. Adebiyi OO, Adebiyi OA, Owira P. Naringin improves zidovudine- and stavudine-induced skeletal muscle complications in rats. Hum Exp Toxicol. 2016.

31. Yin FM, Xiao LB, Zhang Y. [Research progress on Drynaria fortunei naringin on inflammation and bone activity]. Zhongguo Gu Shang. 2015;28(2):182-6.

32. Kawaguchi K, Maruyama H, Hasunuma R, Kumazawa Y. Suppression of inflammatory responses after onset of collagen-induced arthritis in mice by oral administration of the Citrus flavanone naringin. Immunopharmacol Immunotoxicol. 2011;33(4):723-9.

33. Ahmad SF, Zoheir KM, Abdel-hamied HE, et al. Amelioration of autoimmune arthritis by naringin through modulation of T regulatory cells and Th1/Th2 cytokines. Cell Immunol. 2014;287(2):112-20.

34. Lee JH, Kim GH. Evaluation of antioxidant and inhibitory activities for different subclasses flavonoids on enzymes for rheumatoid arthritis. J Food Sci. 2010;75(7):H212-7.

35. Yin FM, Xiao LB, Zhang Y. [Research progress on Drynaria fortunei naringin on inflammation and bone activity]. Zhongguo Gu Shang. 2015;28(2):182-6.

36. Xu T, Wang L, Tao Y, Ji Y, Deng F, Wu XH. The Function of Naringin in Inducing Secretion of Osteoprotegerin and Inhibiting Formation of Osteoclasts. Evid Based Complement Alternat Med. 2016;2016:8981650.

37. Epasinghe DJ, Yiu C, Burrow MF. Effect of flavonoids on remineralization of artificial root caries. Aust Dent J. 2015.

38. Zhao Y, Li Z, Wang W, et al. Naringin Protects Against Cartilage Destruction in Osteoarthritis Through Repression of NF-κB Signaling Pathway. Inflammation. 2016;39(1):385-92.

39. Chtourou Y, Gargouri B, Kebieche M, Fetoui H. Naringin Abrogates Cisplatin-Induced Cognitive Deficits and Cholinergic Dysfunction Through the Down-Regulation of AChE Expression and iNOS Signaling Pathways in Hippocampus of Aged Rats. J Mol Neurosci. 2015;56(2):349-62.

40. Chtourou Y, Aouey B, Kebieche M, Fetoui H. Protective role of naringin against cisplatin induced oxidative stress, inflammatory response and apoptosis in rat striatum via suppressing ROS-mediated NF-κB and P53 signaling pathways. Chem Biol Interact. 2015;239:76-86.

41. Ramalingayya GV, Nampoothiri M, Nayak PG, et al. Naringin and Rutin Alleviates Episodic Memory Deficits in Two Differentially Challenged Object Recognition Tasks. Pharmacogn Mag. 2016;12(Suppl 1):S63-70.

42. Wang DM, Yang YJ, Zhang L, Zhang X, Guan FF, Zhang LF. Naringin Enhances CaMKII Activity and Improves Long-Term Memory in a Mouse Model of Alzheimer's Disease. Int J Mol Sci. 2013;14(3):5576-86.

43. Wang D, Gao K, Li X, et al. Long-term naringin consumption reverses a glucose uptake defect and improves cognitive deficits in a mouse model of Alzheimer's disease. Pharmacol Biochem Behav. 2012;102(1):13-20.

44. Kim HD, Jeong KH, Jung UJ, Kim SR. Naringin treatment induces neuroprotective effects in a mouse model of Parkinson's disease in vivo, but not enough to restore the lesioned dopaminergic system. J Nutr Biochem. 2016;28:140-6.

45. Leem E, Nam JH, Jeon MT, et al. Naringin protects the nigrostriatal dopaminergic projection through induction of GDNF in a neurotoxin model of Parkinson's disease. J Nutr Biochem. 2014;25(7):801-6.

46. Jung UJ, Kim SR. Effects of naringin, a flavanone glycoside in grapefruits and citrus fruits, on the nigrostriatal dopaminergic projection in the adult brain. Neural Regen Res. 2014;9(16):1514-7.

47. Sachdeva AK, Kuhad A, Chopra K. Naringin ameliorates memory deficits in experimental paradigm of Alzheimer's disease by attenuating mitochondrial dysfunction. Pharmacol Biochem Behav. 2014;127:101-10.

48. Golechha M, Sarangal V, Bhatia J, Chaudhry U, Saluja D, Arya DS. Naringin ameliorates pentylenetetrazol-induced seizures and associated oxidative stress, inflammation, and cognitive impairment in rats: possible mechanisms of neuroprotection. Epilepsy Behav. 2014;41:98-102.

49. Adebiyi OA, Adebiyi OO, Owira PM. Naringin Reduces Hyperglycemia-Induced Cardiac Fibrosis by Relieving Oxidative Stress. PLoS ONE. 2016;11(3):e0149890.

50. Dhanya R, Arun KB, Nisha VM, et al. Preconditioning L6 Muscle Cells with Naringin Ameliorates Oxidative Stress and Increases Glucose Uptake. PLoS ONE. 2015;10(7):e0132429.

51. Wang D, Yan J, Chen J, Wu W, Zhu X, Wang Y. Naringin Improves Neuronal Insulin Signaling, Brain Mitochondrial Function, and Cognitive Function in High-Fat Diet-Induced Obese Mice. Cell Mol Neurobiol. 2015;35(7):1061-71.

52. Chen F, Zhang N, Ma X, et al. Naringin Alleviates Diabetic Kidney Disease through Inhibiting Oxidative Stress and Inflammatory Reaction. PLoS ONE. 2015;10(11):e0143868.

53. Sun X, Li F, Ma X, et al. The Effects of Combined Treatment with Naringin and Treadmill Exercise on Osteoporosis in Ovariectomized Rats. Sci Rep. 2015;5:13009.

54. Anuja GI, Latha PG, Suja SR, et al. Anti-inflammatory and analgesic properties of Drynaria quercifolia (L.) J. Smith. J Ethnopharmacol. 2010;132(2):456-60.

55. Kandhare AD, Alam J, Patil MV, Sinha A, Bodhankar SL. Wound healing potential of naringin ointment formulation via regulating the expression of inflammatory, apoptotic and growth mediators in experimental rats. Pharm Biol. 2016;54(3):419-32.

56. Chanet A, Milenkovic D, Deval C, et al. Naringin, the major grapefruit flavonoid, specifically affects atherosclerosis development in diet-induced hypercholesterolemia in mice. J Nutr Biochem. 2012;23(5):469-77.

57. Etxeberria U, De la garza AL, Martíinez JA, Milagro I. Biocompounds Attenuating the Development of Obesity and Insulin Resistance Produced by a High-fat Sucrose Diet. Nat Prod Commun. 2015;10(8):1417-20.

58. Nakajima VM, Madeira JV, Macedo GA, Macedo JA. Biotransformation effects on anti lipogenic activity of citrus extracts. Food Chem. 2016;197 Pt B:1046-53.

59. Stohs SJ, Badmaev V. A Review of Natural Stimulant and Non-stimulant Thermogenic Agents. Phytother Res. 2016;30(5):732-40.

60. Manna K, Das U, Das D, et al. Naringin inhibits gamma radiation-induced oxidative DNA damage and inflammation, by modulating p53 and NF-κB signaling pathways in murine splenocytes. Free Radic Res. 2015;49(4):422-39.

61. Ren X, Shi Y, Zhao D, et al. Naringin protects ultraviolet B-induced skin damage by regulating p38 MAPK signal pathway. J Dermatol Sci. 2016;82(2):106-14.

62. Takekoshi S, Nagata H, Kitatani K. Flavonoids enhance melanogenesis in human melanoma cells. Tokai J Exp Clin Med. 2014;39(3):116-21.

63. Jiao HY, Su WW, Li PB, et al. Therapeutic effects of naringin in a guinea pig model of ovalbumin-induced cough-variant asthma. Pulm Pharmacol Ther. 2015;33:59-65.

64. Casey SC, Amedei A, Aquilano K, et al. Cancer prevention and therapy through the modulation of the tumor microenvironment. Semin Cancer Biol. 2015;35 Suppl:S199-223.

65. Sun Y, Gu J. [Study on effect of naringenin in inhibiting migration and invasion of breast cancer cells and its molecular mechanism]. Zhongguo Zhong Yao Za Zhi. 2015;40(6):1144-50.

66. Song HM, Park GH, Eo HJ, et al. Anti-Proliferative Effect of Naringenin through p38-Dependent Downregulation of Cyclin D1 in Human Colorectal Cancer Cells. Biomol Ther (Seoul). 2015;23(4):339-44.

67. Yen HR, Liu CJ, Yeh CC. Naringenin suppresses TPA-induced tumor invasion by suppressing multiple signal transduction pathways in human hepatocellular carcinoma cells. Chem Biol Interact. 2015;235:1-9.

68. Maggioni D, Nicolini G, Rigolio R, et al. Myricetin and naringenin inhibit human squamous cell carcinoma proliferation and migration in vitro. Nutr Cancer. 2014;66(7):1257-67.

69. Liao AC, Kuo CC, Huang YC, et al. Naringenin inhibits migration of bladder cancer cells through downregulation of AKT and MMP-2. Mol Med Rep. 2014;10(3):1531-6.

70. Lou C, Zhang F, Yang M, et al. Naringenin decreases invasiveness and metastasis by inhibiting TGF-β-induced epithelial to mesenchymal transition in pancreatic cancer cells. PLoS ONE. 2012;7(12).

71. Bao L, Liu F, Guo HB, et al. Naringenin inhibits proliferation, migration, and invasion as well as induces apoptosis of gastric cancer SGC7901 cell line by downregulation of AKT pathway. Tumour Biol. 2016.

72. Song HM, Park GH, Eo HJ, Jeong JB. Naringenin-Mediated ATF3 Expression Contributes to Apoptosis in Human Colon Cancer. Biomol Ther (Seoul). 2016;24(2):140-6.

73. Abaza MS, Orabi KY, Al-quattan E, Al-attiyah RJ. Growth inhibitory and chemo-sensitization effects of naringenin, a natural flavanone purified from Thymus vulgaris, on human breast and colorectal cancer. Cancer Cell Int. 2015;15:46.

74. Ayob Z, Mohd bohari SP, Abd samad A, Jamil S. Cytotoxic Activities against Breast Cancer Cells of Local Justicia gendarussa Crude Extracts. Evid Based Complement Alternat Med. 2014.

75. Li RF, Feng YQ, Chen JH, Ge LT, Xiao SY, Zuo XL. Naringenin suppresses K562 human leukemia cell proliferation and ameliorates Adriamycin-induced oxidative damage in polymorphonuclear leukocytes. Exp Ther Med. 2015;9(3):697-706.

76. Ahamad MS, Siddiqui S, Jafri A, Ahmad S, Afzal M, Arshad M. Induction of apoptosis and antiproliferative activity of naringenin in human epidermoid carcinoma cell through ROS generation and cell cycle arrest. PLoS ONE. 2014;9(10):e110003.

77. Arul D, Subramanian P. Naringenin (citrus flavonone) induces growth inhibition, cell cycle arrest and apoptosis in human hepatocellular carcinoma cells. Pathol Oncol Res. 2013;19(4):763-70.

78. Ekambaram G, Rajendran P, Magesh V, Sakthisekaran D. Naringenin reduces tumor size and weight lost in N-methyl-N'-nitro-N-nitrosoguanidine-induced gastric carcinogenesis in rats. Nutr Res. 2008;28(2):106-12.

79. Qin L, Jin L, Lu L, et al. Naringenin reduces lung metastasis in a breast cancer resection model. Protein Cell. 2011;2(6):507-16.

80. Sabarinathan D, Mahalakshmi P, Vanisree AJ. Naringenin, a flavanone inhibits the proliferation of cerebrally implanted C6 glioma cells in rats. Chem Biol Interact. 2011;189(1-2):26-36.

81. Bodduluru LN, Kasala ER, Madhana RM, et al. Naringenin ameliorates inflammation and cell proliferation in benzo(a)pyrene induced pulmonary carcinogenesis by modulating CYP1A1, NFκB and PCNA expression. Int Immunopharmacol. 2016;30:102-10.

82. Sabarinathan D, Mahalakshmi P, Vanisree AJ. Naringenin promote apoptosis in cerebrally implanted C6 glioma cells. Mol Cell Biochem. 2010;345(1-2):215-22.

83. Shi D, Xu Y, Du X, et al. Co-treatment of THP-1 cells with naringenin and curcumin induces cell cycle arrest and apoptosis via numerous pathways. Mol Med Rep. 2015;12(6):8223-8.

84. Torricelli P, Ricci P, Provenzano B, Lentini A, Tabolacci C. Synergic effect of α-tocopherol and naringenin in transglutaminase-induced differentiation of human prostate cancer cells. Amino Acids. 2011;41(5):1207-14.

85. Bulzomi P, Bolli A, Galluzzo P, Acconcia F, Ascenzi P, Marino M. The naringenin-induced proapoptotic effect in breast cancer cell lines holds out against a high bisphenol a background. IUBMB Life. 2012;64(8):690-6.

86. Kumar SP, Birundha K, Kaveri K, Devi KT. Antioxidant studies of chitosan nanoparticles containing naringenin and their cytotoxicity effects in lung cancer cells. Int J Biol Macromol. 2015;78:87-95.

87. Fouad AA, Albuali WH, Jresat I. Protective Effect of Naringenin against Lipopolysaccharide-Induced Acute Lung Injury in Rats. Pharmacology. 2016;97(5-6):224-32.

88. Mostafa Hel-S, Abd el-baset SA, Kattaia AA, Zidan RA, Al sadek MM. Efficacy of naringenin against permethrin-induced testicular toxicity in rats. Int J Exp Pathol. 2016;97(1):37-49.

89. Chtourou Y, Slima AB, Gdoura R, Fetoui H. Naringenin Mitigates Iron-Induced Anxiety-Like Behavioral Impairment, Mitochondrial Dysfunctions, Ectonucleotidases and Acetylcholinesterase Alteration Activities in Rat Hippocampus. Neurochem Res. 2015;40(8):1563-75.

90. Sachdeva S, Pant SC, Kushwaha P, Bhargava R, Flora SJ. Sodium tungstate induced neurological alterations in rat brain regions and their response to antioxidants. Food Chem Toxicol. 2015;82:64-71.

91. Lin JL, Wang YD, Ma Y, et al. Protective effects of naringenin eye drops on N-methyl-N-nitrosourea-induced photoreceptor cell death in rats. Int J Ophthalmol. 2014;7(3):391-6.

92. Nahmias Y, Goldwasser J, Casali M, et al. Apolipoprotein B-dependent hepatitis C virus secretion is inhibited by the grapefruit flavonoid naringenin. Hepatology. 2008;47(5):1437-45.

93. Paredes A, Alzuru M, Mendez J, Rodríguez-ortega M. Anti-Sindbis activity of flavanones hesperetin and naringenin. Biol Pharm Bull. 2003;26(1):108-9.

94. Pinho-ribeiro FA, Zarpelon AC, Fattori V, et al. Naringenin reduces inflammatory pain in mice. Neuropharmacology. 2016;105:508-519.

95. Manchope MF, Calixto-campos C, Coelho-silva L, et al. Naringenin Inhibits Superoxide Anion-Induced Inflammatory Pain: Role of Oxidative Stress, Cytokines, Nrf-2 and the NO-cGMP-PKG-KATPChannel Signaling Pathway. PLoS ONE. 2016;11(4).

96. Oršolić N, Goluža E, Dikić D, et al. Role of flavonoids on oxidative stress and mineral contents in the retinoic acid-induced bone loss model of rat. Eur J Nutr. 2014;53(5):1217-27.

97. La VD, Tanabe S, Grenier D. Naringenin inhibits human osteoclastogenesis and osteoclastic bone resorption. J Periodont Res. 2009;44(2):193-8.

98. Ming LG, Lv X, Ma XN, et al. The prenyl group contributes to activities of phytoestrogen 8-prenynaringenin in enhancing bone formation and inhibiting bone resorption in vitro. Endocrinology. 2013;154(3):1202-14.

99. Ming LG, Ge BF, Wang MG, Chen KM. Comparison between 8-prenylnarigenin and narigenin concerning their activities on promotion of rat bone marrow stromal cells' osteogenic differentiation in vitro. Cell Prolif. 2012;45(6):508-15.

100. Amat-ur-rasool H, Ahmed M. Designing Second Generation Anti-Alzheimer Compounds as Inhibitors of Human Acetylcholinesterase: Computational Screening of Synthetic Molecules and Dietary Phytochemicals. PLoS ONE. 2015;10(9).

101. Ghofrani S, Joghataei MT, Mohseni S, et al. Naringenin improves learning and memory in an Alzheimer's disease rat model: Insights into the underlying mechanisms. Eur J Pharmacol. 2015;764:195-201.

102. Chtourou Y, Fetoui H, Gdoura R. Protective effects of naringenin on iron-overload-induced cerebral cortex neurotoxicity correlated with oxidative stress. Biol Trace Elem Res. 2014;158(3):376-83.

103. Zbarsky V, Datla KP, Parkar S, Rai DK, Aruoma OI, Dexter DT. Neuroprotective properties of the natural phenolic antioxidants curcumin and naringenin but not quercetin and fisetin in a 6-OHDA model of Parkinson's disease. Free Radic Res. 2005;39(10):1119-25.

104. Lim W, Song G. Naringenin-induced migration of embrynoic trophectoderm cells is mediated via PI3K/AKT and ERK1/2 MAPK signaling cascades. Mol Cell Endocrinol. 2016;428:28-37.

105. Yi LT, Li CF, Zhan X, et al. Involvement of monoaminergic system in the antidepressant-like effect of the flavonoid naringenin in mice. Prog Neuropsychopharmacol Biol Psychiatry. 2010;34(7):1223-8.

106. Yi LT, Liu BB, Li J, et al. BDNF signaling is necessary for the antidepressant-like effect of naringenin. Prog Neuropsychopharmacol Biol Psychiatry. 2014;48:135-41.

107. Yi LT, Li J, Li HC, et al. Antidepressant-like behavioral, neurochemical and neuroendocrine effects of naringenin in the mouse repeated tail suspension test. Prog Neuropsychopharmacol Biol Psychiatry. 2012;39(1):175-81.

108. Ozkaya A, Sahin Z, Dag U, Ozkaraca M. Effects of Naringenin on Oxidative Stress and Histopathological Changes in the Liver of Lead Acetate Administered Rats. J Biochem Mol Toxicol. 2016;30(5):243-8.

109. Roy S, Ahmed F, Banerjee S, Saha U. Naringenin ameliorates streptozotocin-induced diabetic rat renal impairment by downregulation of TGF-β1 and IL-1 via modulation of oxidative stress correlates with decreased apoptotic events. Pharm Biol. 2016;:1-12.

110. Ren B, Qin W, Wu F, et al. Apigenin and naringenin regulate glucose and lipid metabolism, and ameliorate vascular dysfunction in type 2 diabetic rats. Eur J Pharmacol. 2016;773:13-23.

111. Bhattacharya S, Oksbjerg N, Young JF, Jeppesen PB. Caffeic acid, naringenin and quercetin enhance glucose-stimulated insulin secretion and glucose sensitivity in INS-1E cells. Diabetes Obes Metab. 2014;16(7):602-12.

112. Habauzit V, Verny MA, Milenkovic D, et al. Flavanones protect from arterial stiffness in postmenopausal women consuming grapefruit juice for 6 mo: a randomized, controlled, crossover trial. Am J Clin Nutr. 2015;102(1):66-74.

113. Orhan IE, Nabavi SF, Daglia M, Tenore GC, Mansouri K, Nabavi SM. Naringenin and atherosclerosis: a review of literature. Curr Pharm Biotechnol. 2015;16(3):245-51.

114. Zhang N, Yang Z, Yuan Y, et al. Naringenin attenuates pressure overload-induced cardiac hypertrophy. Exp Ther Med. 2015;10(6):2206-2212.

115. Li YR, Chen DY, Chu CL, et al. Naringenin inhibits dendritic cell maturation and has therapeutic effects in a murine model of collagen-induced arthritis. J Nutr Biochem. 2015;26(12):1467-78.

116. Du G, Jin L, Han X, Song Z, Zhang H, Liang W. Naringenin: a potential immunomodulator for inhibiting lung fibrosis and metastasis. Cancer Res. 2009;69(7):3205-12.

117. Qin L, Jin L, Lu L, et al. Naringenin reduces lung metastasis in a breast cancer resection model. Protein Cell. 2011;2(6):507-16.

118. Nasr-bouzaiene N, Sassi A, Bedoui A, Krifa M, Chekir-ghedira L, Ghedira K. Immunomodulatory and cellular antioxidant activities of pure compounds from Teucrium ramosissimum Desf. Tumour Biol. 2015.

119. Kim JH, Lee JK. Naringenin enhances NK cell lysis activity by increasing the expression of NKG2D ligands on Burkitt's lymphoma cells. Arch Pharm Res. 2015;38(11):2042-8.

120. Farzaei MH, Rahimi R, Abdollahi M. The role of dietary polyphenols in the management of inflammatory bowel disease. Curr Pharm Biotechnol. 2015;16(3):196-210.

121. Al-rejaie SS, Abuohashish HM, Al-enazi MM, Al-assaf AH, Parmar MY, Ahmed MM. Protective effect of naringenin on acetic acid-induced ulcerative colitis in rats. World J Gastroenterol. 2013;19(34):5633-44.

122. Azuma T, Shigeshiro M, Kodama M, Tanabe S, Suzuki T. Supplemental naringenin prevents intestinal barrier defects and inflammation in colitic mice. J Nutr. 2013;143(6):827-34.

123. Chattopadhyay D, Sen S, Chatterjee R, Roy D, James J, Thirumurugan K. Context- and dose-dependent modulatory effects of naringenin on survival and development of Drosophila melanogaster. Biogerontology. 2016;17(2):383-93.

124. Assini JM, Mulvihill EE, Burke AC, et al. Naringenin prevents obesity, hepatic steatosis, and glucose intolerance in male mice independent of fibroblast growth factor 21. Endocrinology. 2015;156(6):2087-102.

125. Ke JY, Cole RM, Hamad EM, et al. Citrus flavonoid, naringenin, increases locomotor activity and reduces diacylglycerol accumulation in skeletal muscle of obese ovariectomized mice. Mol Nutr Food Res. 2016;60(2):313-24.

126. Kumar S, Tiku AB. Biochemical and Molecular Mechanisms of Radioprotective Effects of Naringenin, a Phytochemical from Citrus Fruits. J Agric Food Chem. 2016;64(8):1676-85.

127. Jung SK, Ha SJ, Jung CH, et al. Naringenin targets ERK2 and suppresses UVB-induced photoaging. J Cell Mol Med. 2016;20(5):909-19.

128. Martinez RM, Pinho-ribeiro FA, Steffen VS, et al. Topical Formulation Containing Naringenin: Efficacy against Ultraviolet B Irradiation-Induced Skin Inflammation and Oxidative Stress in Mice. PLoS ONE. 2016;11(1):e0146296.

129. Martinez RM, Pinho-ribeiro FA, Steffen VS, et al. Naringenin Inhibits UVB Irradiation-Induced Inflammation and Oxidative Stress in the Skin of Hairless Mice. J Nat Prod. 2015;78(7):1647-55.

130. Kawakami CM, Gaspar LR. Mangiferin and naringenin affect the photostability and phototoxicity of sunscreens containing avobenzone. J Photochem Photobiol B, Biol. 2015;151:239-47.

131. Nasr bouzaiene N, Chaabane F, Sassi A, Chekir-ghedira L, Ghedira K. Effect of apigenin-7-glucoside, genkwanin and naringenin on tyrosinase activity and melanin synthesis in B16F10 melanoma cells. Life Sci. 2016;144:80-5.

132. Liu Y, Wang P, Chen F, et al. Role of plant polyphenols in acrylamide formation and elimination. Food Chem. 2015;186:46-53.

133. Keiler AM, Dörfelt P, Chatterjee N, et al. Assessment of the effects of naringenin-type flavanones in uterus and vagina. J Steroid Biochem Mol Biol. 2015;145:49-57.

134. Lee CJ, Wilson L, Jordan MA, Nguyen V, Tang J, Smiyun G. Hesperidin suppressed proliferations of both human breast cancer and androgen-dependent prostate cancer cells. Phytother Res. 2010;24 Suppl 1:S15-9.

135. Choi EJ. Hesperetin induced G1-phase cell cycle arrest in human breast cancer MCF-7 cells: involvement of CDK4 and p21. Nutr Cancer. 2007;59(1):115-9.

136. Bracke M, Vyncke B, Opdenakker G, Foidart JM, De pestel G, Mareel M. Effect of catechins and citrus flavonoids on invasion in vitro. Clin Exp Metastasis. 1991;9(1):13-25.

137. Banjerdpongchai R, Wudtiwai B, Khaw-on P, Rachakhom W, Duangnil N, Kongtawelert P. Hesperidin from Citrus seed induces human hepatocellular carcinoma HepG2 cell apoptosis via both mitochondrial and death receptor pathways. Tumour Biol. 2016;37(1):227-37.

138. Nazari M, Ghorbani A, Hekmat-doost A, Jeddi-tehrani M, Zand H. Inactivation of nuclear factor-κB by citrus flavanone hesperidin contributes to apoptosis and chemo-sensitizing effect in Ramos cells. Eur J Pharmacol. 2011;650(2-3):526-33.

139. Park HJ, Kim MJ, Ha E, Chung JH. Apoptotic effect of hesperidin through caspase3 activation in human colon cancer cells, SNU-C4. Phytomedicine. 2008;15(1-2):147-51.

140. Ghorbani A, Nazari M, Jeddi-tehrani M, Zand H. The citrus flavonoid hesperidin induces p53 and inhibits NF-κB activation in order to trigger apoptosis in NALM-6 cells: involvement of PPARγ-dependent mechanism. Eur J Nutr. 2012;51(1):39-46.

141. Adan A, Baran Y. The pleiotropic effects of fisetin and hesperetin on human acute promyelocytic leukemia cells are mediated through apoptosis, cell cycle arrest, and alterations in signaling networks. Tumour Biol. 2015;36(11):8973-84.

142. Yumnam S, Hong GE, Raha S, et al. Mitochondrial Dysfunction and Ca(2+) Overload Contributes to Hesperidin Induced Paraptosis in Hepatoblastoma Cells, HepG2. J Cell Physiol. 2016;231(6):1261-8.

143. Birsu cincin Z, Unlu M, Kiran B, Sinem bireller E, Baran Y, Cakmakoglu B. Anti-proliferative, apoptotic and signal transduction effects of hesperidin in non-small cell lung cancer cells. Cell Oncol (Dordr). 2015;38(3):195-204.

144. Palit S, Kar S, Sharma G, Das PK. Hesperetin Induces Apoptosis in Breast Carcinoma by Triggering Accumulation of ROS and Activation of ASK1/JNK Pathway. J Cell Physiol. 2015;230(8):1729-39.

145. Tanaka T, Makita H, Kawabata K, et al. Chemoprevention of azoxymethane-induced rat colon carcinogenesis by the naturally occurring flavonoids, diosmin and hesperidin. Carcinogenesis. 1997;18(5):957-65.

146. Kamaraj S, Anandakumar P, Jagan S, Ramakrishnan G, Devaki T. Modulatory effect of hesperidin on benzo(a)pyrene induced experimental lung carcinogenesis with reference to COX-2, MMP-2 and MMP-9. Eur J Pharmacol. 2010;649(1-3):320-7.

147. Yang M, Tanaka T, Hirose Y, Deguchi T, Mori H, Kawada Y. Chemopreventive effects of diosmin and hesperidin on N-butyl-N-(4-hydroxybutyl)nitrosamine-induced urinary-bladder carcinogenesis in male ICR mice. Int J Cancer. 1997;73(5):719-24.

148. Tanaka T, Makita H, Ohnishi M, et al. Chemoprevention of 4-nitroquinoline 1-oxide-induced oral carcinogenesis by dietary curcumin and hesperidin: comparison with the protective effect of beta-carotene. Cancer Res. 1994;54(17):4653-9.

149. Tanaka T, Makita H, Ohnishi M, et al. Chemoprevention of 4-nitroquinoline 1-oxide-induced oral carcinogenesis in rats by flavonoids diosmin and hesperidin, each alone and in combination. Cancer Res. 1997;57(2):246-52.

150. Tanaka T, Makita H, Kawabata K, et al. Modulation of N-methyl-N-amylnitrosamine-induced rat oesophageal tumourigenesis by dietary feeding of diosmin and hesperidin, both alone and in combination. Carcinogenesis. 1997;18(4):761-9.

151. Zhang J, Wu D, Vikash, et al. Hesperetin Induces the Apoptosis of Gastric Cancer Cells via Activating Mitochondrial Pathway by Increasing Reactive Oxygen Species. Dig Dis Sci. 2015;60(10):2985-95.

152. Saiprasad G, Chitra P, Manikandan R, Sudhandiran G. Hesperidin induces apoptosis and triggers autophagic markers through inhibition of Aurora-A mediated phosphoinositide-3-kinase/Akt/mammalian target of rapamycin and glycogen synthase kinase-3 beta signalling cascades in experimental colon carcinogenesis. Eur J Cancer. 2014;50(14):2489-507.

153. Gwiazdowska D, Juś K, Jasnowska-małecka J, Kluczyńska K. The impact of polyphenols on Bifidobacterium growth. Acta Biochim Pol. 2015;62(4):895-901.

154. Abuelsaad AS, Allam G, Al-solumani AA. Hesperidin inhibits inflammatory response induced by Aeromonas hydrophila infection and alters CD4+/CD8+ T cell ratio. Mediators Inflamm. 2014;2014:393217.

155. Siddiqi A, Nafees S, Rashid S, Sultana S, Saidullah B. Hesperidin ameliorates trichloroethylene-induced nephrotoxicity by abrogation of oxidative stress and apoptosis in wistar rats. Mol Cell Biochem. 2015;406(1-2):9-20.

156. Anandan R, Subramanian P. Renal protective effect of hesperidin on gentamicin-induced acute nephrotoxicity in male Wistar albino rats. Redox Rep. 2012;17(5):219-26.

157. Sahu BD, Kuncha M, Sindhura GJ, Sistla R. Hesperidin attenuates cisplatin-induced acute renal injury by decreasing oxidative stress, inflammation and DNA damage. Phytomedicine. 2013;20(5):453-60.

ORANGES

158. Kamel KM, Abd el-raouf OM, Metwally SA, Abd el-latif HA, El-sayed ME. Hesperidin and rutin, antioxidant citrus flavonoids, attenuate cisplatin-induced nephrotoxicity in rats. J Biochem Mol Toxicol. 2014;28(7):312-9.

159. Polat N, Ciftci O, Cetin A, Yılmaz T. Toxic effects of systemic cisplatin on rat eyes and the protective effect of hesperidin against this toxicity. Cutan Ocul Toxicol. 2016;35(1):1-7.

160. Kaya K, Ciftci O, Cetin A, Doğan H, Başak N. Hesperidin protects testicular and spermatological damages induced by cisplatin in rats. Andrologia. 2015;47(7):793-800.

161. Omar HA, Mohamed WR, Arafa el-SA, et al. Hesperidin alleviates cisplatin-induced hepatotoxicity in rats without inhibiting its antitumor activity. Pharmacol Rep. 2016;68(2):349-56.

162. Saha RK, Takahashi T, Suzuki T. Glucosyl hesperidin prevents influenza a virus replication in vitro by inhibition of viral sialidase. Biol Pharm Bull. 2009;32(7):1188-92.

163. Carvalho OV, Botelho CV, Ferreira CG, et al. In vitro inhibition of canine distemper virus by flavonoids and phenolic acids: implications of structural differences for antiviral design. Res Vet Sci. 2013;95(2):717-24.

164. Bae EA, Han MJ, Lee M, Kim DH. In vitro inhibitory effect of some flavonoids on rotavirus infectivity. Biol Pharm Bull. 2000;23(9):1122-4.

165. Panasiak W, Wleklik M, Oraczewska A, Luczak M. Influence of flavonoids on combined experimental infections with EMC virus and Staphylococcus aureus in mice. Acta Microbiol Pol. 1989;38(2):185-8.

166. Ahmed YM, Messiha BA, Abo-saif AA. Protective Effects of Simvastatin and Hesperidin against Complete Freund's Adjuvant-Induced Rheumatoid Arthritis in Rats. Pharmacology. 2015;96(5-6):217-25.

167. Li R, Cai L, Xie XF, Yang F, Li J. Hesperidin suppresses adjuvant arthritis in rats by inhibiting synoviocyte activity. Phytother Res. 2010;24 Suppl 1:S71-6.

168. Martin BR, Mccabe GP, Mccabe L, et al. Effect of Hesperidin With and Without a Calcium (Calcilock) Supplement on Bone Health in Postmenopausal Women. J Clin Endocrinol Metab. 2016;101(3):923-7.

169. Chiba H, Kim H, Matsumoto A, et al. Hesperidin prevents androgen deficiency-induced bone loss in male mice. Phytother Res. 2014;28(2):289-95.

170. Habauzit V, Sacco SM, Gil-izquierdo A, et al. Differential effects of two citrus flavanones on bone quality in senescent male rats in relation to their bioavailability and metabolism. Bone. 2011;49(5):1108-16.

171. Tamilselvam K, Braidy N, Manivasagam T, et al. Neuroprotective effects of hesperidin, a plant flavanone, on rotenone-induced oxidative stress and apoptosis in a cellular model for Parkinson's disease. Oxid Med Cell Longev. 2013;2013:102741.

172. Khan MH, Parvez S. Hesperidin ameliorates heavy metal induced toxicity mediated by oxidative stress in brain of Wistar rats. J Trace Elem Med Biol. 2015;31:53-60.

173. Wang D, Liu L, Zhu X, Wu W, Wang Y. Hesperidin alleviates cognitive impairment, mitochondrial dysfunction and oxidative stress in a mouse model of Alzheimer's disease. Cell Mol Neurobiol. 2014;34(8):1209-21.

174. Antunes MS, Goes AT, Boeira SP, Prigol M, Jesse CR. Protective effect of hesperidin in a model of Parkinson's disease induced by 6-hydroxydopamine in aged mice. Nutrition. 2014;30(11-12):1415-22.

175. El-marasy SA, Abdallah HM, El-shenawy SM, El-khatib AS, El-shabrawy OA, Kenawy SA. Anti-depressant effect of hesperidin in diabetic rats. Can J Physiol Pharmacol. 2014;92(11):945-52.

176. Donato F, De gomes MG, Goes AT, et al. Hesperidin exerts antidepressant-like effects in acute and chronic treatments in mice: possible role of l-arginine-NO-cGMP pathway and BDNF levels. Brain Res Bull. 2014;104:19-26.

177. Cai L, Li R, Wu QQ, Wu TN. [Effect of hesperidin on behavior and HPA axis of rat model of chronic stress-induced depression]. Zhongguo Zhong Yao Za Zhi. 2013;38(2):229-33.

178. Sharma M, Akhtar N, Sambhav K, Shete G, Bansal AK, Sharma SS. Emerging potential of citrus flavanones as an antioxidant in diabetes and its complications. Curr Top Med Chem. 2015;15(2):187-95.

179. De oliveira DM, Dourado GK, Cesar TB. Hesperidin associated with continuous and interval swimming improved biochemical and oxidative biomarkers in rats. J Int Soc Sports Nutr. 2013;10:27.

180. Dimpfel W. Different anticonvulsive effects of hesperidin and its aglycone hesperetin on electrical activity in the rat hippocampus in-vitro. J Pharm Pharmacol. 2006;58(3):375-9.

181. Zanotti simoes dourado GK, De abreu ribeiro LC, Zeppone carlos I, Borges césar T. Orange juice and hesperidin promote differential innate immune response in macrophages ex vivo. Int J Vitam Nutr Res. 2013;83(3):162-7.

182. Kamboh AA, Hang SQ, Khan MA, Zhu WY. In vivo immunomodulatory effects of plant flavonoids in lipopolysaccharide-challenged broilers. Animal. 2016;:1-7.

183. Amiot MJ, Riva C, Vinet A. Effects of dietary polyphenols on metabolic syndrome features in humans: a systematic review. Obes Rev. 2016.

184. Assini JM, Mulvihill EE, Huff MW. Citrus flavonoids and lipid metabolism. Curr Opin Lipidol. 2013;24(1):34-40.

185. Pradeep K, Ko KC, Choi MH, Kang JA, Chung YJ, Park SH. Protective effect of hesperidin, a citrus flavanoglycone, against γ-radiation-induced tissue damage in Sprague-Dawley rats. J Med Food. 2012;15(5):419-27.

186. Martinez RM, Pinho-ribeiro FA, Steffen VS, et al. Topical formulation containing hesperidin methyl chalcone inhibits skin oxidative stress and inflammation induced by ultraviolet B irradiation. Photochem Photobiol Sci. 2016;15(4):554-63.

187. Madduma hewage SR, Piao MJ, Kang KA, et al. Hesperidin Attenuates Ultraviolet B-Induced Apoptosis by Mitigating Oxidative Stress in Human Keratinocytes. Biomol Ther (Seoul). 2016;24(3):312-9.

188. Said UZ, Saada HN, Abd-alla MS, Elsayed ME, Amin AM. Hesperidin attenuates brain biochemical changes of irradiated rats. Int J Radiat Biol. 2012;88(8):613-8.

189. Lee YR, Jung JH, Kim HS. Hesperidin partially restores impaired immune and nutritional function in irradiated mice. J Med Food. 2011;14(5):475-82.

190. Giannini I, Amato A, Basso L, et al. Flavonoids mixture (diosmin, troxerutin, hesperidin) in the treatment of acute hemorrhoidal disease: a prospective, randomized, triple-blind, controlled trial. Tech Coloproctol. 2015;19(6):339-45.

191. Man G, Mauro TM, Zhai Y, et al. Topical hesperidin enhances epidermal function in an aged murine model. J Invest Dermatol. 2015;135(4):1184-7.

192. Usach I, Taléns-visconti R, Magraner-pardo L, Peris JE. Hesperetin induces melanin production in adult human epidermal melanocytes. Food Chem Toxicol. 2015;80:80-4.

193. Kurata Y, Fukushima S, Hagiwara A, Ito H, Ogawa K, Ito N. Carcinogenicity study of methyl hesperidin in B6C3F1 mice. Food Chem Toxicol. 1990;28(9):613-8.

194. Carpenter KJ. The discovery of vitamin C. Ann Nutr Metab. 2012;61(3):259-64.

195. Padayatty SJ, Levine M. Vitamin C: the known, the unknown, and Goldilocks. Oral Dis. 2016;

196. Shaw JH, Phillips PH, Elvehjem CA. Acute and chronic ascorbic acid deficiencies in the rhesus monkey. J. Nutr. 1945; vol 29. No. 6:365-372.

197. Mastrangelo D, Massai L, Lo coco F, et al. Cytotoxic effects of high concentrations of sodium ascorbate on human myeloid cell lines. Ann Hematol. 2015;94(11):1807-16.

198. Sertkaya A, Wong HH, Jessup A, Beleche T. Key cost drivers of pharmaceutical clinical trials in the United States. Sage Journals. 2016; vol 13, issue 2.

199. PDQ Cancer Information Summaries – High-dose Vitamin C. 2015. [Available] http://www.ncbi.nlm.nih.gov/books/NBK127724/#CDR0000742253__1 [May 11, 2016].

200. Venturelli S, Sinnberg TW, Niessner H, Busch C. Molecular mechanisms of pharmacological doses of ascorbate on cancer cells. Wien Med Wochenschr. 2015;165(11-12):251-7.

201. Cameron E. Vitamin C and cancer: an overview. Int J Vitam Nutr Res Suppl. 1982;23:115-27.

202. Malavolti M, Malagoli C, Fiorentini C, et al. Association between dietary vitamin C and risk of cutaneous melanoma in a population of Northern Italy. Int J Vitam Nutr Res. 2013;83(5):291-8.

203. Vance TM, Wang Y, Su LJ, et al. Dietary Total Antioxidant Capacity is Inversely Associated with Prostate Cancer Aggressiveness in a Population-Based Study. Nutr Cancer. 2016;68(2):214-24.

204. Kong P, Cai Q, Geng Q, et al. Vitamin intake reduce the risk of gastric cancer: meta-analysis and systematic review of randomized and observational studies. PLoS ONE. 2014;9(12):e116060.

205. Benade L, Howard T, Burk D. Synergistic killing of Ehrlich ascites carcinoma cells by ascorbate and 3-amino-1,2,4,-triazole. Oncology. 1969;23(1):33-43.

206. Pires AS, Marques CR, Encarnação JC, et al. Ascorbic acid and colon cancer: an oxidative stimulus to cell death depending on cell profile. Eur J Cell Biol. 2016;

207. Uetaki M, Tabata S, Nakasuka F, Soga T, Tomita M. Metabolomic alterations in human cancer cells by vitamin C-induced oxidative stress. Sci Rep. 2015;5:13896.

208. Serrano OK, Parrow NL, Violet PC, et al. Antitumor effect of pharmacologic ascorbate in the B16 murine melanoma model. Free Radic Biol Med. 2015;87:193-203.

209. Mastrangelo D, Massai L, Lo coco F, et al. Cytotoxic effects of high concentrations of sodium ascorbate on human myeloid cell lines. Ann Hematol. 2015;94(11):1807-16.

210. Chen N, Yin S, Song X, Fan L, Hu H. Vitamin B_2 Sensitizes Cancer Cells to Vitamin-C-Induced Cell Death via Modulation of Akt and Bad Phosphorylation. J Agric Food Chem. 2015;63(30):6739-48.

211. Campbell EJ, Vissers MC, Bozonet S, Dyer A, Robinson BA, Dachs GU. Restoring physiological levels of ascorbate slows tumor growth and moderates HIF-1 pathway activity in Gulo(-/-) mice. Cancer Med. 2015;4(2):303-14.

212. Chen Q, Espey MG, Sun AY, et al. Pharmacologic doses of ascorbate act as a prooxidant and decrease growth of aggressive tumor xenografts in mice. Proc Natl Acad Sci USA. 2008;105(32):11105-9.

213. Takemura Y, Satoh M, Satoh K, Hamada H, Sekido Y, Kubota S. High dose of ascorbic acid induces cell death in mesothelioma cells. Biochem Biophys Res Commun. 2010;394(2):249-53.

214. Yun J, Mullarky E, Lu C, et al. Vitamin C selectively kills KRAS and BRAF mutant colorectal cancer cells by targeting GAPDH. Science. 2015;350(6266):1391-6.

215. Yeom CH, Lee G, Park JH, et al. High dose concentration administration of ascorbic acid inhibits tumor growth in BALB/C mice implanted with sarcoma 180 cancer cells via the restriction of angiogenesis. J Transl Med. 2009;7:70.

216. Casciari JJ, Riordan HD, Miranda-massari JR, Gonzalez MJ. Effects of high dose ascorbate administration on L-10 tumor growth in guinea pigs. P R Health Sci J. 2005;24(2):145-50.

217. Roomi MW, Cha J, Kalinovsky T, Roomi N, Niedzwiecki A, Rath M. Effect of a nutrient mixture on the localization of extracellular matrix proteins in HeLa human cervical cancer xenografts in female nude mice. Exp Ther Med. 2015;10(3):901-906.

218. Ambattu LA, Rekha MR. Collagen synthesis promoting pullulan-PEI-ascorbic acid conjugate as an efficient anti-cancer gene delivery vector. Carbohydr Polym. 2015;126:52-61.

219. Güney G, Kutlu HM, Genç L. Preparation and characterization of ascorbic acid loaded solid lipid nanoparticles and investigation of their apoptotic effects. Colloids Surf B Biointerfaces. 2014;121:270-80.

220. Gustafson CB, Yang C, Dickson KM, et al. Epigenetic reprogramming of melanoma cells by vitamin C treatment. Clin Epigenetics. 2015;7(1):51.

221. Robinson AB, Hunsberger A, Westall FC. Suppression of squamous cell carcinoma in hairless mice by dietary nutrient variation. Mech Ageing Dev. 1994;76(2-3):201-14.

222. Cameron E, Pauling L. Supplemental ascorbate in the supportive treatment of cancer: Prolongation of survival times in terminal human cancer. Proc Natl Acad Sci USA. 1976;73(10):3685-9.

223. Raymond YC, Glenda CS, Meng LK. Effects of High Doses of Vitamin C on Cancer Patients in Singapore: Nine Cases. Integr Cancer Ther. 2015;

224. Vollbracht C, Schneider B, Leendert V, Weiss G, Auerbach L, Beuth J. Intravenous vitamin C administration improves quality of life in breast cancer patients during chemo-/radiotherapy and aftercare: results of a retrospective, multicentre, epidemiological cohort study in Germany. In Vivo. 2011;25(6):983-90.

225. Yeom CH, Jung GC, Song KJ. Changes of terminal cancer patients' health-related quality of life after high dose vitamin C administration. J Korean Med Sci. 2007;22(1):7-11.

226. Mikirova N, Casciari J, Rogers A, Taylor P. Effect of high-dose intravenous vitamin C on inflammation in cancer patients. J Transl Med. 2012;10:189.

227. Mateen S, Moin S, Khan AQ, Zafar A, Fatima N. Increased Reactive Oxygen Species Formation and Oxidative Stress in Rheumatoid Arthritis. PLoS ONE. 2016;11(4):e0152925.

228. Mohamed R, Shivaprasad HV, Jameel NM, Shekar MA, Vishwanath BS. Neutralization of local toxicity induced by vipera russelli phospholipase A2 by lipophilic derivative of ascorbic acid. Curr Top Med Chem. 2011;11(20):2531-9.

229. Laing MD. A cure for mushroom poisoning. S Afr Med J. 1984;65(15):590.

230. Pavlovic V, Cekic S, Kamenov B, Ciric M, Krtinic D. The Effect of Ascorbic Acid on Mancozeb-Induced Toxicity in Rat Thymocytes. Folia Biol (Praha). 2015;61(3):116-23.

231. Ozmen O. Endosulfan splenic pathology and amelioration by vitamin C in New Zealand rabbit. J Immunotoxicol. 2015;:1-6.

232. Guo W, Huen K, Park JS, et al. Vitamin C intervention may lower the levels of persistent organic pollutants in blood of healthy women - A pilot study. Food Chem Toxicol. 2016;92:197-204.

233. Roderique JD, Josef CS, Newcomb AH, Reynolds PS, Somera LG, Spiess BD. Preclinical evaluation of injectable reduced hydroxocobalamin as an antidote to acute carbon monoxide poisoning. J Trauma Acute Care Surg. 2015;79(4 Suppl 2):S116-20.

234. Abe S, Tanaka Y, Fujise N, et al. An antioxidative nutrient-rich enteral diet attenuates lethal activity and oxidative stress induced by lipopolysaccharide in mice. JPEN J Parenter Enteral Nutr. 2007;31(3):181-7.

235. Berger MM, Oudemans-van straaten HM. Vitamin C supplementation in the critically ill patient. Curr Opin Clin Nutr Metab Care. 2015;18(2):193-201.

236. Arslan M, Sezen SC, Turgut HC, et al. Vitamin C ameliorates high dose Dexmedetomidine induced liver injury. Bratisl Lek Listy. 2016;117(1):36-40.

237. Farombi EO, Onyema OO. Monosodium glutamate-induced oxidative damage and genotoxicity in the rat: modulatory role of vitamin C, vitamin E and quercetin. Hum Exp Toxicol. 2006;25(5):251-9.

238. Mozhdeganloo Z, Jafari AM, Koohi MK, Heidarpour M. Methylmercury-induced oxidative stress in rainbow trout (Oncorhynchus mykiss) liver: ameliorating effect of vitamin C. Biol Trace Elem Res. 2015;165(1):103-9.

239. Gulec M, Gurel A, Armutcu F. Vitamin E protects against oxidative damage caused by formaldehyde in the liver and plasma of rats. Mol Cell Biochem. 2006;290(1-2):61-7.

240. Rezvanjoo B, Rashidi S, Jouyban A, Beheshtiha SH, Samini M. Effects of vitamin C and melatonin on cysteamine-induced duodenal ulcer in a cholestatic rat model: A controlled experimental study. Curr Ther Res Clin Exp. 2010;71(5):322-30.

241. Kim SR, Ha YM, Kim YM, et al. Ascorbic acid reduces HMGB1 secretion in lipopolysaccharide-activated RAW 264.7 cells and improves survival rate in septic mice by activation of Nrf2/HO-1 signals. Biochem Pharmacol. 2015;95(4):279-89.

242. Tokuda Y, Miura N, Kobayashi M, et al. Ascorbic acid deficiency increases endotoxin influx to portal blood and liver inflammatory gene expressions in ODS rats. Nutrition. 2015;31(2):373-9.

243. Fisher BJ, Kraskauskas D, Martin EJ, et al. Attenuation of sepsis-induced organ injury in mice by vitamin C. JPEN J Parenter Enteral Nutr. 2014;38(7):825-39.

244. Abhilash PA, Harikrishnan R, Indira M. Ascorbic acid suppresses endotoxemia and NF-κB signaling cascade in alcoholic liver fibrosis in guinea pigs: a mechanistic approach. Toxicol Appl Pharmacol. 2014;274(2):215-24.

245. Lowes DA, Webster NR, Galley HF. Dehydroascorbic acid as pre-conditioner: protection from lipopolysaccharide induced mitochondrial damage. Free Radic Res. 2010;44(3):283-92.

246. Fisher BJ, Seropian IM, Kraskauskas D, et al. Ascorbic acid attenuates lipopolysaccharide-induced acute lung injury. Crit Care Med. 2011;39(6):1454-60.

247. Mckinnon RL, Lidington D, Tyml K. Ascorbate inhibits reduced arteriolar conducted vasoconstriction in septic mouse cremaster muscle. Microcirculation. 2007;14(7):697-707.

248. Kanter M, Coskun O, Armutcu F, Uz YH, Kizilay G. Protective effects of vitamin C, alone or in combination with vitamin A, on endotoxin-induced oxidative renal tissue damage in rats. Tohoku J Exp Med. 2005;206(2):155-62.

249. Chen MF, Yang CM, Su CM, Hu ML. Vitamin C protects against cisplatin-induced nephrotoxicity and damage without reducing its effectiveness in C57BL/6 mice xenografted with Lewis lung carcinoma. Nutr Cancer. 2014;66(7):1085-91.

250. Al-asmari AK, Khan AQ, Al-masri N. Mitigation of 5-fluorouracil-induced liver damage in rats by vitamin C via targeting redox-sensitive transcription factors. Hum Exp Toxicol. 2016;

251. Peng LJ, Lu DX, Qi RB, Zhang T, Wang Z, Sun Y. [Therapeutic effect of intravenous high-dose vitamin C on implanted hepatoma in rats]. Nan Fang Yi Ke Da Xue Xue Bao. 2009;29(2):264-6.

252. Cheng LL, Liu YY, Li B, Li SY, Ran PX. [An in vitro study on the pharmacological ascorbate treatment of influenza virus]. Zhonghua Jie He He Hu Xi Za Zhi. 2012;35(7):520-3.

253. Wintergerst ES, Maggini S, Hornig DH. Immune-enhancing role of vitamin C and zinc and effect on clinical conditions. Ann Nutr Metab. 2006;50(2):85-94.

254. Harakeh S, Jariwalla RJ. Comparative study of the anti-HIV activities of ascorbate and thiol-containing reducing agents in chronically HIV-infected cells. Am J Clin Nutr. 1991;54(6 Suppl):1231S-1235S.

255. Dalton WL. Massive Doses of Vitamin C in the Treatment of Viral Diseases. Journal of the Indiana State Medical Association. 1962.

256. Riordan Clinic. *High-dose Intravenous Vitamin C as a Successful Treatment of Viral Infections.* [Available] https://riordanclinic.org/2014/02/high-dose-intravenous-vitamin-c-as-a-successful-treatment-of-viral-infections [May 11, 2016].

257. Mikirova N, Hunninghake R. Effect of high dose vitamin C on Epstein-Barr viral infection. Med Sci Monit. 2014;20:725-32.

258. Jahan K, Ahmad K, Ali MA. Effect of ascorbic acid in the treatment of tetanus. Bangladesh Med Res Counc Bull. 1984;10(1):24-8.

259. Hemilä H, Koivula TT. Vitamin C for preventing and treating tetanus. Cochrane Database Syst Rev. 2008;(2):CD006665.

260. Gonzalez MJ, Miranda-massari JR, Berdiel MJ, et al. High Dose Intraveneous Vitamin C and Chikungunya Fever: A Case Report. J Orthomol Med. 2014;29(4):154-156.

261. Chin KY, Ima-nirwana S. Vitamin C and Bone Health: Evidence from Cell, Animal and Human Studies. Curr Drug Targets. 2015;

262. Kim YA, Kim KM, Lim S, et al. Favorable effect of dietary vitamin C on bone mineral density in postmenopausal women (KNHANES IV, 2009): discrepancies regarding skeletal sites, age, and vitamin D status. Osteoporos Int. 2015;26(9):2329-37.

263. Hart A, Cota A, Makhdom A, Harvey EJ. The Role of Vitamin C in Orthopedic Trauma and Bone Health. Am J Orthop. 2015;44(7):306-11.

264. Sun LL, Li BL, Xie HL, et al. Associations between the dietary intake of antioxidant nutrients and the risk of hip fracture in elderly Chinese: a case-control study. Br J Nutr. 2014;112(10):1706-14.

265. Zhu LL, Cao J, Sun M, et al. Vitamin C prevents hypogonadal bone loss. PLoS ONE. 2012;7(10):e47058.

266. Torbergsen AC, Watne LO, Wyller TB, et al. Micronutrients and the risk of hip fracture: Case-control study. Clin Nutr. 2015.

267. Huang YN, Yang LY, Wang JY, Lai CC, Chiu CT, Wang JY. L-Ascorbate Protects Against Methamphetamine-Induced Neurotoxicity of Cortical Cells via Inhibiting Oxidative Stress, Autophagy, and Apoptosis. Mol Neurobiol. 2016.

268. Ozkan F, Gündüz SG, Berköz M, Hunt AO, Yalın S. The protective role of ascorbic acid (vitamin C) against chlorpyrifos-induced oxidative stress in Oreochromis niloticus. Fish Physiol Biochem. 2012;38(3):635-43.

269. Altuntas I, Delibas N, Sutcu R. The effects of organophosphate insecticide methidathion on lipid peroxidation and anti-oxidant enzymes in rat erythrocytes: role of vitamins E and C. Hum Exp Toxicol. 2002;21(12):681-5.

270. Shah SA, Yoon GH, Kim HO, Kim MO. Vitamin C neuroprotection against dose-dependent glutamate-induced neurodegeneration in the postnatal brain. Neurochem Res. 2015;40(5):875-84.

271. Warner TA, Kang JQ, Kennard JA, Harrison FE. Low brain ascorbic acid increases susceptibility to seizures in mouse models of decreased brain ascorbic acid transport and Alzheimer's disease. Epilepsy Res. 2015;110:20-5.

272. Ide K, Yamada H, Umegaki K, et al. Lymphocyte vitamin C levels as potential biomarker for progression of Parkinson's disease. Nutrition. 2015;31(2):406-8.

273. Schjoldager JG, Paidi MD, Lindblad MM, et al. Maternal vitamin C deficiency during pregnancy results in transient fetal and placental growth retardation in guinea pigs. Eur J Nutr. 2015;54(4):667-76.

274. Rafiee B, Morowvat MH, Rahimi-ghalati N. Comparing the Effectiveness of Dietary Vitamin C and Exercise Interventions on Fertility Parameters in Normal Obese Men. Urol J. 2016;13(2):2635-9.

275. Vijayprasad S, Bb G, Bb N. Effect of vitamin C on male fertility in rats subjected to forced swimming stress. J Clin Diagn Res. 2014;8(7):HC05-8.

276. De oliveira IJ, De souza VV, Motta V, Da-silva SL. Effects of Oral Vitamin C Supplementation on Anxiety in Students: A Double-Blind, Randomized, Placebo-Controlled Trial. Pak J Biol Sci. 2015;18(1):11-8.

277. Ebuehi OA, Ogedegbe RA, Ebuehi OM. Oral administration of vitamin C and vitamin E ameliorates lead-induced hepatotoxicity and oxidative stress in the rat brain. Nig Q J Hosp Med. 2012;22(2):85-90.

278. Tabatabaei-malazy O, Nikfar S, Larijani B, Abdollahi M. Influence of ascorbic acid supplementation on type 2 diabetes mellitus in observational and randomized controlled trials; a systematic review with meta-analysis. J Pharm Pharm Sci. 2014;17(4):554-82.

279. Maged AM, Torky H, Fouad MA, et al. Role of antioxidants in gestational diabetes mellitus and relation to fetal outcome: a randomized controlled trial. J Matern Fetal Neonatal Med. 2016;:1-6.

280. Mason SA, Della gatta PA, Snow RJ, Russell AP, Wadley GD. Ascorbic acid supplementation improves skeletal muscle oxidative stress and insulin sensitivity in people with type 2 diabetes: Findings of a randomized controlled study. Free Radic Biol Med. 2016;93:227-38.

281. Kim HJ, Song W, Jin EH, et al. Combined Low-Intensity Exercise and Ascorbic Acid Attenuates Kainic Acid-Induced Seizure and Oxidative Stress in Mice. Neurochem Res. 2016;41(5):1035-41.

282. Tutkun E, Arslan G, Soslu R, Ayyildiz M, Agar E. Long-term ascorbic acid administration causes anticonvulsant activity during moderate and long-duration swimming exercise in experimental epilepsy. Acta Neurobiol Exp (Wars). 2015;75(2):192-9.

283. Richards JC, Crecelius AR, Larson DG, Dinenno FA. Acute ascorbic acid ingestion increases skeletal muscle blood flow and oxygen consumption via local vasodilation during graded handgrip exercise in older adults. Am J Physiol Heart Circ Physiol. 2015;309(2):H360-8.

284. Chayasirisobhon S. Efficacy of Pinus radiata bark extract and vitamin C combination product as a prophylactic therapy for recalcitrant migraine and long-term results. Acta Neurol Taiwan. 2013;22(1):13-21.

285. Kim JE, Cho HS, Yang HS, et al. Depletion of ascorbic acid impairs NK cell activity against ovarian cancer in a mouse model. Immunobiology. 2012;217(9):873-81.

286. Li K, Wang J, Shi M, et al. Prescription consisting of Vitamin C and Baicalin inhibits tumor growth by enhancing the antioxidant capacity in vivo. J BUON. 2015;20(5):1368-72.

287. Maggini S, Wenzlaff S, Hornig D. Essential role of vitamin C and zinc in child immunity and health. J Int Med Res. 2010;38(2):386-414.

288. Ströhle A, Hahn A. [Vitamin C and immune function]. Med Monatsschr Pharm. 2009;32(2):49-54.

289. Huijskens MJ, Walczak M, Sarkar S, et al. Ascorbic acid promotes proliferation of natural killer cell populations in culture systems applicable for natural killer cell therapy. Cytotherapy. 2015;17(5):613-20.

290. Toliopoulos IK, Simos YV, Daskalou TA, Verginadis II, Evangelou AM, Karkabounas SC. Inhibition of platelet aggregation and immunomodulation of NK lymphocytes by administration of ascorbic acid. Indian J Exp Biol. 2011;49(12):904-8.

291. Atasever B, Ertan NZ, Erdem-kuruca S, Karakas Z. In vitro effects of vitamin C and selenium on NK activity of patients with beta-thalassemia major. Pediatr Hematol Oncol. 2006;23(3):187-97.

292. Kim JE, Cho HS, Yang HS, et al. Depletion of ascorbic acid impairs NK cell activity against ovarian cancer in a mouse model. Immunobiology. 2012;217(9):873-81.

293. Choi MK, Song HJ, Paek YJ, Lee HJ. Gender differences in the relationship between vitamin C and abdominal obesity. Int J Vitam Nutr Res. 2013;83(6):377-84.

294. Adaramoye O, Ogungbenro B, Anyaegbu O, Fafunso M. Protective effects of extracts of Vernonia amygdalina, Hibiscus sabdariffa and vitamin C against radiation-induced liver damage in rats. J Radiat Res. 2008;49(2):123-31.

295. Vasilyeval IN, Bespalov VG. [Release of Extracellular DNA after Administration of Radioprotective Combination of α-Tocopherol and Ascorbic Acid]. Radiats Biol Radioecol. 2015;55(5):495-500.

296. Rostami A, Moosavi SA, Dianat moghadam H, Bolookat ER. Micronuclei Assessment of The Radioprotective Effects of Melatonin and Vitamin C in Human Lymphocytes. Cell J. 2016;18(1):46-51.

297. Mortazavi SM, Rahimi S, Mosleh-shirazi MA, et al. A Comparative Study on the Life-Saving Radioprotective Effects of Vitamins A, E, C and Over-the-Counter Multivitamins. J Biomed Phys Eng. 2015;5(2):59-66.

298. Domina EA, Pylypchuk OP, Mikhailenko VM. Destabilization of human cell genome under the combined effect of radiation and ascorbic acid. Exp Oncol. 2014;36(4):236-40.

299. Fujii Y, Kato TA, Ueno A, Kubota N, Fujimori A, Okayasu R. Ascorbic acid gives different protective effects in human cells exposed to X-rays and heavy ions. Mutat Res. 2010;699(1-2):58-61.

300. Mhaidat NM, Alzoubi KH, Khabour OF, Tashtoush NH, Banihani SA, Abdul-razzak KK. Exploring the effect of vitamin C on sleep deprivation induced memory impairment. Brain Res Bull. 2015;113:41-7.

301. Mohammed BM, Fisher BJ, Kraskauskas D, et al. Vitamin C promotes wound healing through novel pleiotropic mechanisms. Int Wound J. 2015;

302. Murray EL. Burning mouth syndrome response to high-dose vitamin C. Headache. 2014;54(1):169.

303. Dawood MA, Koshio S, Ishikawa M, Yokoyama S. Immune responses and stress resistance in red sea bream, Pagrus major, after oral administration of heat-killed Lactobacillus plantarum and vitamin C. Fish Shellfish Immunol. 2016;54:266-275.

304. Sadeghpour A, Alizadehasl A, Kyavar M, et al. Impact of vitamin C supplementation on post-cardiac surgery ICU and hospital length of stay. Anesth Pain Med. 2015;5(1):e25337.

305. Yang M, Barak OF, Dujic Z, et al. Ascorbic acid supplementation diminishes microparticle elevations and neutrophil activation following SCUBA diving. Am J Physiol Regul Integr Comp Physiol. 2015;309(4):R338-44.

306. Besse JL, Gadeyne S, Galand-desmé S, Lerat JL, Moyen B. Effect of vitamin C on prevention of complex regional pain syndrome type I in foot and ankle surgery. Foot Ankle Surg. 2009;15(4):179-82.

307. Lane DJ, Richardson DR. The active role of vitamin C in mammalian iron metabolism: much more than just enhanced iron absorption!. Free Radic Biol Med. 2014;75:69-83.

308. May JM, Qu ZC, Mendiratta S. Role of ascorbic acid in transferrin-independent reduction and uptake of iron by U-937 cells. Biochem Pharmacol. 1999;57(11):1275-82.

309. Lane DJ, Chikhani S, Richardson V, Richardson DR. Transferrin iron uptake is stimulated by ascorbate via an intracellular reductive mechanism. Biochim Biophys Acta. 2013;1833(6):1527-41.

310. Mojić M, Bogdanović pristov J, Maksimović-ivanić D, et al. Extracellular iron diminishes anticancer effects of vitamin C: an in vitro study. Sci Rep. 2014;4:5955.

311. Angelucci E, Pilo F. Management of iron overload before, during, and after hematopoietic stem cell transplantation for thalassemia major. Ann N Y Acad Sci. 2016;

312. Grenier D, Huot MP, Mayrand D. Iron-chelating activity of tetracyclines and its impact on the susceptibility of Actinobacillus actinomycetemcomitans to these antibiotics. Antimicrob Agents Chemother. 2000;44(3):763-6.

313. National Institutes of Health. (2008). *Vitamin C Injections Slow Tumor Growth in Mice.* [Available] https://www.nih.gov/news-events/news-releases/vitamin-c-injections-slow-tumor-growth-mice [May 11, 2016].

314. Hickey, S., & Saul, A. W. (2008). *Vitamin C: The real story: The remarkable and controversial healing factor.* Laguna Beach, CA: Basic Health Publications.

315. Jackson CL, Dreaden TM, Theobald LK, et al. Pectin induces apoptosis in human prostate cancer cells: correlation of apoptotic function with pectin structure. Glycobiology. 2007;17(8):805-19.

316. Zhang L, Ye X, Xue SJ, et al. Effect of high-intensity ultrasound on the physicochemical properties and nanostructure of citrus pectin. J Sci Food Agric. 2013;93(8):2028-36.

317. Leclere L, Fransolet M, Cambier P, et al. Identification of a cytotoxic molecule in heat-modified citrus pectin. Carbohydr Polym. 2016;137:39-51.

318. Glinsky VV, Raz A. Modified citrus pectin anti-metastatic properties: one bullet, multiple targets. Carbohydr Res. 2009;344(14):1788-91.

319. Huang ZL, Liu HY. [Expression of galectin-3 in liver metastasis of colon cancer and the inhibitory effect of modified citrus pectin]. Nan Fang Yi Ke Da Xue Xue Bao. 2008;28(8):1358-61.

320. Hsieh TC, Wu JM. Changes in cell growth, cyclin/kinase, endogenous phosphoproteins and nm23 gene expression in human prostatic JCA-1 cells treated with modified citrus pectin. Biochem Mol Biol Int. 1995;37(5):833-41.

321. Leclere L, Fransolet M, Cote F, et al. Heat-modified citrus pectin induces apoptosis-like cell death and autophagy in HepG2 and A549 cancer cells. PLoS ONE. 2015;10(3):e0115831.

322. Yan J, Katz A. PectaSol-C modified citrus pectin induces apoptosis and inhibition of proliferation in human and mouse androgen-dependent and- independent prostate cancer cells. Integr Cancer Ther. 2010;9(2):197-203.

323. Hao M, Yuan X, Cheng H, et al. Comparative studies on the anti-tumor activities of high temperature- and pH-modified citrus pectins. Food Funct. 2013;4(6):960-71.

324. Jiang J, Eliaz I, Sliva D. Synergistic and additive effects of modified citrus pectin with two polybotanical compounds, in the suppression of invasive behavior of human breast and prostate cancer cells. Integr Cancer Ther. 2013;12(2):145-52.

325. Wang Y, Nangia-makker P, Balan V, Hogan V, Raz A. Calpain activation through galectin-3 inhibition sensitizes prostate cancer cells to cisplatin treatment. Cell Death Dis. 2010;1:e101.

326. Hossein G, Keshavarz M, Ahmadi S, Naderi N. Synergistic effects of PectaSol-C modified citrus pectin an inhibitor of Galectin-3 and paclitaxel on apoptosis of human SKOV-3 ovarian cancer cells. Asian Pac J Cancer Prev. 2013;14(12):7561-8.

327. Inohara H, Raz A. Effects of natural complex carbohydrate (citrus pectin) on murine melanoma cell properties related to galectin-3 functions. Glycoconj J. 1994;11(6):527-32.

328. Nangia-makker P, Hogan V, Honjo Y, et al. Inhibition of human cancer cell growth and metastasis in nude mice by oral intake of modified citrus pectin. J Natl Cancer Inst. 2002;94(24):1854-62.

329. Pienta KJ, Naik H, Akhtar A, et al. Inhibition of spontaneous metastasis in a rat prostate cancer model by oral administration of modified citrus pectin. J Natl Cancer Inst. 1995;87(5):348-53.

330. Platt D, Raz A. Modulation of the lung colonization of B16-F1 melanoma cells by citrus pectin. J Natl Cancer Inst. 1992;84(6):438-42.

331. Liu HY, Huang ZL, Yang GH, Lu WQ, Yu NR. Inhibitory effect of modified citrus pectin on liver metastases in a mouse colon cancer model. World J Gastroenterol. 2008;14(48):7386-91.

332. Hayashi A, Gillen AC, Lott JR. Effects of daily oral administration of quercetin chalcone and modified citrus pectin on implanted colon-25 tumor growth in Balb-c mice. Altern Med Rev. 2000;5(6):546-52.

333. Ma Z, Han Q, Wang X, Ai Z, Zheng Y. Galectin-3 Inhibition Is Associated with Neuropathic Pain Attenuation after Peripheral Nerve Injury. PLoS ONE. 2016;11(2):e0148792.

334. Abu-elsaad NM, Elkashef WF. Modified citrus pectin stops progression of liver fibrosis by inhibiting galectin-3 and inducing apoptosis of stellate cells. Can J Physiol Pharmacol. 2016;94(5):554-62.

335. Kolatsi-joannou M, Price KL, Winyard PJ, Long DA. Modified citrus pectin reduces galectin-3 expression and disease severity in experimental acute kidney injury. PLoS ONE. 2011;6(4):e18683.

336. Chen CH, Sheu MT, Chen TF, et al. Suppression of endotoxin-induced proinflammatory responses by citrus pectin through blocking LPS signaling pathways. Biochem Pharmacol. 2006;72(8):1001-9.

337. Arad U, Madar-balakirski N, Angel-korman A, et al. Galectin-3 is a sensor-regulator of toll-like receptor pathways in synovial fibroblasts. Cytokine. 2015;73(1):30-5.

338. Eliaz I, Hotchkiss AT, Fishman ML, Rode D. The effect of modified citrus pectin on urinary excretion of toxic elements. Phytother Res. 2006;20(10):859-64.

339. Zhao ZY, Liang L, Fan X, et al. The role of modified citrus pectin as an effective chelator of lead in children hospitalized with toxic lead levels. Altern Ther Health Med. 2008;14(4):34-8.

340. Eliaz I, Weil E, Wilk B. Integrative medicine and the role of modified citrus pectin/alginates in heavy metal chelation and detoxification--five case reports. Forsch Komplementmed. 2007;14(6):358-64.

341. Vergaro G, Prud'homme M, Fazal L, et al. Inhibition of Galectin-3 Pathway Prevents Isoproterenol-Induced Left Ventricular Dysfunction and Fibrosis in Mice. Hypertension. 2016;67(3):606-12.

342. Martínez-martínez E, López-Andrés N, Jurado-lópez R, et al. Galectin-3 Participates in Cardiovascular Remodeling Associated With Obesity. Hypertension. 2015;66(5):961-9.

343. Martínez-martínez E, Calvier L, Fernández-celis A, et al. Galectin-3 blockade inhibits cardiac inflammation and fibrosis in experimental hyperaldosteronism and hypertension. Hypertension. 2015;66(4):767-75.

344. Calvier L, Martinez-martinez E, Miana M, et al. The impact of galectin-3 inhibition on aldosterone-induced cardiac and renal injuries. JACC Heart Fail. 2015;3(1):59-67.

345. Mackinnon AC, Liu X, Hadoke PW, Miller MR, Newby DE, Sethi T. Inhibition of galectin-3 reduces atherosclerosis in apolipoprotein E-deficient mice. Glycobiology. 2013;23(6):654-63.

346. Ramachandran C, Wilk BJ, Hotchkiss A, Chau H, Eliaz I, Melnick SJ. Activation of human T-helper/inducer cell, T-cytotoxic cell, B-cell, and natural killer (NK)-cells and induction of natural killer cell activity against K562 chronic myeloid leukemia cells with modified citrus pectin. BMC Complement Altern Med. 2011;11:59.

347. Martínez-martínez E, Calvier L, Rossignol P, et al. Galectin-3 inhibition prevents adipose tissue remodelling in obesity. Int J Obes (Lond). 2016;

348. Dourado GK, Stanilka JM, Percival SS, Cesar TB. Chemopreventive Actions of Blond and Red-Fleshed Sweet Orange Juice on the Loucy Leukemia Cell Line. Asian Pac J Cancer Prev. 2015;16(15):6491-9.

349. So FV, Guthrie N, Chambers AF, Moussa M, Carroll KK. Inhibition of human breast cancer cell proliferation and delay of mammary tumorigenesis by flavonoids and citrus juices. Nutr Cancer. 1996;26(2):167-81.

350. Tanaka T, Kohno H, Murakami M, et al. Suppression of azoxymethane-induced colon carcinogenesis in male F344 rats by mandarin juices rich in beta-cryptoxanthin and hesperidin. Int J Cancer. 2000;88(1):146-50.

351. Miyagi Y, Om AS, Chee KM, Bennink MR. Inhibition of azoxymethane-induced colon cancer by orange juice. Nutr Cancer. 2000;36(2):224-9.

352. Tanaka T, Tanaka T, Tanaka M, Kuno T. Cancer chemoprevention by citrus pulp and juices containing high amounts of β-cryptoxanthin and hesperidin. J Biomed Biotechnol. 2012;2012:516981.

353. Oikeh EI, Omoregie ES, Oviasogie FE, Oriakhi K. Phytochemical, antimicrobial, and antioxidant activities of different citrus juice concentrates. Food Sci Nutr. 2016;4(1):103-9.

354. Buscemi S, Rosafio G, Arcoleo G, et al. Effects of red orange juice intake on endothelial function and inflammatory markers in adult subjects with increased cardiovascular risk. Am J Clin Nutr. 2012;95(5):1089-95.

355. Ko SH, Choi SW, Ye SK, Cho BL, Kim HS, Chung MH. Comparison of the antioxidant activities of nine different fruits in human plasma. J Med Food. 2005;8(1):41-6.

356. Constans J, Bennetau-pelissero C, Martin JF, et al. Marked antioxidant effect of orange juice intake and its phytomicronutrients in a preliminary randomized cross-over trial on mild hypercholesterolemic men. Clin Nutr. 2015;34(6):1093-100.

357. Lee SG, Yang M, Wang Y, et al. Impact of orange juice consumption on bone health of the U.S. population in the national health and nutrition examination survey 2003-2006. J Med Food. 2014;17(10):1142-50.

358. Deyhim F, Garica K, Lopez E, et al. Citrus juice modulates bone strength in male senescent rat model of osteoporosis. Nutrition. 2006;22(5):559-63.

359. Pittaluga M, Sgadari A, Tavazzi B, et al. Exercise-induced oxidative stress in elderly subjects: the effect of red orange supplementation on the biochemical and cellular response to a single bout of intense physical activity. Free Radic Res. 2013;47(3):202-11.

360. Aptekmann NP, Cesar TB. Orange juice improved lipid profile and blood lactate of overweight middle-aged women subjected to aerobic training. Maturitas. 2010;67(4):343-7.

361. Escudero-lópez B, Berná G, Ortega Á, et al. Consumption of orange fermented beverage reduces cardiovascular risk factors in healthy mice. Food Chem Toxicol. 2015;78:78-85.

362. Zanotti simoes dourado GK, De abreu ribeiro LC, Zeppone carlos I, Borges césar T. Orange juice and hesperidin promote differential innate immune response in macrophages ex vivo. Int J Vitam Nutr Res. 2013;83(3):162-7.

363. Wang Y, Lloyd B, Yang M, et al. Impact of orange juice consumption on macronutrient and energy intakes and body composition in the US population. Public Health Nutr. 2012;15(12):2220-7.

364. O'neil CE, Nicklas TA, Rampersaud GC, Fulgoni VL. 100% orange juice consumption is associated with better diet quality, improved nutrient adequacy, decreased risk for obesity, and improved biomarkers of health in adults: National Health and Nutrition Examination Survey, 2003-2006. Nutr J. 2012;11:107.

365. Salamone F, Li volti G, Titta L, et al. Moro orange juice prevents fatty liver in mice. World J Gastroenterol. 2012;18(29):3862-8.

366. Azik M. Phytochemicals in citrus. Florida Department of Citrus. 2010. Available: http://fdocgrower.com/wp-content/uploads/2010/11/Flavonoids_Orange.pdf. [February 5, 2017].

367. Better Health Publishing. New Research: Modified Citrus Pectin – A potent anti-cancer therapy. *PR Newswire*. 2013.

368. Stone I. On the genetic etiology of scurvy. Acta Genet Med Gemellol (Roma). 1966;15(4):345-50.

369. Jiao Y, Wilkinson J, Di X, et al. Curcumin, a cancer chemopreventive and chemotherapeutic agent, is a biologically active iron chelator. Blood. 2009;113(2):462-9.

CHAPTER 8

COCONUT OIL

COCONUT IS A fruit, a seed and a nut that grows on palm trees in over 90 different countries worldwide.[1] Its meat, juice, milk and oil have been staples in the diets of many cultures for generations.[2]

The word *coconut* is derived from the 16th century Portuguese and Spanish word *coco,* meaning "head" or "skull," because the three indentations on its hairy shell resemble a face.[3]

Coconut oil consists of about 93% saturated fat, 4% monounsaturated fat and 3% unsaturated fat.[4] Understanding the role of dietary fat in health and disease is essential for understanding cancer.

SATURATED VS. UNSATURATED FAT

Due to its high content of saturated fatty acids, coconut oil is stable and protected from reacting with oxygen (oxidation). Romanian researchers tested the stability of coconut oil in 2012 by storing it at room temperature for one full year. When the year was up, they analyzed the coconut oil and found, "The physic-chemical oxidation of this oil keeped [sic] at room temperature was negligible."[5] In other words, coconut oil can sit at room temperature for *at least* a year without becoming rancid, making it "suitable for the preservation of medicinal plants and for wound treatment"[6] and desirable to commercial interests such as baking industries, processed foods, infant formulae, pharmaceuticals and cosmetics.[7] Since coconut oil is one of the least vulnerable dietary oils to oxidation and free-radical formation, "...it is therefore the safest to use in cooking," wrote scientists from Columbia University in 1992.[8]

Conversely, unsaturated fatty acids are highly unstable and easily react with oxygen.[9] When an unsaturated fatty acid is oxidized, a number of toxic breakdown products can be formed;[10] including prostaglandin E2, which "dominantly enables progressive tumor growth."[11,12] Unsaturated fats include oils that are liquid at room temperature like corn, soy, canola, hemp, flax, sunflower, safflower, peanut and fish oil. In 1990, researchers demonstrated that feeding 20% corn oil diets to rats produced more prostaglandin E2 than feeding them diets containing 19% coconut oil and 1% corn oil.[13]

Interestingly, the most unsaturated of all dietary fats – omega-3 and omega-6 – are the ones that health 'authorities' (and corporations selling them) claim are essential. In 1981, researchers from the University of Texas Health Science Center discovered that by not feeding mice any 'essential' fatty acids, autoimmune disease was prevented and their lifespans were increased.[14] Looking at the immune system, we find that unsaturated fats inhibit anti-cancer immunity and saturated fats promote anti-cancer immunity.[95,250]

Experiments have shown that unsaturated fatty acids inhibit the growth of the human fetus[15] and, in the absence of omega-3 and omega-6, both short-term and long-term memory of the fetus are improved.[16] In a 2016 study, Taiwanese scientists reported that 'essential' unsaturated fats from fish oil (omega-3) are toxic to the aging brain,[17] and as it turns out: fish oil isn't even good for fish! Researchers who fed salmon highly unsaturated fat diets "enriched" with DHA or EPA in an experiment from 2003 discovered, "an increased incidence of oxidative stress" in the livers of the fish.[18]

162

The detrimental effects of unsaturated fats on the heart build an even stronger case for its dietary avoidance. "Atherosclerotic plaques readily incorporate n-3 [omega-3] PUFAs from fish-oil supplementation"[19] and continued consumption leads to a linear increase in arterial plaque buildup.[20] "Men advised to eat oily fish, and particularly those supplied with fish oil capsules, had a higher risk of cardiac death,"[21] reported UK researchers in 2003.

To put it into perspective, New Zealand researchers conducted a 2014 review on the use of fish oil supplements based on 18 random controlled trials and 6 meta-analysis' published between January 2005 and December 2012. Of 16 publications that focused on the relationship between fish oil supplementation and cardiovascular health, only two reported benefits from fish oil.[22]

SATURATED FAT PROTECTS THE HEART

One of the many popular myths taught in school and on television is that saturated fat causes heart disease. Examining the diets and subsequent health of native cultures worldwide reveals a very different reality. People living in the country of Azerbaijan are famous for being long-lived; the most famous among them, according to Soviet authorities, was Shirali Muslimov, who died at the age of 168 in 1973.[23] A 1991 study on the Azerbaijani people revealed their dietary staples were fresh fruit, vegetables and fermented milk products. Perhaps most importantly, their diets contained a low ratio of unsaturated to saturated fats.[24]

The island-dwelling Polynesian populations near the equator known as Pukapuka and Tokelau obtain 63% and 34% of their nutrition from coconut, respectively. A 1981 study revealed that despite consumption of large quantities of saturated fat, their rates of cardiovascular disease were nearly non-existent. "Vascular disease is uncommon in both populations and there is no evidence of the high saturated fat intake having a harmful effect in these populations."[25]

In 1978, Sri Lankan's were consuming coconut oil as their main dietary fat and had the lowest death rate from ischemic heart disease in the world.[26] "All available population studies show that dietary coconut oil does not lead to high serum cholesterol nor to high coronary heart disease mortality or morbidity rate," concluded American and Filipino researchers in 1992.[27]

For decades, the belief that 'saturated fat causes heart disease' has been echoed as if it were fact, yet scientific studies have never proven a link between saturated fat intake and cardiovascular disease.[28]   In 2013, Cardiologist Dr. Aseem Malhotra of the Croydon University Hospital in London, England wrote, "The mantra that saturated fat must be removed to reduce the risk of cardiovascular disease has dominated dietary advice and guidelines for almost four decades. Yet scientific evidence shows that this advice has, paradoxically, increased our cardiovascular risks."[29] Two years later, another study was published in the highly-esteemed *British Medical Journal* that concluded, "Saturated fats are not associated with all-cause mortality, cardiovascular disease, coronary heart disease, stroke, or type 2 diabetes..."[30] Dietary saturated fats protect the heart and reduce the risk of cardiovascular disease.[31]

COCONUT OIL VS. CANCER

It has been known since at least 1945 that unsaturated fats are strong promoters of tumors and that saturated fats, like coconut oil, protect against tumor formation. When scientists from the University of Wisconsin fed rats a 5% corn oil diet for 6 months, 80% of the rats developed tumors. When they fed another group of rats a diet containing 4.7% hydrogenated (100% saturated) coconut oil, "no liver tumors developed by 6 months."[32]

A few decades later, researchers compared the effects of either 20% safflower oil or 20% coconut oil diets on tumor growth in mice. After four months, "the high-oleic safflower oil group had significantly more tumors than did the coconut oil group."[33] Since then, research has repeatedly demonstrated that tumor-induced animals fed the least amount of unsaturated fats formed the least amount of tumors.[36,39-42,90-92,95]

A CLOSER LOOK...

- A 1992 review from Michigan State University reported, "as the fat content of the diet is increased from a low or standard level to a high level, a consistent and substantial increase in the development of rodent mammary gland tumors is observed." This effect was found to be largely dependent on the type of fat consumed. "High dietary levels of unsaturated fats (e.g., corn oil, sunflower-seed oil) stimulate this tumorigenic process more than high levels of saturated fats (e.g., beef tallow, coconut oil)."[40]

- A group of researchers from the University of South Carolina examined the effects of high fat diets on rats induced with colon cancer in 2016. Published in the *American Journal of Physiology*, "we found an inverse association between SF [saturated fat] content and tumor burden." In other words, the more saturated the fat fed to rats, the less colon tumors they developed. Furthermore, "we found that high SF [saturated fat] content was protective," and "there was a decrease in mortality in mice consuming the highest concentration of SFAs [saturated fatty acids]."[42]

Both the type and the amount of fat are important considerations when devising a cancer-preventive diet. Low fat diets and high saturated fat diets both represent a low intake of unsaturated fat and are therefore similarly effective in preventing tumor formation; the less unsaturated fat in the diet, the less likely a tumor will form.

Beginning in 1978, a series of studies were published in the *Journal of the National Cancer Institute* that looked at the effects of dietary fat on tumor growth. Their conclusions were as follows:

1978: "Compared to animals fed diets rich in safflower oil, animals that ate coconut oil-rich diets survived longer."[34]

1981: "...the higher tumor yields were associated with increased unsaturation of mammary tissue phospholipids."[35]

1984: High-fat corn or safflower oil diets produced more colon tumors in mice than low-fat corn or safflower oil diets. Olive oil, coconut oil and MCT had "no promoting effect on tumor incidence"[37]

1986: Rats fed high-fat safflower or corn oil diets "exhibited enhanced mammary tumor yields" compared to animals fed high-fat olive, coconut or low-fat diets.[38]

The National Cancer Institute, "the nation's leader in cancer research,"[251] published these studies in what was at the time their official journal. Why wasn't the public notified of these findings? If they had been, tens of millions of lives could have been saved and the "war on cancer" would be long over. The blood cannot be washed from their hands.

SUCCESS STORIES

Entrepreneur Julie Figueroa of Maryland, Ohio was running a computer company in New York and owned an internet company in the Philippines in 1998. That same year she had an annual checkup with her doctor and was given a clean bill of health. "A few months later I began feeling a strange sensation in my breast late October that developed into a sharp pain." She went back to her doctor and was immediately referred to an oncologist for testing. "I was told I had a very aggressive form of breast cancer and needed surgery immediately." With no history of cancer in Julie's family, this news came as a shock to her. "Before going through with the mastectomy I wanted a second opinion."

Julie went to a second specialist but they told her the same thing. She kept trying to find a doctor who would give her a better option and "finally, the fifth doctor told it to me straight, 'you don't have a choice. We don't even know if we can still save you. You are at stage 4, the most serious stage, we need to do the surgery immediately.'"

Julie went through with the operation to remove her breast and afterwards underwent several months of chemotherapy. Doctors told her the cancer was under control but wasn't completely gone so they kept her on medication afterwards. Julie decided to go back to the Philippines where she owned a farm that happened to be filled with coconut palm trees.

In 2011, she began to experience painful headaches; "They became so severe that I felt like the bones in my skull were being fractured." She went to her doctor in the Philippines and had an x-ray taken. When she went back the next day for her results, several doctors met with her and said they had never seen anything like the cancer she had. "Almost half my skull looks like cheese that had been eaten by rats," described Julie. When she asked what her chances of survival were, they replied, "In the Philippines, at your stage... none."

Julie took the next flight back to the United States and went to see her doctor that same day, who scheduled her for emergency surgery to remove the hairline cancer close to the main artery of her brain. Unfortunately, 20% of the cancer was in the back of her skull over her main artery and could not be removed. "My chances of survival were grim. I knew I'd better make the most of the time I had remaining."

After several months of recovery following surgery, Julie returned to her farm in the Philippines to visit her family. "I was really weak and would just sit on the hill watching the farmers work among the coconut trees planting coffee seedlings." She knew she needed to do something to strengthen her immune system and wanted to plant a medicinal herb garden. "I started doing research on what medicinal plants I should grow that would boost my immune system...Just about that time, I came across some research on coconut oil." She read about the clinical trials in the Philippines where coconut oil was used to cure AIDS patients and figured it might also work for her.

"I started taking 3 to 4 tablespoons of oil a day plus whatever I used in preparing my meals," she explained. "I would add it to my oatmeal in the morning, put it in my hot chocolate, cook my meals in it. I also snacked on fresh coconut and drank coconut juice."

By July, Julie hadn't been back for a checkup in nearly six months and was asked to return home. She flew back to the US and to the complete surprise of her doctors, her cancer was in remission. They asked her what she had done. "I told them I found a cure: virgin coconut oil."

As a child, Julie had grown up around coconut trees in the Philippines. Her grandmother used to make coconut oil from fresh coconuts, but she never used it because she was told saturated fats were unhealthy. So instead her family used corn and soybean oil. "I had coconut oil around me all my life. It took getting cancer and a desperate search for a cure that made me rediscover this miracle oil."[43]

ADDITIONAL HEALTH EFFECTS

Antibacterial:

- Lipolyzed coconut oil inhibits growth of clostridium difficile bacteria[44]
- Coconut oil inhibits growth of staphylococcus aureus bacteria[45]

Antifungal:

- Coconut oil exhibits "significant antifungal activity"[46,47]

Antioxidant:

- Coconut oil increases antioxidant status in rats[48,49]
- Coconut oil reduces damage caused by numerous poisons,[50-52] including chemotherapy[53]

Antiviral:

- Coconut oil reduces viral load of HIV patients[54,55]

Arthritis:

- Coconut oil reduces inflammation in arthritis-induced rats[56]

Bone Health:

- Coconut oil maintains bone structure and prevents bone loss[57,58]

Brain Health:

- Coconut oil improves brain function in patients with Alzheimer's disease[59]
- Coconut oil drastically improves life of 74-year-old man with Parkinson's[60]

Dental Health:

- Coconut oil pulling decreases plaque formation and gingivitis[62,64]
- Coconut oil pulling inhibits streptococcus mutans in saliva[63]

Diabetes:

- Coconut oil prevents diabetes in rats chemically-induced with diabetes[65]

- Virgin coconut oil prevents insulin-resistance in rats[66]

Exercise:

- Coconut oil with exercise training improves impaired baroreflex sensitivity[67]

Eyes:

- Virgin coconut oil can safely be used as eye drops[68]

Farming:

- Coconut oil improves skeletal growth and fecal scores in jersey calves[69]
- Replacing 75% of dietary soybean oil with coconut oil reduces fat in broiler chickens[70]

Food Industry:

- Ionizing radiation (used for food preservation) "had little effect on the fatty acid compositions of saturated fats (lard and coconut oil)... but caused destruction of 98% of the highly unsaturated acids..."[71]

Hair:

- Coconut oil prewash conditioner prevents cuticle damage caused by wet combing[72]
- Coconut oil conditioner prevents hair damage caused by bleaching and exposing hair to boiling water for 2 hours[73]
- Coconut oil and anise spray "significantly more effective" than the most commonly used lice shampoo permethrin[74]

Healing:

- Coconut oil applied topically to wounds accelerates healing[75]

Heart Health:

- Coconut oil prevents blood pressure elevation and improves blood vessel function[76]

Immune System:

- Unsaturated fat inhibits anti-cancer immunity[95,250]

- Coconut oil maintains anti-cancer immunity[95,250]

Liver Health:

- Coconut oil protects liver from chemical damage[249]

Metabolism:

- Coconut oil helps maintain a healthy metabolism[77]

Obesity:

- Coconut oil (2 tablespoons per day for 12 weeks) reduces waist circumference;[78,79] body weight, body mass index and neck circumference[80,81]

Radiation Protective:

- Coconut oil blocks out about 20% of UV rays[82]

Reproduction:

- Coconut oil massage improves weight gain in newborns[61]

Sexual Health:

- Coconut oil increases testosterone[253]

Skin:

- Coconut oil topically treats patients with atopic dermatitis[83]

Sleep:

- Partially-hydrogenated coconut oil diet more-than doubles sleeping time in sleep-deficient mice[84]

Tumor Microenvironment:

- Coconut oil decreases free radicals[259]
- Coconut oil decreases serum free fatty acids[140]
- Coconut oil decreases prostaglandins[254]
- Coconut oil decreases nitric oxide[254]
- Coconut oil decreases tumor necrosis factor alpha[103,254]
- Coconut oil decreases interleukin-1[260]

- Coconut oil decreases interleukin-6[254]
- Coconut oil decreases interleukin-8[106]
- Coconut oil decreases nuclear factor kappa b[230]
- Coconut oil decreases estrogen[255]
- Coconut oil decreases lactic acid[256]
- Coconut oil decreases serotonin[257]
- Coconut oil decreases histamine[258]

MEDIUM-CHAIN TRIGLYCERIDES

Depending on growing conditions, anywhere from 55-72% of coconut fat consists of medium-chain triglycerides (MCTs). The four types of MCTs in coconut oil are caproic (0-0.8%), caprylic (5-9%), capric (6-10%), and lauric acids (44-52%).[85,86]

Medium-chain triglycerides have been described as fats that are rapidly absorbed and oxidized.[87-89] The fact that they can be used by the body as efficiently as glucose[87] makes them a great alternative fuel source. "Because of their smaller molecular size, MCTs require less bile and pancreatic juices for digestion and absorption than LCTs [Long Chain Triglycerides]." Aside from coconut and palm kernel oils, MCTs are found in only one other place in nature – milk.[87]

MEDIUM-CHAIN TRIGLYCERIDES VS. CANCER

Tumor-bearing mice fed diets high in MCTs were found to have reduced levels of the enzyme fatty acid synthase and also reduced acetyl CoA, similar to tumor free mice, suggesting cancer cell metabolism was restored back to that of normal cells.[94]

Inflammatory cytokines nuclear factor kappa b (NF-κB) and tumor necrosis factor alpha (TNF-a) both play major roles in the development of cancer.[99-101] A single dose of corn oil "rapidly activates" NF-κB, which "triggers production of low levels" of TNF-a.[102] Interestingly, replacing just 50% of unsaturated fatty acids with MCTs is enough to inhibit the production of TNF-a.[103]

Interleukin-8 (IL-8), a well-known tumor-growth promoting inflammatory cytokine[104] is "substantially increased" in a number of different types of cancer cells.[105] "We found for the first time that caprylic acid and MCT suppress IL-8 secretion by Caco-2 cells [colon cancer cells]," reported Japanese researchers in 2002.[106]

Up to 90% of patients with advanced cancer are affected by anorexia and many also suffer from muscle-wasting (cachexia).[252] In mice with induced colon tumors, MCTs shrank tumors and prevented muscle-wasting.[91,93]

Vitamin D3 dissolved in MCT inhibits the growth of cancer in vitro and in dogs "significantly greater" than Vitamin D3 alone.[96,97]

And in cancer patients following surgery for gastrointestinal cancer, MCT and protein-enriched nutrition enhanced recovery and reduced their length of hospital stay.[98]

SAFETY

Studies suggest that about 25-30 grams of MCTs can be tolerated at a single meal and that larger amounts may cause gastrointestinal symptoms, including nausea, vomiting, bloating, gastrointestinal discomfort, abdominal cramps and diarrhea.[222] In MCT-treated patients with Alzheimer's disease, "adverse events observed were mild and included minor gastrointestinal problems such as diarrhea, dyspepsia, and flatulence."[128]

In one study, 56 grams of MCTs were consumed every day for 24 weeks with no reported side effects,[135] and several clinical trials have reported the safety of MCT consumption as high as 1g/kg.[223]

SUCCESS STORIES

- A 24-year-old woman had a tumor of her lymph nodes that was blocking her lymphatic system and resulted in a recurrent milky fluid leaking into her abdominal cavity (chylous ascites). She was told to restrict fat in her diet and was supplemented with medium-chain triglycerides. At the time her case study was published, she was alive and had been free of abdominal leakage for 2 years.[107]

- Two female brain cancer patients were put on diets containing 60% medium-chain triglycerides for 8 weeks at the University Hospital of Cleveland. Within one week, the growth, spread and progression of cancer in both patients was halted by the diet. "One patient exhibited significant clinical improvements in mood and new skill development during the study. She continued the ketogenic diet for an additional twelve months and remained free of disease progression."[108]

ADDITIONAL HEALTH EFFECTS

Alcoholism:

- MCTs prevent free radical formation caused by alcohol[109]
- MCTs prevent alcohol-induced liver injury[110,111]
- "A diet enriched in saturated fatty acids effectively reverses alcohol-induced necrosis, inflammation, and fibrosis despite continued alcohol consumption." [112]

Antibacterial:

- MCTs inhibit staphylococcus aureus,[113] escherichia coli,[113] and clostridium difficile bacteria[114]

Antifungal:

- MCTs inhibit malassezia fungi[116]

Antioxidant:

- MCTs prevent death caused by lipopolysaccharide (LPS) in rats; "All rats given corn oil died after LPS administration" [117]
- MCTs reduce oxidative stress caused by surgery[118]

Antiviral:

- MCTs inactivate HIV-1,[119] HIV-2,[119] herpes simplex virus type 1,[115] respiratory syncytial virus,[115] group b streptococcus virus[115] and haemophilus influenza virus.[115]
- MCTs prevent diarrhea/wasting caused by HIV virus[120,121]

Autism:

- MCTs reduce seizures, obesity, improve brain function and behavior, increase IQ 70-points and cure child of autism[123]

Bone Health:

- MCTs improve calcium absorption[124,125]

Brain Health:

- MCTs have "long-lasting cognition-enhancing effects in aged dogs" [126,127]
- MCTs enhance memory[131] and cognition[132] in humans
- MCTs improve brain function in patients with Alzheimer's disease[128-130,133]

Dental Health:

- MCTs inhibit periodontal pathogens[135]

Detoxification:

- MCTs detoxify drugs from bloodstream[136]

Diabetes:

- MCTs improve insulin sensitivity[137-139]
- MCTs stimulate insulin secretion[141-143]

Exercise:

- MCTs and exercise synergistically reduce visceral and subcutaneous fat accumulation[144]

The effects of MCTs on exercise performance in animals and humans have been thoroughly tested, yet the results are extraordinarily inconclusive. Taken before or during endurance exercise and with or without carbohydrates - three studies showed MCTs increase performance,[146-148] four showed MCTs provide no performance enhancement,[148-151] and two showed MCTs actually have a negative effect on performance.[152,153]

As I understand it, a healthy person will store carbohydrates in their liver and muscles (called glycogen), and after carbohydrates in the blood have been used up during exercise, glycogen stores will be used for fuel. Once glycogen has been depleted, the body will begin breaking down its own muscle and fat tissues for fuel. Like strapping a hybrid fuel tank onto a car, the question is - can MCT ingestion delay the depletion of glycogen and thereby expand the body's useable energy supply?

Four studies found that MCT ingestion before or during exercise reduces glycogen depletion,[154-157] and five found that MCT ingestion during exercise doesn't reduce glycogen depletion and thus has no additive effect on overall energy reserves.[158-162]

South African researchers conducted a review on MCTs for performance enhancement in 1998 and concluded, "In the search for strategies to improve athletic performance, recent interest has focused on several nutritional procedures which may theoretically promote FA [fatty acid] oxidation, attenuate the rate of muscle glycogen depletion and improve exercise capacity... At present, there is insufficient scientific evidence to recommend that athletes either ingest fat, in the form of MCTs, during exercise..."[163]

Farming:

- Feeding pigs diets containing 15% MCTs "resulted in a lower mortality of newborns and better development, particularly of underweight piglets" [164]

Healing:

- MCTs enhance wound healing[165]
- MCTs help young male survive point-blank .32 caliber gunshot wound[166]

Heart Health:

- MCTs improve heart function[168-172]

Immune System:

- MCTs enhance immune system[173,176]
- MCTs prevent immune system damage caused by soybean oil[174,175]

Inflammation:

- MCTs reduce inflammation caused by fish oil[122]

Intestinal Health:

- MCTs reduce incidence of colitis in mice[177,178]
- MCTs decrease gut inflammation[179,180,183]
- MCTs reduce mortality and improve symptoms of Waldmann's disease[181,182]

Obesity:

- MCTs cause weight loss in cats[193]
- MCTs increase satiety and reduce food intake[196,197]
- MCTs reduce body fat accumulation[194,195,198,199,200-205]

Medium-chain triglycerides have been demonstrated to increase resting energy expenditure (metabolism) in all animal studies[184-186] and most human studies,[187-191] for up to 24 hours;[192] meaning additional energy will be burnt for a full 24-hours by doing nothing other than eating MCTs.

Radiation protective:

- MCTs reduce damage caused by ionizing radiation[206]
- MCTs eliminate chylous ascites caused by pelvic irradiation[207]

Reproduction:

- MCTs during pregnancy reduce chances of obesity in offspring later in life[134]
- MCTs heal cardiomyopathy and normalize liver function in a newborn baby[167]
- MCTs increase metabolic rate, cheek skin temperature and total sleep time in newborn babies[219]

Seizures:

- MCTs significantly reduce seizures in animals, children and adults[208-216]

Skin:

- MCTs increase skin hydration[217]

Thyroid:

- MCTs increase thermogenesis in rodents;[87] (thyroid hormone is responsible for thermogenesis[221])

Other:

- MCTs stop eye bleeding after retinal surgery[220]
- MCTs preserve dissolved drugs and increase transdermal drug delivery[218]

LAURIC ACID

While only 2-5% of the fatty acids in cow's milk are lauric acid, coconut oil is comprised of almost 50% lauric acid.[224-226]

LAURIC ACID VS. CANCER

All saturated fatty acids have antimicrobial properties to varying degrees;[233] and lauric acid has a greater antimicrobial potency than all other saturated fatty acids found in nature.[234]

Studies testing lauric acid specifically on cancer are limited, but the ones that have been conducted are promising. Australian researchers from the University of Adelaide compared the effects of lauric acid vs. short-chain fatty acid butyrate (a saturated fat found in butter) on two types of colon cancer cells in 2013. The results showed, "Lauric acid induced apoptosis in Caco-2 ($p < 0.05$) and IEC-6 cells" while butyrate did not. [227]

In 2012, Chinese researchers from Wuhan University reported that overexpression of the gene Cytochrome P450 promotes the growth of human breast cancer cells and that lauric and myristic acid suppress the overexpression of this gene.[228]

One method of reducing cancer growth is to inhibit the pro-inflammatory cytokine nuclear factor kappa b (NF-κB)[229] and lauric acid happens to be a NF-κB inhibitor.[230]

ADDITIONAL HEALTH EFFECTS

Acne:

- Lauric acid is effective for treating acne[231,232]

Antibacterial:

- Lauric acid inhibits heliobacter pylori[235]

Antifungal:

- Lauric acid inhibits growth of candida albicans[236,237]

Antioxidant:

- Lauric acid-enriched rice bran oil a more potent antioxidant than rice bran oil alone[238]

Antiviral:

- Lauric acid inhibits vesicular stomatitis virus[239]
- Lauric acid inhibits junin virus[240]

Dental Health:

- Lauric acid inhibits oral bacteria[242]

Depression:

- Lauric acid reduces depression[241]

Diabetes:

- Lauric acid "may protect against diabetes-induced dyslipidemia"[243]

Electricity:

- Lauric acid enhances sustainable power generation of microbial fuel cell by 3.9-times[244]

Farming:

- Lauric acid and myristic acid increase breast muscle size of broiler chickens[245]

- Lauric and oleic acids improve yolk quality of laying hens[246]

Seizures:

- Lauric, capric, myristic, palmitic and stearic acids prevent seizures[247]

Skin:

- Lauric acid enhances absorption of medication through shed snake skin[248]

REFERENCES

1. Ridgeway, S. (2016). *Different Uses for a Coconut.* [Online]. Available: https://caloriebee.com/nutrition/Different-Uses-for-a-Coconut. [November 6, 2016].

2. Debmandal M, Mandal S. Coconut (Cocos nucifera L.: Arecaceae): in health promotion and disease prevention. Asian Pac J Trop Med. 2011;4(3):241-7.

3. Delgado, S.R. 1982. *Glossário luso-asiático, Part 1.* Buske Verlag.

4. Marina, A.M., Che Man, Y.B., Nazimah, S.A.H. et al. Physicochemical properties of virgin coconut oil extracted from different processing methods. J Am Oil Chem Soc. 2009;86: 301.

5. Moigradean D, Poiana MA, Gogoasa I. Quality characteristics and oxidative stability of coconut oil during storage. J Agro. Proc. & Tech. 2012; 18(4):272-276.

6. Sachs M, Von eichel J, Asskali F. [Wound management with coconut oil in Indonesian folk medicine]. Chirurg. 2002;73(4):387-92.

7. Krishna GAG, Gaurav R, Singh BA, Prasanth PKK, Preeti C. Coconut oil: Chemistry, production and its applications – a review. Agris. 2010.

8. Kaunitz H. Coconut oil consumption and coronary heart disease. Agris. 1992.

9. Marina AM, Che Man YB, Nazimah SAH, Amin I. Chemical properties of virgin coconut oil. J. Amer. Oil. Chem. Soc. 2009; 86(4):301-307.

10. Srivastava KC, Awasthi KK, Lindegård P, Tiwari KP. Effect of some saturated and unsaturated fatty acids on prostaglandin biosynthesis in washed human blood platelets from (1-14 C)arachidonic acid. Prostaglandins Leukot Med. 1982;8(3):219-37.

11. Zelenay S, Reis e sousa C. Reducing prostaglandin E2 production to raise cancer immunogenicity. Oncoimmunology. 2016;5(5):e1123370.

12. Bellamkonda K, Chandrashekar NK, Osman J, Selvanesan BC, Savari S, Sjölander A. The eicosanoids leukotriene D4 and prostaglandin E2 promote the tumorigenicity of colon cancer-initiating cells in a xenograft mouse model. BMC Cancer. 2016;16:425.

13. Bibby DC, Grimble RF. Tumour necrosis factor-alpha and endotoxin induce less prostaglandin E2 production from hypothalami of rats fed coconut oil than from hypothalami of rats fed maize oil. Clin Sci. 1990;79(6):657-62.

14. Hurd ER, Johnston JM, Okita JR, Macdonald PC, Ziff M, Gilliam JW. Prevention of glomerulonephritis and prolonged survival in New Zealand Black/New Zealand White F1 hybrid mice fed an essential fatty acid-deficient diet. J Clin Invest. 1981;67(2):476-85.

15. Dirix CE, Kester AD, Hornstra G. Associations between term birth dimensions and prenatal exposure to essential and trans fatty acids. Early Hum Dev. 2009;85(8):525-30.

16. Dirix CE, Hornstra G, Nijhuis JG. Fetal learning and memory: weak associations with the early essential polyunsaturated fatty acid status. Prostaglandins Leukot Essent Fatty Acids. 2009;80(4):207-12.

17. Hsu YM, Yin MC. EPA or DHA enhanced oxidative stress and aging protein expression in brain of d-galactose treated mice. Biomedicine (Taipei). 2016;6(3):17.

18. Kjaer MA, Todorcević M, Torstensen BE, Vegusdal A, Ruyter B. Dietary n-3 HUFA affects mitochondrial fatty acid beta-oxidation capacity and susceptibility to oxidative stress in Atlantic salmon. Lipids. 2008;43(9):813-27.

19. Thies F, Garry JM, Yaqoob P, et al. Association of n-3 polyunsaturated fatty acids with stability of atherosclerotic plaques: a randomised controlled trial. Lancet. 2003;361(9356):477-85.

20. Rapp JH, Connor WE, Lin DS, Porter JM. Dietary eicosapentaenoic acid and docosahexaenoic acid from fish oil. Their incorporation into advanced human atherosclerotic plaques. Arterioscler Thromb. 1991;11(4):903-11.

21. Burr ML, Ashfield-watt PA, Dunstan FD, et al. Lack of benefit of dietary advice to men with angina: results of a controlled trial. Eur J Clin Nutr. 2003;57(2):193-200.

22. Grey A, Bolland M. Clinical trial evidence and use of fish oil supplements. JAMA Intern Med. 2014;174(3):460-2.

23. Gasimov, C., Hashimova, U., Abbasov, A., Ismayilova, A. (1994). *Centenarians in Azerbaijan*. [Online]. Available: http://www.azer.com/aiweb/categories/magazine/23_folder/23_articles/23_centenarians.html. [November 6, 2016].

24. Grigorov IuG, Kozlovskaia SG, Semes'ko TM, Asadov ShA. [Characteristics of actual nutrition of the long-lived population of Azerbaijan]. Vopr Pitan. 1991;(2):36-40.

25. Prior IA, Davidson F, Salmond CE, Czochanska Z. Cholesterol, coconuts, and diet on Polynesian atolls: a natural experiment: the Pukapuka and Tokelau island studies. Am J Clin Nutr. 1981;34(8):1552-61.

26. Kaunitz H. Medium chain triglycerides (MCT) in aging and arteriosclerosis. J Environ Pathol Toxicol Oncol. 1986;6(3-4):115-21.

27. Kaunitz H. Coconut oil consumption and coronary heart disease. Phillip. J. Int. Med. 1992;30(3):165-171.

28. Siri-tarino PW, Sun Q, Hu FB, Krauss RM. Meta-analysis of prospective cohort studies evaluating the association of saturated fat with cardiovascular disease. Am J Clin Nutr. 2010;91(3):535-46.

29. Malhotra A. Saturated fat is not the major issue. BMJ. 2013;347:f6340.

30. De souza RJ, Mente A, Maroleanu A, et al. Intake of saturated and trans unsaturated fatty acids and risk of all cause mortality, cardiovascular disease, and type 2 diabetes: systematic review and meta-analysis of observational studies. BMJ. 2015;351:h3978.

31. Mozaffarian D, Rimm EB, Herrington DM. Dietary fats, carbohydrate, and progression of coronary atherosclerosis in postmenopausal women. Am J Clin Nutr. 2004;80(5):1175-84.

32. Kline BE, Miller JA. The carcinogenicity of p-dimethylaminoazobenzene in diets containing the fatty acids of hydrogenated coconut oil or of corn oil. Cancer Res. 1946;6:1-4.

33. Dayton S, Hashimoto S, Wollman J. Effect of high-oleic and high-linoleic safflower oils on mammary tumors induced in rats by 7,12-dimethylbenz(alpha)anthracene. J Nutr. 1977;107(8):1353-60.

34. Burns CP, Luttenegger DG, Spector AA. Effect of dietary fat saturation on survival of mice with L1210 leukemia. J Natl Cancer Inst. 1978;61(2):513-5.

35. Hopkins GJ, Kennedy TG, Carroll KK. Polyunsaturated fatty acids as promoters of mammary carcinogenesis induced in Sprague-Dawley rats by 7,12-dimethylbenz[a]anthracene. J Natl Cancer Inst. 1981;66(3):517-22.

36. Ip C, Sinha DK. Enhancement of mammary tumorigenesis by dietary selenium deficiency in rats with a high polyunsaturated fat intake. Cancer Res. 1981;41(1):31-4.

37. Reddy BS, Maeura Y. Tumor promotion by dietary fat in azoxymethane-induced colon carcinogenesis in female F344 rats: influence of amount and source of dietary fat. J Natl Cancer Inst. 1984;72(3):745-50.

38. Cohen LA, Thompson DO, Maeura Y, Choi K, Blank ME, Rose DP. Dietary fat and mammary cancer. I. Promoting effects of different dietary fats on N-nitrosomethylurea-induced rat mammary tumorigenesis. J Natl Cancer Inst. 1986;77(1):33-42.

39. Cohen LA. Fat and endocrine-responsive cancer in animals. Prev Med. 1987;16(4):468-74.

40. Welsch CW. Dietary fat, calories, and mammary gland tumorigenesis. Adv Exp Med Biol. 1992;322:203-22.

41. Craig-schmidt M, White MT, Teer P, Johnson J, Lane HW. Menhaden, coconut, and corn oils and mammary tumor incidence in BALB/c virgin female mice treated with DMBA. Nutr Cancer. 1993;20(2):99-106.

42. Enos RT, Velázquez KT, Mcclellan JL, et al. High-fat diets rich in saturated fat protect against azoxymethane/dextran sulfate sodium-induced colon cancer. Am J Physiol Gastrointest Liver Physiol. 2016;310(11):G906-19.

43. Figueroa, J. (2015). *Coconut Oil Cures Cancer.* [Online]. Available: http://revelation12.ca/?p=2110. [November 6, 2016].

44. Shilling M, Matt L, Rubin E, et al. Antimicrobial effects of virgin coconut oil and its medium-chain fatty acids on Clostridium difficile. J Med Food. 2013;16(12):1079-85.

45. Verallo-rowell VM, Dillague KM, Syah-tjundawan BS. Novel antibacterial and emollient effects of coconut and virgin olive oils in adult atopic dermatitis. Dermatitis. 2008;19(6):308-15.

46. Shino B, Peedikayil FC, Jaiprakash SR, Ahmed bijapur G, Kottayi S, Jose D. Comparison of Antimicrobial Activity of Chlorhexidine, Coconut Oil, Probiotics, and Ketoconazole on Candida albicans Isolated in Children with Early Childhood Caries: An In Vitro Study. Scientifica (Cairo). 2016;2016:7061587.

47. Ogbolu DO, Oni AA, Daini OA, Oloko AP. In vitro antimicrobial properties of coconut oil on Candida species in Ibadan, Nigeria. J Med Food. 2007;10(2):384-7.

48. Marina AM, Man YB, Nazimah SA, Amin I. Antioxidant capacity and phenolic acids of virgin coconut oil. Int J Food Sci Nutr. 2009;60 Suppl 2:114-23.

49. Yeap SK, Beh BK, Ali NM, et al. Antistress and antioxidant effects of virgin coconut oil in vivo. Exp Ther Med. 2015;9(1):39-42.

50. Otuechere CA, Madarikan G, Simisola T, Bankole O, Osho A. Virgin coconut oil protects against liver damage in albino rats challenged with the anti-folate combination, trimethoprim-sulfamethoxazole. J Basic Clin Physiol Pharmacol. 2014;25(2):249-53.

51. Nair SS, Manalil JJ, Ramavarma SK, Suseela IM, Thekkepatt A, Raghavamenon AC. Virgin coconut oil supplementation ameliorates cyclophosphamide-induced systemic toxicity in mice. Hum Exp Toxicol. 2016;35(2):205-12.

52. Shadnia S, Rahimi M, Pajoumand A, Rasouli MH, Abdollahi M. Successful treatment of acute aluminium phosphide poisoning: possible benefit of coconut oil. Hum Exp Toxicol. 2005;24(4):215-8.

53. Law KS, Azman N, Omar EA, et al. The effects of virgin coconut oil (VCO) as supplementation on quality of life (QOL) among breast cancer patients. Lipids Health Dis. 2014;13:139.

54. Coconut oil in health and disease: Its and monolaurin's potential as cure for aids. Unknown journal. Date   unknown.   Available: https://www.researchgate.net/publication/237233256_COCONUT_OIL_IN_HEALTH_AND_DISE ASE_ITS_AND_MONOLAURIN%27S_POTENTIAL_AS_CURE_FOR_HIVAIDS_By. [February 15, 2017].

55. Interviews and anecdotal reports. Posit Health News. 1998;(No 16):13-5.

56. Vysakh A, Ratheesh M, Rajmohanan TP, et al. Polyphenolics isolated from virgin coconut oil inhibits adjuvant induced arthritis in rats through antioxidant and anti-inflammatory action. Int Immunopharmacol. 2014;20(1):124-30.

57. Hayatullina Z, Muhammad N, Mohamed N, Soelaiman IN. Virgin coconut oil supplementation prevents bone loss in osteoporosis rat model. Evid Based Complement Alternat Med. 2012;2012:237236.

58. Abujazia MA, Muhammad N, Shuid AN, Soelaiman IN. The effects of virgin coconut oil on bone oxidative status in ovariectomised rat. Evid Based Complement Alternat Med. 2012;2012:525079.

59. Hu yang I, De la rubia ortí JE, Selvi sabater P, et al. [Coconut Oil: Non-Alternative Drug Treatment Against Alzheimer's Disease]. Nutr Hosp. 2015;32(6):2822-7.

60. Newport, S. (2013). *Coconut Oil has Improved My Life.* [Online]. Available: https://healthunlocked.com/parkinsonsmovement/posts/1170627/coconut-oil-has-improved-my-life [November 6, 2016].

61. Sankaranarayanan K, Mondkar JA, Chauhan MM, Mascarenhas BM, Mainkar AR, Salvi RY. Oil massage in neonates: an open randomized controlled study of coconut versus mineral oil. Indian Pediatr. 2005;42(9):877-84.

62. Peedikayil FC, Sreenivasan P, Narayanan A. Effect of coconut oil in plaque related gingivitis - A preliminary report. Niger Med J. 2015;56(2):143-7.

63. Kaushik M, Reddy P, Sharma R, Udameshi P, Mehra N, Marwaha A. The Effect of Coconut Oil pulling on Streptococcus mutans Count in Saliva in Comparison with Chlorhexidine Mouthwash. J Contemp Dent Pract. 2016;17(1):38-41.

64. Singla N, Acharya S, Martena S, Singla R. Effect of oil gum massage therapy on common pathogenic oral microorganisms - A randomized controlled trial. J Indian Soc Periodontol. 2014;18(4):441-6.

65. Houssay BA, Martínez C. Experimental Diabetes and Diet. Science. 1947;105(2734):548-9.

66. Narayanankutty A, Mukesh RK, Ayoob SK, et al. Virgin coconut oil maintains redox status and improves glycemic conditions in high fructose fed rats. J Food Sci Technol. 2016;53(1):895-901.

67. Alves NF, Porpino SK, Monteiro MM, Gomes ER, Braga VA. Coconut oil supplementation and physical exercise improves baroreflex sensitivity and oxidative stress in hypertensive rats. Appl Physiol Nutr Metab. 2015;40(4):393-400.

68. Mutalib HA, Kaur S, Ghazali AR, Chinn hooi N, Safie NH. A pilot study: the efficacy of virgin coconut oil as ocular rewetting agent on rabbit eyes. Evid Based Complement Alternat Med. 2015;2015:135987.

69.   Bowen yoho WS, Swank VA, Eastridge ML, O'diam KM, Daniels KM. Jersey calf performance in response to high-protein, high-fat liquid feeds with varied fatty acid profiles: intake and performance. J Dairy Sci. 2013;96(4):2494-506.

70.   Wang J, Wang X, Li J, Chen Y, Yang W, Zhang L. Effects of Dietary Coconut Oil as a Medium-chain Fatty Acid Source on Performance, Carcass Composition and Serum Lipids in Male Broilers. Asian-australas J Anim Sci. 2015;28(2):223-30.

71.   Hammer CT, Wills ED. The effect of ionizing radiation on the fatty acid composition of natural fats and on lipid peroxide formation. Int J Radiat Biol Relat Stud Phys Chem Med. 1979;35(4):323-32.

72.   Rele AS, Mohile RB. Effect of mineral oil, sunflower oil, and coconut oil on prevention of hair damage. J Cosmet Sci. 2003;54(2):175-92.

73.   Rele AS, Mohile RB. Effect of coconut oil on prevention of hair damage. Part 1. J. Cosmet. Sci. 1999; 50:327-339.

74.   Burgess IF, Brunton ER, Burgess NA. Clinical trial showing superiority of a coconut and anise spray over permethrin 0.43% lotion for head louse infestation, ISRCTN96469780. Eur J Pediatr. 2010;169(1):55-62.

75.   Nevin KG, Rajamohan T. Effect of topical application of virgin coconut oil on skin components and antioxidant status during dermal wound healing in young rats. Skin Pharmacol Physiol. 2010;23(6):290-7.

76.   Nurul-iman BS, Kamisah Y, Jaarin K, Qodriyah HM. Virgin coconut oil prevents blood pressure elevation and improves endothelial functions in rats fed with repeatedly heated palm oil. Evid Based Complement Alternat Med. 2013;2013:629329.

77.   Deol P, Evans JR, Dhahbi J, et al. Soybean Oil Is More Obesogenic and Diabetogenic than Coconut Oil and Fructose in Mouse: Potential Role for the Liver. PLoS ONE. 2015;10(7):e0132672.

78.   Assunção ML, Ferreira HS, Dos santos AF, Cabral CR, Florêncio TM. Effects of dietary coconut oil on the biochemical and anthropometric profiles of women presenting abdominal obesity. Lipids. 2009;44(7):593-601.

79.   Liau KM, Lee YY, Chen CK, Rasool AH. An open-label pilot study to assess the efficacy and safety of virgin coconut oil in reducing visceral adiposity. ISRN Pharmacol. 2011;2011:949686.

80.   Cardoso DA, Moreira AS, De oliveira GM, Raggio luiz R, Rosa G. A Coconut Extra Virgin Oil-Rich Diet Increases HDL Cholesterol And Decreases Waist Circumference And Body Mass In Coronary Artery Disease Patients. Nutr Hosp. 2015;32(5):2144-52.

81.   Lawrence GD. Dietary fats and health: dietary recommendations in the context of scientific evidence. Adv Nutr. 2013;4(3):294-302.

82.   Korać RR, Khambholja KM. Potential of herbs in skin protection from ultraviolet radiation. Pharmacogn Rev. 2011;5(10):164-73.

83.   Evangelista MT, Abad-casintahan F, Lopez-villafuerte L. The effect of topical virgin coconut oil on SCORAD index, transepidermal water loss, and skin capacitance in mild to moderate pediatric atopic dermatitis: a randomized, double-blind, clinical trial. Int J Dermatol. 2014;53(1):100-8.

84.   Aloia RC, Mlekusch W. The effect of a saturated fat diet on pentobarbital induced sleeping time and phospholipid composition of mouse brain and liver. Pharmazie. 1988;43(7):496-8.

85.   Chempro. *Top-notch technology in production of oils and fats*. Available at: http://www.chempro.in/fattyacid.htm. [February 6, 2016].

86.   Magalhães MS, Fechine FV, Macedo RN, et al. Effect of a combination of medium chain triglycerides, linoleic acid, soy lecithin and vitamins A and E on wound healing in rats. Acta Cir Bras. 2008;23(3):262-9.

87. Bach AC, Babayan VK. Medium-chain triglycerides: an update. Am J Clin Nutr. 1982;36(5):950-62.

88. Bach A, Phan T, Metais P. Influence of a long or medium chain triglyceride diet on intermediary hepatic metabolism of the rat. Nutr Metab. 1975;19(1-2):103-10.

89. Bach A, Schirardin H, Weryha A, Bauer M. Ketogenic response to medium-chain triglyceride load in the rat. J Nutr. 1977;107(10):1863-70.

90. Cohen LA, Thompson DO, Maeura Y, Weisburger JH. Influence of dietary medium-chain triglycerides on the development of N-methylnitrosourea-induced rat mammary tumors. Cancer Res. 1984;44(11):5023-8.

91. Tisdale MJ, Brennan RA, Fearon KC. Reduction of weight loss and tumour size in a cachexia model by a high fat diet. Br J Cancer. 1987;56(1):39-43.

92. Cohen LA, Thompson DO. The influence of dietary medium chain triglycerides on rat mammary tumor development. Lipids. 1987;22(6):455-61.

93. Tisdale MJ, Brennan RA. A comparison of long-chain triglycerides and medium-chain triglycerides on weight loss and tumour size in a cachexia model. Br J Cancer. 1988;58(5):580-3.

94. Tisdale MJ, Leung YC. Changes in host liver fatty acid synthase in tumour-bearing mice. Cancer Lett. 1988;42(3):231-5.

95. Kimoto Y, Tanji Y, Taguchi T, et al. Antitumor effect of medium-chain triglyceride and its influence on the self-defense system of the body. Cancer Detect Prev. 1998;22(3):219-24.

96. Pourgholami MH, Akhter J, Morris DL. In vitro antiproliferative activity of a medium-chain triglyceride solution of 1,25-dihydroxyvitamin D3 in HepG2 cells. Anticancer Res. 2000;20(6B):4257-60.

97. Kaewsakhorn T, Kisseberth WC, Capen CC, Hayes KA, Calverley MJ, Inpanbutr N. Effects of calcitriol, seocalcitol, and medium-chain triglyceride on a canine transitional cell carcinoma cell line. Anticancer Res. 2005;25(4):2689-96.

98. Wang X, Pan L, Zhang P, et al. Enteral nutrition improves clinical outcome and shortens hospital stay after cancer surgery. J Invest Surg. 2010;23(6):309-13.

99. Nomura A, Majumder K, Giri B, et al. Inhibition of NF-kappa B pathway leads to deregulation of epithelial-mesenchymal transition and neural invasion in pancreatic cancer. Lab Invest. 2016.

100. Wu L, Zhang X, Zhang B, et al. Exosomes derived from gastric cancer cells activate NF-κB pathway in macrophages to promote cancer progression. Tumour Biol. 2016;37(9):12169-12180.

101. Wang X, Lin Y. Tumor necrosis factor and cancer, buddies or foes?. Acta Pharmacol Sin. 2008;29(11):1275-88.

102. Rusyn I, Bradham CA, Cohn L, et al. Corn oil rapidly activates nuclear factor-kappaB in hepatic Kupffer cells by oxidant-dependent mechanisms. Carcinogenesis. 1999;20(11):2095-100.

103. Gogos CA, Zoumbos N, Makri M, Kalfarentzos F. Medium- and long-chain triglycerides have different effects on the synthesis of tumor necrosis factor by human mononuclear cells in patients under total parenteral nutrition. J Am Coll Nutr. 1994;13(1):40-4.

104. Bussard KM, Mutkus L, Stumpf K, Gomez-manzano C, Marini FC. Tumor-associated stromal cells as key contributors to the tumor microenvironment. Breast Cancer Res. 2016;18(1):84.

105. Ha NH, Park DG, Woo BH, et al. Porphyromonas gingivalis increases the invasiveness of oral cancer cells by upregulating IL-8 and MMPs. Cytokine. 2016;86:64-72.

106. Hoshimoto A, Suzuki Y, Katsuno T, Nakajima H, Saito Y. Caprylic acid and medium-chain triglycerides inhibit IL-8 gene transcription in Caco-2 cells: comparison with the potent histone deacetylase inhibitor trichostatin A. Br J Pharmacol. 2002;136(2):280-6.

107. Calabrese PR, Frank HD, Taubin HL. Lymphangiomyomatosis with chylous ascites: treatment with dietary fat restriction and medium chain triglycerides. Cancer. 1977;40(2):895-7.

108. Nebeling LC, Miraldi F, Shurin SB, Lerner E. Effects of a ketogenic diet on tumor metabolism and nutritional status in pediatric oncology patients: two case reports. J Am Coll Nutr. 1995;14(2):202-8.

109. Kono H, Enomoto N, Connor HD, et al. Medium-chain triglycerides inhibit free radical formation and TNF-alpha production in rats given enteral ethanol. Am J Physiol Gastrointest Liver Physiol. 2000;278(3):G467-76.

110. Zhong W, Li Q, Xie G, et al. Dietary fat sources differentially modulate intestinal barrier and hepatic inflammation in alcohol-induced liver injury in rats. Am J Physiol Gastrointest Liver Physiol. 2013;305(12):G919-32.

111. Ronis MJ, Korourian S, Zipperman M, Hakkak R, Badger TM. Dietary saturated fat reduces alcoholic hepatotoxicity in rats by altering fatty acid metabolism and membrane composition. J Nutr. 2004;134(4):904-12.

112. Nanji AA, Jokelainen K, Tipoe GL, Rahemtulla A, Dannenberg AJ. Dietary saturated fatty acids reverse inflammatory and fibrotic changes in rat liver despite continued ethanol administration. J Pharmacol Exp Ther. 2001;299(2):638-44.

113. Khoramnia A, Ebrahimpour A, Ghanbari R, Ajdari Z, Lai OM. Improvement of medium chain fatty acid content and antimicrobial activity of coconut oil via solid-state fermentation using a Malaysian Geotrichum candidum. Biomed Res Int. 2013;2013:954542.

114. Shilling M, Matt L, Rubin E, et al. Antimicrobial effects of virgin coconut oil and its medium-chain fatty acids on Clostridium difficile. J Med Food. 2013;16(12):1079-85.

115. Isaacs CE, Litov RE, Thormar H. Antimicrobial activity of lipids added to human milk, infant formula, and bovine milk. J Nutr Biochem. 1995;6(7):362-366.

116. Papavassilis C, Mach KK, Mayser PA. Medium-chain triglycerides inhibit growth of Malassezia: implications for prevention of systemic infection. Crit Care Med. 1999;27(9):1781-6.

117. Kono H, Fujii H, Asakawa M, et al. Protective effects of medium-chain triglycerides on the liver and gut in rats administered endotoxin. Ann Surg. 2003;237(2):246-55.

118. Lin MT, Yeh SL, Kuo ML, et al. Effects of medium-chain triglyceride in parenteral nutrition on rats undergoing gastrectomy. Clin Nutr. 2002;21(1):39-43.

119. Isaacs CE, Kim KS, Thormar H. Inactivation of enveloped viruses in human bodily fluids by purified lipids. Ann N Y Acad Sci. 1994;724:457-64.

120. Wanke C. Single-agent/combination therapy of human immunodeficiency virus-related wasting. Semin Oncol. 1998;25(2 Suppl 6):98-103.

121. Wanke CA, Pleskow D, Degirolami PC, Lambl BB, Merkel K, Akrabawi S. A medium chain triglyceride-based diet in patients with HIV and chronic diarrhea reduces diarrhea and malabsorption: a prospective, controlled trial. Nutrition. 1996;12(11-12):766-71.

122. Carlson SJ, Nandivada P, Chang MI, et al. The addition of medium-chain triglycerides to a purified fish oil-based diet alters inflammatory profiles in mice. Metab Clin Exp. 2015;64(2):274-82.

123. Herbert MR, Buckley JA. Autism and dietary therapy: case report and review of the literature. J Child Neurol. 2013;28(8):975-82.

124. Kehayoglou K, Hadziyannis S, Kostamis P, Malamos B. The effect of medium-chain triglyceride on 47 calcium absorption in patients with primary biliary cirrhosis. Gut. 1973;14(8):653-6.

125. Kehayoglou AK, Williams HS, Whimster WF, Holdsworth CD. Calcium absorption in the normal, bile-duct ligated, and cirrhotic rat, with observations on the effect of long- and medium-chain triglycerides. Gut. 1968;9(5):597-603.

126. Pan Y, Larson B, Araujo JA, et al. Dietary supplementation with medium-chain TAG has long-lasting cognition-enhancing effects in aged dogs. Br J Nutr. 2010;103(12):1746-54.

127. Manteca X. Nutrition and behavior in senior dogs. Top Companion Anim Med. 2011;26(1):33-6.

128. Sharma A, Bemis M, Desilets AR. Role of Medium Chain Triglycerides (Axona®) in the Treatment of Mild to Moderate Alzheimer's Disease. Am J Alzheimers Dis Other Demen. 2014;29(5):409-14.

129. Ohnuma T, Toda A, Kimoto A, et al. Benefits of use, and tolerance of, medium-chain triglyceride medical food in the management of Japanese patients with Alzheimer's disease: a prospective, open-label pilot study. Clin Interv Aging. 2016;11:29-36.

130. Cunnane SC, Courchesne-loyer A, St-pierre V, et al. Can ketones compensate for deteriorating brain glucose uptake during aging? Implications for the risk and treatment of Alzheimer's disease. Ann N Y Acad Sci. 2016;1367(1):12-20.

131. Rebello CJ, Keller JN, Liu AG, Johnson WD, Greenway FL. Pilot feasibility and safety study examining the effect of medium chain triglyceride supplementation in subjects with mild cognitive impairment: A randomized controlled trial. BBA Clin. 2015;3:123-5.

132. Page KA, Williamson A, Yu N, et al. Medium-chain fatty acids improve cognitive function in intensively treated type 1 diabetic patients and support in vitro synaptic transmission during acute hypoglycemia. Diabetes. 2009;58(5):1237-44.

133. Reger MA, Henderson ST, Hale C, et al. Effects of beta-hydroxybutyrate on cognition in memory-impaired adults. Neurobiol Aging. 2004;25(3):311-4.

134. Dong YM, Li Y, Ning H, Wang C, Liu JR, Sun CH. High dietary intake of medium-chain fatty acids during pregnancy in rats prevents later-life obesity in their offspring. J Nutr Biochem. 2011;22(8):791-7.

135. Laverty G, Gilmore BF, Jones DS, Coyle L, Folan M, Breathnach R. Antimicrobial efficacy of an innovative emulsion of medium chain triglycerides against canine and feline periodontopathogens. J Small Anim Pract. 2015;56(4):253-63.

136. Dhanikula AB, Khalid NM, Lee SD, et al. Long circulating lipid nanocapsules for drug detoxification. Biomaterials. 2007;28(6):1248-57.

137. Han J, Hamilton JA, Kirkland JL, Corkey BE, Guo W. Medium-chain oil reduces fat mass and down-regulates expression of adipogenic genes in rats. Obes Res. 2003;11(6):734-44.

138. Eckel RH, Hanson AS, Chen AY, Berman JN, Yost TJ, Brass EP. Dietary substitution of medium-chain triglycerides improves insulin-mediated glucose metabolism in NIDDM subjects. Diabetes. 1992;41(5):641-7.

139. Yost TJ, Eckel RH. Hypocaloric feeding in obese women: metabolic effects of medium-chain triglyceride substitution. Am J Clin Nutr. 1989;49(2):326-30.

140. Gola A, Bochenek W, Molin I. Effects of medium chain triglycerides on plasma free fatty acids in normal subjects. Arch Immunol Ther Exp (Warsz). 1974;22(6):797-802.

141. Perret JP, Guiffray N, Mottaz P. [Stimulation of insulin secretion by medium-chain fatty acids in the diet of young rabbits]. Ann Nutr Metab. 1983;27(2):153-61.

142. Greenberger NJ, Tzagournis M, Graves TM. Stimulation of insulin secretion in man by medium chain triglycerides. Metab Clin Exp. 1968;17(9):796-801.

143. Valls E, Herrera E, Díaz M, Barreiro P, Valls A. [Modifications of insulin and growth hormone after medium chain triglycerides ingestion (author's transl)]. An Esp Pediatr. 1978;11(10):675-82.

144. Ooyama K, Wu J, Nosaka N, Aoyama T, Kasai M. Combined intervention of medium-chain triacylglycerol diet and exercise reduces body fat mass and enhances energy expenditure in rats. J Nutr Sci Vitaminol. 2008;54(2):136-41.

145. Fushiki T, Matsumoto K, Inoue K, Kawada T, Sugimoto E. Swimming endurance capacity of mice is increased by chronic consumption of medium-chain triglycerides. J Nutr. 1995;125(3):531-9.

146. Van zyl CG, Lambert EV, Hawley JA, Noakes TD, Dennis SC. Effects of medium-chain triglyceride ingestion on fuel metabolism and cycling performance. J Appl Physiol. 1996;80(6):2217-25.

147. Nosaka N, Suzuki Y, Nagatoishi A, Kasai M, Wu J, Taguchi M. Effect of ingestion of medium-chain triacylglycerols on moderate- and high-intensity exercise in recreational athletes. J Nutr Sci Vitaminol. 2009;55(2):120-5.

148. Misell LM, Lagomarcino ND, Schuster V, Kern M. Chronic medium-chain triacylglycerol consumption and endurance performance in trained runners. J Sports Med Phys Fitness. 2001;41(2):210-5.

149. Angus DJ, Hargreaves M, Dancey J, Febbraio MA. Effect of carbohydrate or carbohydrate plus medium-chain triglyceride ingestion on cycling time trial performance. J Appl Physiol. 2000;88(1):113-9.

150. Goedecke JH, Elmer-english R, Dennis SC, Schloss I, Noakes TD, Lambert EV. Effects of medium-chain triaclyglycerol ingested with carbohydrate on metabolism and exercise performance. Int J Sport Nutr. 1999;9(1):35-47.

151. Satabin P, Portero P, Defer G, Bricout J, Guezennec CY. Metabolic and hormonal responses to lipid and carbohydrate diets during exercise in man. Med Sci Sports Exerc. 1987;19(3):218-23.

152. Goedecke JH, Clark VR, Noakes TD, Lambert EV. The effects of medium-chain triacylglycerol and carbohydrate ingestion on ultra-endurance exercise performance. Int J Sport Nutr Exerc Metab. 2005;15(1):15-27.

153. Jeukendrup AE, Thielen JJ, Wagenmakers AJ, Brouns F, Saris WH. Effect of medium-chain triacylglycerol and carbohydrate ingestion during exercise on substrate utilization and subsequent cycling performance. Am J Clin Nutr. 1998;67(3):397-404.

154. Lambert EV, Hawley JA, Goedecke J, Noakes TD, Dennis SC. Nutritional strategies for promoting fat utilization and delaying the onset of fatigue during prolonged exercise. J Sports Sci. 1997;15(3):315-24.

155. Behrend AM, Harding CO, Shoemaker JD, et al. Substrate oxidation and cardiac performance during exercise in disorders of long chain fatty acid oxidation. Mol Genet Metab. 2012;105(1):110-5.

156. Jeukendrup AE, Saris WH, Schrauwen P, Brouns F, Wagenmakers AJ. Metabolic availability of medium-chain triglycerides coingested with carbohydrates during prolonged exercise. J Appl Physiol. 1995;79(3):756-62.

157. Hawley JA. Effect of increased fat availability on metabolism and exercise capacity. Med Sci Sports Exerc. 2002;34(9):1485-91.

158. Auclair E, Satabin P, Servan E, Guezennec CY. Metabolic effects of glucose, medium chain triglyceride and long chain triglyceride feeding before prolonged exercise in rats. Eur J Appl Physiol Occup Physiol. 1988;57(1):126-31.

159. Horowitz JF, Mora-rodriguez R, Byerley LO, Coyle EF. Preexercise medium-chain triglyceride ingestion does not alter muscle glycogen use during exercise. J Appl Physiol. 2000;88(1):219-25.

160. Jeukendrup AE, Saris WH, Brouns F, Halliday D, Wagenmakers JM. Effects of carbohydrate (CHO) and fat supplementation on CHO metabolism during prolonged exercise. Metab Clin Exp. 1996;45(7):915-21.

161. Décombaz J, Arnaud MJ, Milon H, et al. Energy metabolism of medium-chain triglycerides versus carbohydrates during exercise. Eur J Appl Physiol Occup Physiol. 1983;52(1):9-14.

162. Massicotte D, Péronnet F, Brisson GR, Hillaire-marcel C. Oxidation of exogenous medium-chain free fatty acids during prolonged exercise: comparison with glucose. J Appl Physiol. 1992;73(4):1334-9.

163. Hawley JA, Brouns F, Jeukendrup A. Strategies to enhance fat utilisation during exercise. Sports Med. 1998;25(4):241-57.

164. Zentek J, Buchheit-renko S, Ferrara F, Vahjen W, Van kessel AG, Pieper R. Nutritional and physiological role of medium-chain triglycerides and medium-chain fatty acids in piglets. Anim Health Res Rev. 2011;12(1):83-93.

165. Steinbrenner I, Houdek P, Pollok S, Brandner JM, Daniels R. Influence of the Oil Phase and Topical Formulation on the Wound Healing Ability of a Birch Bark Dry Extract. PLoS ONE. 2016;11(5):e0155582.

166. Rudich MD, Rowland MC, Seibel RW, Border J. Survival following a gunshot wound of the abdominal aorta and inferior vena cava. J Trauma. 1978;18(7):548-9.

167. Duran M, Wanders RJ, De jager JP, et al. 3-Hydroxydicarboxylic aciduria due to long-chain 3-hydroxyacyl-coenzyme A dehydrogenase deficiency associated with sudden neonatal death: protective effect of medium-chain triglyceride treatment. Eur J Pediatr. 1991;150(3):190-5.

168. Finck BN, Han X, Courtois M, et al. A critical role for PPARalpha-mediated lipotoxicity in the pathogenesis of diabetic cardiomyopathy: modulation by dietary fat content. Proc Natl Acad Sci USA. 2003;100(3):1226-31.

169. Footitt EJ, Stafford J, Dixon M, et al. Use of a long-chain triglyceride-restricted/medium-chain triglyceride-supplemented diet in a case of malonyl-CoA decarboxylase deficiency with cardiomyopathy. J Inherit Metab Dis. 2010;33 Suppl 3:S253-6.

170. Labarthe F, Khairallah M, Bouchard B, Stanley WC, Des rosiers C. Fatty acid oxidation and its impact on response of spontaneously hypertensive rat hearts to an adrenergic stress: benefits of a medium-chain fatty acid. Am J Physiol Heart Circ Physiol. 2005;288(3):H1425-36.

171. Shimojo N, Miyauchi T, Iemitsu M, et al. Effects of medium-chain triglyceride (MCT) application to SHR on cardiac function, hypertrophy and expression of endothelin-1 mRNA and other genes. J Cardiovasc Pharmacol. 2004;44 Suppl 1:S181-5.

172. Iemitsu M, Shimojo N, Maeda S, et al. The benefit of medium-chain triglyceride therapy on the cardiac function of SHRs is associated with a reversal of metabolic and signaling alterations. Am J Physiol Heart Circ Physiol. 2008;295(1):H136-44.

173. Kono H, Fujii H, Asakawa M, et al. Medium-chain triglycerides enhance secretory IgA expression in rat intestine after administration of endotoxin. Am J Physiol Gastrointest Liver Physiol. 2004;286(6):G1081-9.

174. Sedman PC, Somers SS, Ramsden CW, Brennan TG, Guillou PJ. Effects of different lipid emulsions on lymphocyte function during total parenteral nutrition. Br J Surg. 1991;78(11):1396-9.

175. Gogos CA, Kalfarentzos FE, Zoumbos NC. Effect of different types of total parenteral nutrition on T-lymphocyte subpopulations and NK cells. Am J Clin Nutr. 1990;51(1):119-22.

176. Hinton PS, Peterson CA, Mccarthy DO, Ney DM. Medium-chain compared with long-chain triacylglycerol emulsions enhance macrophage response and increase mucosal mass in parenterally fed rats. Am J Clin Nutr. 1998;67(6):1265-72.

177. Kono H, Fujii H, Ishii K, Hosomura N, Ogiku M. Dietary medium-chain triglycerides prevent chemically induced experimental colitis in rats. Transl Res. 2010;155(3):131-41.

178. Mañé J, Pedrosa E, Lorén V, et al. Partial replacement of dietary (n-6) fatty acids with medium-chain triglycerides decreases the incidence of spontaneous colitis in interleukin-10-deficient mice. J Nutr. 2009;139(3):603-10.

179. Cabré E, Gassull MA. Nutritional and metabolic issues in inflammatory bowel disease. Curr Opin Clin Nutr Metab Care. 2003;6(5):569-76.

180. Cabré E, Domènech E. Impact of environmental and dietary factors on the course of inflammatory bowel disease. World J Gastroenterol. 2012;18(29):3814-22.

181. Eisenberh BC. Congenital lymphangiectasia and atopy. Ann Allergy. 1976;36(5):342-50.

182. Desai AP, Guvenc BH, Carachi R. Evidence for medium chain triglycerides in the treatment of primary intestinal lymphangiectasia. Eur J Pediatr Surg. 2009;19(4):241-5.

183. Li R, Ma J, Yu K, Wang L. Dietary or enteral medium-chain triglyceride usage in a Chinese general hospital. Asia Pac J Clin Nutr. 2015;24(3):387-93.

184. Lasekan JB, Rivera J, Hirvonen MD, Keesey RE, Ney DM. Energy expenditure in rats maintained with intravenous or intragastric infusion of total parenteral nutrition solutions containing medium- or long-chain triglyceride emulsions. J Nutr. 1992;122(7):1483-92.

185. Mabayo RT, Furuse M, Murai A, Okumura J. Interactions between medium-chain and long-chain triacylglycerols in lipid and energy metabolism in growing chicks. Lipids. 1994;29(2):139-44.

186. Rothwell NJ, Stock MJ. Stimulation of thermogenesis and brown fat activity in rats fed medium chain triglyceride. Metab Clin Exp. 1987;36(2):128-30.

187. Scalfi L, Coltorti A, Contaldo F. Postprandial thermogenesis in lean and obese subjects after meals supplemented with medium-chain and long-chain triglycerides. Am J Clin Nutr. 1991;53(5):1130-3.

188. Seaton TB, Welle SL, Warenko MK, Campbell RG. Thermic effect of medium-chain and long-chain triglycerides in man. Am J Clin Nutr. 1986;44(5):630-4.

189. Hill JO, Peters JC, Yang D, et al. Thermogenesis in humans during overfeeding with medium-chain triglycerides. Metab Clin Exp. 1989;38(7):641-8.

190. White MD, Papamandjaris AA, Jones PJ. Enhanced postprandial energy expenditure with medium-chain fatty acid feeding is attenuated after 14 d in premenopausal women. Am J Clin Nutr. 1999;69(5):883-9.

191. Kasai M, Nosaka N, Maki H, et al. Comparison of diet-induced thermogenesis of foods containing medium- versus long-chain triacylglycerols. J Nutr Sci Vitaminol. 2002;48(6):536-40.

192. Dulloo AG, Fathi M, Mensi N, Girardier L. Twenty-four-hour energy expenditure and urinary catecholamines of humans consuming low-to-moderate amounts of medium-chain triglycerides: a dose-response study in a human respiratory chamber. Eur J Clin Nutr. 1996;50(3):152-8.

193. Macdonald ML, Rogers QR, Morris JG. Aversion of the cat to dietary medium-chain triglycerides and caprylic acid. Physiol Behav. 1985;35(3):371-5.

194. Lee YY, Tang TK, Ab karim NA, Alitheen NB, Lai OM. Short term and dosage influences of palm based medium- and long-chain triacylglycerols on body fat and blood parameters in C57BL/6J mice. Food Funct. 2014;5(1):57-64.

195. Geliebter A, Torbay N, Bracco EF, Hashim SA, Van itallie TB. Overfeeding with medium-chain triglyceride diet results in diminished deposition of fat. Am J Clin Nutr. 1983;37(1):1-4.

196. Coleman H, Quinn P, Clegg ME. Medium-chain triglycerides and conjugated linoleic acids in beverage form increase satiety and reduce food intake in humans. Nutr Res. 2016;36(6):526-33.

197. St-onge MP, Mayrsohn B, O'keeffe M, Kissileff HR, Choudhury AR, Laferrère B. Impact of medium and long chain triglycerides consumption on appetite and food intake in overweight men. Eur J Clin Nutr. 2014;68(10):1134-40.

198. Matsuo T, Matsuo M, Kasai M, Takeuchi H. Effects of a liquid diet supplement containing structured medium- and long-chain triacylglycerols on bodyfat accumulation in healthy young subjects. Asia Pac J Clin Nutr. 2001;10(1):46-50.

199. Nosaka N, Maki H, Suzuki Y, et al. Effects of margarine containing medium-chain triacylglycerols on body fat reduction in humans. J Atheroscler Thromb. 2003;10(5):290-8.

200. St-onge MP, Bosarge A. Weight-loss diet that includes consumption of medium-chain triacylglycerol oil leads to a greater rate of weight and fat mass loss than does olive oil. Am J Clin Nutr. 2008;87(3):621-6.

201. Hainer V, Kunesová M, Stich V, Zák A, Parizková J. [The role of oils containing triacylglycerols and medium-chain fatty acids in the dietary treatment of obesity. The effect on resting energy expenditure and serum lipids]. Cas Lek Cesk. 1994;133(12):373-5.

202. Krotkiewski M. Value of VLCD supplementation with medium chain triglycerides. Int J Obes Relat Metab Disord. 2001;25(9):1393-400.

203. St-onge MP, Ross R, Parsons WD, Jones PJ. Medium-chain triglycerides increase energy expenditure and decrease adiposity in overweight men. Obes Res. 2003;11(3):395-402.

204. Xue C, Liu Y, Wang J, et al. Consumption of medium- and long-chain triacylglycerols decreases body fat and blood triglyceride in Chinese hypertriglyceridemic subjects. Eur J Clin Nutr. 2009;63(7):879-86.

205. Han JR, Deng B, Sun J, et al. Effects of dietary medium-chain triglyceride on weight loss and insulin sensitivity in a group of moderately overweight free-living type 2 diabetic Chinese subjects. Metab Clin Exp. 2007;56(7):985-91.

206. Bounous G, Le bel E, Shuster J, Gold P, Tahan WT, Bastin E. Dietary protection during radiation therapy. Strahlentherapie. 1975;149(5):476-83.

207. Sipes SL, Newton M, Lurain JR. Chylous ascites: a sequel of pelvic radiation therapy. Obstet Gynecol. 1985;66(6):832-5.

208. Law TH, Davies ES, Pan Y, Zanghi B, Want E, Volk HA. A randomised trial of a medium-chain TAG diet as treatment for dogs with idiopathic epilepsy. Br J Nutr. 2015;114(9):1438-47.

209. Rosenthal E, Weissman B, Kyllonen K. Use of parenteral medium-chain triglyceride emulsion for maintaining seizure control in a 5-year-old girl with intractable diarrhea. JPEN J Parenter Enteral Nutr. 1990;14(5):543-5.

210. Calandre L, Martínez martin P, Campos castelló J. [Treatment of lennox syndrome with medium chain triglycerides (author's transl)]. An Esp Pediatr. 1978;11(3):189-94.

211. Schiff Y, Lerman-sagie T. [Ketogenic diet--an alternative therapy for epilepsy in adults]. Harefuah. 1998;134(7):529-31, 591.

212. Ros pérez P, Zamarrón cuesta I, Aparicio meix M, Sastre gallego A. [Evaluation of the effectiveness of the ketogenic diet with medium-chain triglycerides, in the treatment of refractory epilepsy in children. Apropos of a series of cases]. An Esp Pediatr. 1989;30(3):155-8.

213. Sills MA, Forsythe WI, Haidukewych D, Macdonald A, Robinson M. The medium chain triglyceride diet and intractable epilepsy. Arch Dis Child. 1986;61(12):1168-72.

214. Chomtho K, Suteerojntrakool O, Chomtho S. Effectiveness of Medium Chain Triglyceride Ketogenic Diet in Thai Children with Intractable Epilepsy. J Med Assoc Thai. 2016;99(2):159-65.

215. Mak SC, Chi CS, Wan CJ. Clinical experience of ketogenic diet on children with refractory epilepsy. Acta Paediatr Taiwan. 1999;40(2):97-100.

216. Azzam R, Azar NJ. Marked Seizure Reduction after MCT Supplementation. Case Rep Neurol Med. 2013;2013:809151.

217. Wiedersberg S, Leopold CS, Guy RH. Effects of various vehicles on skin hydration in vivo. Skin Pharmacol Physiol. 2009;22(3):128-30.

218. Kogan A, Garti N. Microemulsions as transdermal drug delivery vehicles. Adv Colloid Interface Sci. 2006;123-126:369-85.

219. Telliez F, Bach V, Leke A, Chardon K, Libert JP. Feeding behavior in neonates whose diet contained medium-chain triacylglycerols: short-term effects on thermoregulation and sleep. Am J Clin Nutr. 2002;76(5):1091-5.

220. Auriol S, Mahieu L, Brousset P, Malecaze F, Mathis V. Safety of medium-chain triglycerides used as an intraocular tamponading agent in an experimental vitrectomy model rabbit. Retina (Philadelphia, Pa). 2013;33(1):217-23.

221. Broeders EP, Vijgen GH, Havekes B, et al. Thyroid Hormone Activates Brown Adipose Tissue and Increases Non-Shivering Thermogenesis--A Cohort Study in a Group of Thyroid Carcinoma Patients. PLoS ONE. 2016;11(1):e0145049.

222. Jeukendrup AE, Aldred S. Fat supplementation, health, and endurance performance. Nutrition. 2004;20(7-8):678-88.

223. Traul KA, Driedger A, Ingle DL, Nakhasi D. Review of the toxicologic properties of medium-chain triglycerides. Food Chem Toxicol. 2000;38(1):79-98.

224. Nonaka Y, Takagi T, Inai M, et al. Lauric Acid Stimulates Ketone Body Production in the KT-5 Astrocyte Cell Line. J Oleo Sci. 2016;65(8):693-9.

225. Faciola AP, Broderick GA. Effects of feeding lauric acid or coconut oil on ruminal protozoa numbers, fermentation pattern, digestion, omasal nutrient flow, and milk production in dairy cows. J Dairy Sci. 2014;97(8):5088-100.

226. Lieberman S, Enig MG, Preuss HG. A review of monolaurin and lauric acid. Alt. & Complem. Ther. 2006.

227. Fauser JK, Matthews GM, Cummins AG, Howarth GS. Induction of apoptosis by the medium-chain length fatty acid lauric acid in colon cancer cells due to induction of oxidative stress. Chemotherapy. 2013;59(3):214-24.

228. Yu W, Chai H, Li Y, et al. Increased expression of CYP4Z1 promotes tumor angiogenesis and growth in human breast cancer. Toxicol Appl Pharmacol. 2012;264(1):73-83.

229. Saccani A, Schioppa T, Porta C, et al. p50 nuclear factor-kappaB overexpression in tumor-associated macrophages inhibits M1 inflammatory responses and antitumor resistance. Cancer Res. 2006;66(23):11432-40.

230. Huang WC, Tsai TH, Chuang LT, Li YY, Zouboulis CC, Tsai PJ. Anti-bacterial and anti-inflammatory properties of capric acid against Propionibacterium acnes: a comparative study with lauric acid. J Dermatol Sci. 2014;73(3):232-40.

231. Yang D, Pornpattananangkul D, Nakatsuji T, et al. The antimicrobial activity of liposomal lauric acids against Propionibacterium acnes. Biomaterials. 2009;30(30):6035-40.

232. Nakatsuji T, Kao MC, Fang JY, et al. Antimicrobial property of lauric acid against Propionibacterium acnes: its therapeutic potential for inflammatory acne vulgaris. J Invest Dermatol. 2009;129(10):2480-8.

233. Huang CB, Alimova Y, Myers TM, Ebersole JL. Short- and medium-chain fatty acids exhibit antimicrobial activity for oral microorganisms. Arch Oral Biol. 2011;56(7):650-4.

234. Kabara JJ, Swieczkowski DM, Conley AJ, Truant JP. Fatty acids and derivatives as antimicrobial agents. Antimicrob Agents Chemother. 1972;2(1):23-8.

235. Petschow BW, Batema RP, Ford LL. Susceptibility of Helicobacter pylori to bactericidal properties of medium-chain monoglycerides and free fatty acids. Antimicrob Agents Chemother. 1996;40(2):302-6.

236. Souza JL, Da silva AF, Carvalho PH, Pacheco BS, Pereira CM, Lund RG. Aliphatic fatty acids and esters: inhibition of growth and exoenzyme production of Candida, and their cytotoxicity in vitro: anti-Candida effect and cytotoxicity of fatty acids and esters. Arch Oral Biol. 2014;59(9):880-6.

237. Takahashi M, Inoue S, Hayama K, Ninomiya K, Abe S. [Inhibition of Candida mycelia growth by a medium chain fatty acids, capric acid in vitro and its therapeutic efficacy in murine oral candidiasis]. Med Mycol J. 2012;53(4):255-61.

238. Sengupta A, Ghosh M, Bhattacharyya DK. In vitro antioxidant assay of medium chain fatty acid rich rice bran oil in comparison to native rice bran oil. J Food Sci Technol. 2015;52(8):5188-95.

239. Hornung B, Amtmann E, Sauer G. Lauric acid inhibits the maturation of vesicular stomatitis virus. J Gen Virol. 1994;75 (Pt 2):353-61.

240. Bartolotta S, García CC, Candurra NA, Damonte EB. Effect of fatty acids on arenavirus replication: inhibition of virus production by lauric acid. Arch Virol. 2001;146(4):777-90.

241. Irmisch G, Schläfke D, Richter J. Relationships between fatty acids and psychophysiological parameters in depressive inpatients under experimentally induced stress. Prostaglandins Leukot Essent Fatty Acids. 2006;74(2):149-56.

242. Shapiro S. The inhibitory action of fatty acids on oral bacteria. Oral Microbiol Immunol. 1996;11(5):350-5.

243. Kochikuzhyil BM, Devi K, Fattepur SR. Effect of saturated fatty acid-rich dietary vegetable oils on lipid profile, antioxidant enzymes and glucose tolerance in diabetic rats. Indian J Pharmacol. 2010;42(3):142-5.

244. Rajesh PP, Noori MT, Ghangrekar MM. Controlling methanogenesis and improving power production of microbial fuel cell by lauric acid dosing. Water Sci Technol. 2014;70(8):1363-9.

245. Zeitz JO, Fennhoff J, Kluge H, Stangl GI, Eder K. Effects of dietary fats rich in lauric and myristic acid on performance, intestinal morphology, gut microbes, and meat quality in broilers. Poult Sci. 2015;94(10):2404-13.

246. Goldberg EM, Ryland D, Gibson RA, Aliani M, House JD. Designer laying hen diets to improve egg fatty acid profile and maintain sensory quality. Food Sci Nutr. 2013;1(4):324-35.

247. Nakamura J, Miwa T, Sasaki H, Shibasaki J, Kaneto H. Effect of straight chain fatty acids on seizures induced by picrotoxin and pentylenetetrazole in mice. J Pharmacobio-dyn. 1990;13(1):76-81.

248. Kouchak M, Handali S. Effects of various penetration enhancers on penetration of aminophylline through shed snake skin. Jundishapur J Nat Pharm Prod. 2014;9(1):24-9.

249. Otuechere CA, Madarikan G, Simisola T, Bankole O, Osho A. Virgin coconut oil protects against liver damage in albino rats challenged with the anti-folate combination, trimethoprim-sulfamethoxazole. J Basic Clin Physiol Pharmacol. 2014;25(2):249-53.

250. Wallace FA, Neely SJ, Miles EA, Calder PC. Dietary fats affect macrophage-mediated cytotoxicity towards tumour cells. Immunol Cell Biol. 2000;78(1):40-8.

251. American Cancer Society. Homepage slider. (2016). Available at: https://www.cancer.gov [November 28th, 2016].

252. Reuter SE, Martin JH. Pharmacokinetics of Cannabis in Cancer Cachexia-Anorexia Syndrome. Clin Pharmacokinet. 2016;55(7):807-12.

253. Volek JS, Kraemer WJ, Bush JA, Incledon T, Boetes M. Testosterone and cortisol in relationship to dietary nutrients and resistance exercise. Journal of applied physiology (Bethesda, Md. : 1985). 82(1):49-54. 1997.

254. Vysakh A, Ratheesh M, Rajmohanan TP, et al. Polyphenolics isolated from virgin coconut oil inhibits adjuvant induced arthritis in rats through antioxidant and anti-inflammatory action. Int Immunopharmacol. 2014;20(1):124-30.

255. Monteiro R, Azevedo I, Calhau C. Modulation of aromatase activity by diet polyphenolic compounds. J Agric Food Chem. 2006;54(10):3535-40.

256. Otuechere CA, Madarikan G, Simisola T, Bankole O, Osho A. Virgin coconut oil protects against liver damage in albino rats challenged with the anti-folate combination, trimethoprim-sulfamethoxazole. J Basic Clin Physiol Pharmacol. 2014;25(2):249-53.

257. Yeap SK, Beh BK, Ali NM, et al. Antistress and antioxidant effects of virgin coconut oil in vivo. Exp Ther Med. 2015;9(1):39-42.

258. Jing H, Wang Z, Chen Y. Effect of oestradiol on mast cell number and histamine level in the mammary glands of rat. Anat Histol Embryol. 2012;41(3):170-6.

259. Yeap SK, Beh BK, Ali NM, et al. Antistress and antioxidant effects of virgin coconut oil in vivo. Exp Ther Med. 2015;9(1):39-42.

260. Sadeghi S, Wallace FA, Calder PC. Dietary lipids modify the cytokine response to bacterial lipopolysaccharide in mice. Immunology. 1999;96(3):404-10.

CHAPTER 9

SODIUM BICARBONATE

SODIUM BICARBONATE, ALSO known as baking soda, is a type of salt that can be found in crystalline rock formations in nature. Bicarbonate, the acid-neutralizing portion of sodium bicarbonate, is naturally produced by the human body and used to buffer excess acidity.[1]

Since one of the metabolic hallmarks of a cancer cell, as first described by Dr. Otto Warburg in 1930,[2] is elevated production of lactic acid,[3-8] which "directly contributes to tumor growth and progression,"[9] it seems reasonable to predict that cancer patients could benefit from additional bicarbonate.

The *fizz* that captured our amazement as children after adding baking soda and vinegar together was sodium bicarbonate rapidly neutralizing the acid and producing carbon dioxide (CO_2) gas as a result. Similarly, once inside the body, bicarbonate is converted into carbon dioxide;[10] so when we're talking about sodium bicarbonate, essentially what we're dealing with is carbon dioxide, which opens the door to some fascinating lines of research.

The relationship between carbon dioxide and life itself is entirely misunderstood by most people in the medical profession and by society as a whole. We've been told that carbon dioxide is a toxic environmental pollutant causing dangerous increases in temperature that threaten the existence of life on earth. However, like many things we're told by politicians and the media, the reality is far different. One of the best ways to learn about carbon dioxide is to examine what happens to various life forms when they are exposed to increased concentrations of it.

THE NAKED MOLE RAT

Found naturally in the hot, arid regions of eastern Africa, the naked mole rat is a type of rodent that lives strictly underground in large colonies. Remarkably, naked mole rats reproduce for their entire lifespans,[12] they don't feel pain after being burnt with acid,[11] their brains can withstand over 30 minutes without oxygen without damage[137] and in their natural habitats, they are immune to cancer.[13] And while the average lifespan for most rats is less than two years,[14,15] the naked mole rat can live an astounding *30 years,*[16,17] making it the longest-lived rodent known.[18]

The exceptional longevity and disease resistance of the naked mole rat have researchers calling it "a true 'supermodel' for aging research and resistance to chronic age-associated diseases."[19] Yet despite decades of research, scientists still haven't been able to determine the reasons behind the mole rat's longevity, even in the most recent studies.[20-22] Perhaps it's because they're searching for a genetic explanation rather than simply examining the naked mole rat's natural environment.

"They live in burrows that are kept closed, so the percentage of oxygen is lower than in the outside air, and the percentage of carbon dioxide ranges from 0.2% to 5%," explains Dr. Raymond Peat.[23] A 2005 study by Israeli scientists investigated the oxygen and carbon dioxide content in burrows of three species of subterranean mole rats and found that maximal CO_2 levels were 6.1% and minimal O_2 levels were 7.2%.[24]

	Carbon dioxide	Oxygen
Air on Earth	0.04%	20.95%
Mole Rat Burrow	6.1%	7.2%

Researchers at the College of Staten Island in New York re-created these environmental conditions in their laboratory and examined its effects on a colony of naked mole rats in 2010. Although they hypothesized the environment would have a negative impact on the activity, memory and social interaction of the rats, what they found was the complete opposite. When the rats were put into an environment of decreased oxygen (hypoxic) and increased carbon dioxide (hypercapnic) they became more social, had significantly improved brain function and their overall movements increased by 76.8%.[25]

THE QUEEN BEE

In honey bee hives, worker bees carefully regulate the concentration of carbon dioxide, which can be as high at 6%.[26] Remarkably, the lifespan of a queen bee is more than 40-times that of a worker bee.[27] So while the queen is in the hive, protected by high concentrations of carbon dioxide, the worker bees are out breathing regular atmospheric air and consuming pollen, which is high in unsaturated fat and produces large amounts of free radicals in the absence of carbon dioxide.

THE LONG-LIVED SIBERIAN BAT

Bats are physiologically the same as mice and as such are destined to live similar lifespans. However, the oldest-surviving bat ever documented is a tiny bat from Siberia that lived more than 41 years in the wild.[28] Researchers measuring the air quality in caves where bats roost have discovered that carbon dioxide concentrations are significantly higher than in the outside air. For example, in Drum Cave, Bungonia, New South Wales, Australia, "the CO2 concentration rises to over 6% in summer when a nursery colony, which contains more than 1000 unidentified bats, is present..."[29]

HUMANS AT HIGH-ALTITUDES

People living at high altitudes have shown a similar resiliency to the long-lived creatures above, including reduced rates of heart disease[30-34] and cancer[35-39] compared to people living at sea level.

What's the link between living at altitude and carbon dioxide? The decrease in oxygen pressure that occurs at elevation means there is less oxygen pressure pushing carbon dioxide out of cells, allowing the body to retain more carbon dioxide – a phenomenon known as *the Haldane effect*.[40,211]

In 2009, a Swiss study involving 1.64 million people found that the benefits of altitude begin at an elevation of about 900m and that for every 1000m increase in elevation, mortality from heart disease decreases by 22% and mortality from stroke decreases by 12%.[34] San Francisco and Philadelphia researchers reported a 12.7% drop in the incidence of lung cancer for every 1000m increase in elevation.[35]

THE PLANT KINGDOM

For over 100 years, carbon dioxide has been used to increase the productivity of greenhouse crops.[41] In 1978, scientists from the University of British Columbia, Canada, found that tomato plants grown in greenhouses with enhanced CO_2 concentrations, "flowered earlier and produced more marketable fruit than those grown in normal air."[42] Peanuts,[43] rice,[44] ginger,[45] and lettuce[46] have also displayed elevated growth performance when cultivated in environments enriched with CO_2, and these growth-enhancing benefits also extend to grasses,[48] trees,[49-51] tobacco,[52] hemp,[53] roses,[54] algae[55,56] and indeed all plant life on earth. Reviews of plant science literature indicate that boosting greenhouse carbon dioxide levels by just 300 parts per million (ppm) will increase plant growth by 30%.[47]

Even better, elevated concentrations of carbon dioxide can increase the nutrient value of food for humans,[46,57-59] while decreasing its nutrient value for insects. By significantly lowering the radio of nitrogen to carbon in plants, nutrient availability for predatory insects is significantly limited. Furthermore, under increased concentrations of CO_2, the production of natural defensive compounds by plants is increased and the growth and survival of pests are adversely affected.[60,61]

Better still, carbon dioxide enrichment reduces the water requirements of plants by enabling them to use water more efficiently;[62] it makes them better able to survive extreme growing conditions like draught,[63] high temperatures,[64] and excess salinity;[65] it makes them more resistant to bacterial and fungal infections;[66] it suppresses invasive plant species;[48] it increases the number of seeds a plant produces;[67] and it also increases the annual life cycle of plants, extending the growing season.[68]

Once food crops have fully-ripened, packaging them in containers with added carbon dioxide can reduce their decay and significantly prolong shelf-life.[69-71]

The extraordinary disease resistance, longevity and myriad of other benefits imparted to animals, humans and plants inhabiting carbon dioxide-enriched environments have shown us the importance of carbon dioxide. And since organisms that don't require oxygen still need carbon dioxide to survive, we can conclude that carbon dioxide is more fundamental to life than oxygen.[72]

A CLOSER LOOK...

- An experiment from 1980 incubated anaerobic bacteria (bacteria that don't use oxygen) into jars containing a range of carbon dioxide concentrations. The study revealed that contrary to established teaching, "Small supplements of CO2 (0.25%) allowed good growth of the majority of anaerobes studied." Furthermore, some anaerobes had a minimum requirement of at least 1% CO2 for survival and an anaerobe called B. melaninogenicus "needed an atmospheric content of 10--40% CO2 for optimal growth."[72]

Many living creatures, from mole rats to bats to bees, even amphibians like frogs, which burrow in the mud to accumulate a surplus of carbon dioxide, inherently understand the essentiality of CO2 and as such have found ways to intensify their exposures to it. Humans, on the other hand, believe that carbon dioxide is an environmental waste gas and have actually altered their behavior to reduce the amount of it in their environment. (Who is smarter - *man or frog?*)

There's one more thing that must be addressed in order to eliminate the phobia surrounding carbon dioxide.

Is CO2 leading humanity towards climate catastrophe?

It is the duty of every human being alive to question everything we are told by those who claim authority over us, especially when the solutions they advance involve us giving them $226 million more in taxes every year,[74] or when we see the media calling us 'genocidal mass murderers' simply for doing so.[73]

Anytime the subject of climate change is discussed in the media, we are presented with the extreme view that elevated CO_2 is moving humanity towards catastrophe and that all scientists agree on this "fact."[209,210] However, when we read the climate science ourselves, we find that not only is there no consensus among scientists, but there is little to no evidence suggesting any reason to be alarmed at all. An extensive review of 539 climate change studies published in peer-reviewed scientific journals between 2004 and 2007 concluded, "Only one paper refers to 'catastrophic' climate change, but without offering evidence."[89]

So while politicians and the media push their unscientific, alarmist perspectives about climate change onto the public in support of their own political and economic interests, scientists, who base their views on empirical evidence, take into account the large and growing body of research showing that carbon dioxide has little or nothing to do with the earth's surface temperature.[75-87] The surge of peer-reviewed studies, analysis and data error discoveries published in recent years have prompted Dr. Ian Wilson and many others to declare that the fear surrounding man-made global warming "bites the dust."[88]

Rather than catastrophe, the rising levels of natural and man-made carbon dioxide in our environment[208] are sparking a revolution of intensified plant growth and abundance that greens the earth and delivers everything needed by humans and all living creatures to thrive with unprecedented levels of health, intelligence, compassion and longevity.

Now that we've solved all of the world's problems, let's find out what sodium bicarbonate can do for a person with cancer and other diseases.

✳ ✳ ✳

SODIUM BICARBONATE VS CANCER

Many people have claimed that baking soda is a 'quack' treatment with no anti-cancer effects; and if this is your opinion, the research on baking soda and cancer may surprise you.

Investigations using sodium bicarbonate to treat cancer cells *in vitro* are limited, yet promising; published in the *World Journal of Pharmacy and Pharmaceutical Sciences* in 2014 by researchers from North Carolina, the study confirmed that sodium bicarbonate can trigger apoptosis in colon cancer cells.[90]

In 2006, Norwegian researchers discovered that an acidic tumor microenvironment promotes metastasis in mice bearing three different types of tumors.[92] Since sodium bicarbonate mixed in drinking water and consumed orally can effectively raise the pH of tumors,[97] researchers from the University of Arizona administered it to tumor-bearing mice to see if cancer metastasis could be prevented. Results confirmed that baking soda "increases tumor pH and inhibits spontaneous metastases" in mice with breast and prostate tumors.[93]

Dr. Robert J. Gillies and his team from the H. Lee Moffitt Cancer Center & Research Institute in Florida examined the relationship between tumor microenvironment pH and the growth and spread of cancer in vivo. Results were published in the journal *Cancer Research* in 2013 and found that oral administration of sodium bicarbonate inhibited the growth and spread of colon and breast tumors. "In every case... the regions of highest tumor invasion corresponded to areas of lowest pH. Tumor invasion did not occur into regions with normal or near-normal extracellular pH," they wrote.[94] In other words, an acidic tumor environment is essential for cancer metastasis and balancing out the pH using sodium bicarbonate can prevent it from occurring.

One of the mechanisms behind the anti-metastatic effect of sodium bicarbonate was discovered by scientists Ian Robey and Lance Nesbit from the University of Arizona in 2013. Their study found that sodium bicarbonate treatment reduced the number of circulating tumor cells in the blood of tumor-bearing mice to less than half.[95]

Dr. Gillies and his team discovered another mechanism behind sodium bicarbonate's anti-cancer effects in 2016. It is well established that excess acidity impedes immune system function[166-168] and that neutralization of acidity with sodium bicarbonate can amplify the immune response.[169,171] After administering sodium bicarbonate to tumor-bearing mice, the researchers observed an influx of immune cells into tumors, which prevented the growth of numerous tumor types.[170]

One shocking and incredibly rare fact about sodium bicarbonate is that oncologists actually administer it to cancer patients before, during and after chemotherapy and radiotherapy to protect them from the extreme toxicity.[90] "If you want to see how fast a person can hit the floor during chemotherapy just forget to mix in the bicarbonate and get out your stopwatch!" exclaimed Dr. Mark Sircus. "Those who survive the deadly treatment known as chemotherapy were likely saved by the sodium bicarbonate, and not the deadly chemotherapy poison pumped into their bodies."[91]

26 terminal cancer patients suffering from severe pain and side effects caused by failed chemotherapy and radiotherapy treatments were administered sodium bicarbonate dissolved in DMSO intravenously by Vietnamese researchers in 2011. Results showed the treatment considerably eased the pain and discomfort of all patients.[96]

SUCCESS STORIES

Vernon Johnson

In 2008, Vernon Johnson was diagnosed with stage 4 prostate cancer that was so advanced it had already metastasized to his bones. Not wanting to subject himself to toxic cancer therapies, Vernon refused all treatments recommended by his doctor and followed the advice of his brother instead. "When Vernon was diagnosed with the disease, I told him to increase the pH in his body because any type of cancer cannot thrive in an alkaline environment," recalled his brother Larry.

Vernon read that a mixture of baking soda and maple syrup was effective for raising pH, but since he didn't have any in his kitchen at the time, he substituted it for molasses and began self-treatment.

After consuming the mixture multiple times a day for 11 days, Vernon received a medical examination from his doctor and the results showed his prostate and bone cancers had disappeared completely. Vernon's success story made headlines in the California newspaper *Valley News* in 2009.[98]

Loredana

Loredana was diagnosed with a breast tumor in 2010. "I took all the tests requested, and it turned out that I needed to get an operation," she explained. Frightened by the prospect of having to undergo chemotherapy and radiotherapy following surgery, Loredana did some research and found that she had the option to receive sodium bicarbonate therapy following surgery instead. "This got me very interested," exclaimed Loredana.

She found a surgeon willing to follow the sodium bicarbonate protocol of Italian doctor Tullio Simoncini and had her tumor surgically removed. Once the tumor was cut from her breast, the area was washed with sodium bicarbonate and she continued repeating the washes according to the protocol. One year and multiple checkups, ultrasounds and a mammogram later, she was completely free of cancer.[99]

Rod Peterson

In June of 2008, Canadian Rod Peterson was diagnosed with a tumor in his right kidney. Two months later, Rod had his kidney surgically removed and about 6 months post-surgery, cancer was found in his lungs. Rod's oncologist explained that he could undergo surgery, chemotherapy or radiation, but none would really work with the type of cancer he had. "Basically, he told me to go home and enjoy the rest of my life. He gave me a card for the psychologist if I needed him and I left the office. I was fairly numb, so to speak."

Not ready to leave his family behind, Rod started doing some research and found the work of Dr. Tullio Simoncini. After finding his theories convincing, Rod flew to Rome to talk with the doctor in person. Impressed with the meeting and excited to begin, Rod underwent treatment for 6 weeks in August of 2009. "After the treatment I was curious. I came back, I had my CT Scans, and you could clearly see, from past scans where the tumors kept constantly growing, all of a sudden they had shrank, some cases in half.

Of course it was very exciting. My oncologist was ecstatic. He started to say 'this only happens with 1% of the population. If this continues, we're going to have to do a write-up on you.'"

Wanting to see his health improve even more, Rod returned for further treatments with Dr. Simoncini in January of 2010. "I went back for treatment with Simoncini. I had a CT Scan to followup with my oncologist, and after two weeks of a second cycle, my tumors *again* had shrunk in half. I continued again with another two weeks of treatment and came back to Canada. In the CT Scan I got when I returned, the tumors were gone; all there was left was scar tissue." After just three cycles of sodium bicarbonate therapy, doctors confirmed Rod Peterson no longer had cancer. "Because of Dr. Tullio Simoncini I have a second chance at life, and I believe everybody should have that. By meeting Dr. Simoncini, I'm still here today and I am very thankful. I thank God for that."[100]

ADDITIONAL HEALTH EFFECTS

Acidosis:

- Sodium bicarbonate cures metabolic acidosis[101]

Antibacterial:

- Sodium bicarbonate inhibits bacterial growth[102,104,105]
- Sodium bicarbonate prevents growth of spoilage microbes on vegetables[106]
- Sodium bicarbonate and hydrogen peroxide have synergistic antimicrobial effects[107]

Antioxidant:

- Sodium bicarbonate "is central to the treatment of many poisonings"[108,114,115]
- Sodium bicarbonate prevents damage caused by herbicide glyphosate,[109] paraquat,[111] amitriptyline,[159] yew berry poisoning[112] and uranium[136]
- Sodium bicarbonate (topically) reduces redness caused by jellyfish sting[110]
- Sodium bicarbonate effectively treats near-fatal flecainide overdose[113]

Antiviral:

- Sodium bicarbonate inhibits calcivirus[103]

Arthritis:

- Sodium bicarbonate and calcium gluconate solution effective for treating osteoarthritis[116]

Bone Health:

- Sodium bicarbonate prevents bone demineralization caused by acidosis[117]

Brain Health:

- Sodium bicarbonate corrects mental status abnormalities (i.e. confusion, slurred speech) caused by acidosis[118]

Chronic Kidney Disease:

- Sodium bicarbonate improves nutritional status and dramatically slows progression of CKD[119,120]
- Sodium bicarbonate preserves kidney function in patients with CKD[117]
- Sodium bicarbonate resolves abnormal heart rate in patients with CKD[121]
- Sodium bicarbonate mouth rinse restores function of taste buds and relieves other symptoms of CKD[122]

Dental Health:

- Sodium bicarbonate toothpaste provides a 'clean mouth feel,'[123] whitens teeth,[124] enhances plaque removal,[126,127] reduces bleeding[128] and provides "statistically significant improvements in gingival health"[128]
- Sodium bicarbonate mouthwash significantly reduces mineral loss from tooth enamel[125,129-132]
- Sodium bicarbonate chewing gum significantly removes dental plaque and reduces gingivitis[133-135]

Detoxification:

- Sodium bicarbonate eliminates uranium from the body[136]

Diabetes:

- Bicarbonate-rich mineral water increases insulin sensitivity in humans[138]
- Sodium bicarbonate treats diabetic acidosis in children[139]

Environmental Remediation:

- Sodium bicarbonate neutralizes high aluminum concentrations in water[141]
- Sodium bicarbonate removes 92% of uranium from contaminated soil samples[142]
- Sodium bicarbonate removes chemical pollutant polychlorinated biphenyl (PCB) from waterways[140]
- "Mixed with sodium bicarbonate, one metric ton of PCB-tainted soil can be cleansed per hour in a rotary reactor."[143]

Exercise:

- Sodium bicarbonate increases back squat repetitions to failure[144]
- Sodium bicarbonate improves 200m swimming time[145]
- Sodium bicarbonate significantly increases punches landed during 4 rounds of boxing[146]
- Sodium bicarbonate improves cycling performance during repeated sprints[147,148]

Farming:

- Sodium bicarbonate fed to black belly barbados lambs for 10 days significantly improves meat quality[149]
- Sodium bicarbonate corrects acidosis and improves hydration in diarrheal calves[150]
- Sodium bicarbonate improves calcium absorption and eggshell quality of laying hens[153]
- Sodium bicarbonate promotes growth, photosynthesis and biochemical composition of marine algae[151,152]

Healing:

- Sodium bicarbonate prevents excessive inflammation and accelerates healing process[154]

- Bicarbonate-calcium-magnesium water improves skin regeneration[155]

Heart Health:

- Sodium bicarbonate restores abnormal heart rate caused by crack cocaine,[156,157] bupropion[160] and diphenhydramine[161]
- Sodium bicarbonate eliminates seizures and heart abnormalities caused by antidepressant overdose[162,163]
- Carbonated water with a meal reduces risk of cardiovascular disease[164,165]

Immune System:

- Sodium bicarbonate enhances immune system[169]
- Sodium bicarbonate promotes antitumor immunity[170,171]

Inflammation:

- Sodium bicarbonate reduces inflammation[154,174]

Lifespan:

- Sodium bicarbonate significantly increases lifespan of mice[172]

Metabolism:

- Sodium bicarbonate stimulates oxidative metabolism[171]
- Sodium bicarbonate substantially decreases tissue calcification[172]

Obesity:

- Sodium bicarbonate and albumin enhance weight loss effects of anti-obesity herb fenugreek[173]

Radiation:

- Sodium bicarbonate prevents painful ulceration of the mouth caused by radiotherapy[174]

Reproduction:

- Bicarbonate "plays critically important roles during virtually the entire process of reproduction in mammals"[175]

- Sodium bicarbonate effective for simulating embryonic environment during in vitro fertilization[176]
- Sodium bicarbonate improves growth of children[202]

Skin:

- Sodium bicarbonate and acetic acid solution (topically) renews natural immune barrier of skin[177]
- Sodium bicarbonate baths dramatically improve psoriasis in humans[178,179]

Sleep:

- Sodium bicarbonate improves sleep quality[180]

Thyroid:

- Sodium bicarbonate improves thyroid function[181]

Tumor Microenvironment:

- Sodium bicarbonate reduces free radicals[182,183]
- Sodium bicarbonate reduces tumor necrosis factor-alpha[184,185]
- Sodium bicarbonate reduces interleukin-1beta[186,187]
- Sodium bicarbonate reduces interleukin-6[186,188]
- Sodium bicarbonate reduces interleukin-8[187,189]
- Sodium bicarbonate reduces nuclear factor kappa-b[189,190]
- Sodium bicarbonate reduces cortisol[191]
- Sodium bicarbonate reduces prolactin[192,193]
- Sodium bicarbonate reduces nitric oxide[194,195]
- Sodium bicarbonate reduces lactic acid[196,197]
- Sodium bicarbonate reduces prostaglandins[198,199]
- Sodium bicarbonate reduces histamine[200]

Other:

- Sodium bicarbonate softens earwax and aids in its removal[201]
- Sodium bicarbonate dissolves uric acid stones[203,204] and bladder stones[205]
- Sodium bicarbonate effective for treating cystic fibrosis[206]
- Sodium bicarbonate decreases mortality in patients treated for acute respiratory failure[207]

- Sodium bicarbonate increases return of spontaneous circulation during CPR[158]

SAFETY

Considering all the benefits of using sodium bicarbonate therapeutically, and especially when compared to orthodox cancer treatments, side effects are few and exceptionally minor. Some participants in exercise performance-related studies reported upset stomachs and/or diarrhea at doses of 300mg/kg, which is about 22.5 grams of sodium bicarbonate for a 75kg (165lb) man or woman. Athletes loading up on baking soda for performance enhancement have been able to resolve this issue by consuming sodium bicarbonate in multiple, split-doses.

Vernon Johnson cured himself of metastasized prostate cancer using sodium bicarbonate and the only side effects he experienced were the occasional nausea, diarrhea and weakness. All in all, the treatment consisted of less than half a box of sodium bicarbonate, costing less than $1, and all of his symptoms went away after the treatment ended - not bad for completely eliminating his cancer.

VERNON JOHNSTON'S BAKING SODA & MOLASSES PROTOCOL

To give people enough confidence to begin self-treatment with baking soda if they choose, it's useful to know the exact protocol used by Vernon Johnson to cure himself of cancer. Vernon's protocol involved a mixture of baking soda, molasses and water over the course of 11 days.

Here's how he did it:

Days 1-4: Vernon began by consuming 1 cup of water containing 1 teaspoon of baking soda and 1 teaspoon of black strap molasses. Vernon consumed this mixture once daily for the first four days. After noting that he felt fine and his pH was 7.0 (saliva) and 7.5 (urine), he decided to increase his dose.

Day 5: On day five, Vernon doubled his dose and began drinking the same solution twice per day. After reading that cancer cells become dormant at a pH of 7 and dead at a pH of 8.0-8.5, his goal was to achieve a saliva and urine pH between 8.0-8.5 and hold it for four or five days. He used pH test strips to measure his pH and emphasized the importance of taking both saliva and urine pH into consideration, since saliva pH can at times be a poor indicator of blood pH.

Day 6: He continued taking two daily doses of his solution and on day six, his pH averaged out to be 7.25. On this day he felt slightly nauseous and his stool had a yellowish tinge.

Day 7: Vernon took 3 teaspoons of baking soda in water with 1 teaspoon of molasses for his first dose. For his second dose he went back down to the 2 teaspoons of baking soda with molasses in water.

Day 8: Hoping to elevate his pH even more, Vernon took two teaspoons of baking soda in water and molasses three times over the course of day 8.

Day 9: He noticed a little diarrhea and felt a bit weak on day 9, but said he "felt oxygen euphoria throughout the day. Like my body was breathing pure oxygen."

Day 10: Vernon had a persistent headache at this point and noticed body sweats at night. He took 4 pH readings over the course of the day and they were all in the mid 8's. He then cut back his dose on this day to a 2 teaspoon sodium bicarbonate solution in molasses and water, twice daily.

Day 11: On the day before returning to his doctor to assess the condition of his cancerous bones, Vernon experienced diarrhea that was slightly yellow. He reduced his dose to 1.5 teaspoons of the baking soda, molasses and water solution and consumed it twice.

"So there you have it. That was my last day before the scan," said Vernon, before emphasizing the importance of consuming baking soda two hours before or two hours after a meal to maintain the stomach acidity necessary for digestion.[91]

REFERENCES:

1. Scialla JJ, Appel LJ, Astor BC, et al. Estimated net endogenous acid production and serum bicarbonate in African Americans with chronic kidney disease. Clin J Am Soc Nephrol. 2011;6(7):1526-32.

2. Semenza GL, Artemov D, Bedi A, et al. 'The metabolism of tumours': 70 years later. Novartis Found Symp. 2001;240:251-60.

3. Gogvadze V, Orrenius S, Zhivotovsky B. Mitochondria in cancer cells: what is so special about them?. Trends Cell Biol. 2008;18(4):165-73.

4. Boag JM, Beesley AH, Firth MJ, et al. Altered glucose metabolism in childhood pre-B acute lymphoblastic leukaemia. Leukemia. 2006;20(10):1731-7.

5. Seyfried TN, Mukherjee P. Targeting energy metabolism in brain cancer: review and hypothesis. Nutr Metab (Lond). 2005;2:30.

6. Ristow M. Oxidative metabolism in cancer growth. Curr Opin Clin Nutr Metab Care. 2006;9(4):339-45.

7. Gatenby RA, Gillies RJ. Why do cancers have high aerobic glycolysis?. Nat Rev Cancer. 2004;4(11):891-9.

8. Tannock IF, Rotin D. Acid pH in tumors and its potential for therapeutic exploitation. Cancer Res. 1989;49(16):4373-84.

9. Dhup S, Dadhich RK, Porporato PE, Sonveaux P. Multiple biological activities of lactic acid in cancer: influences on tumor growth, angiogenesis and metastasis. Curr Pharm Des. 2012;18(10):1319-30.

10. Goto K. A study of the acidosis, blood urea, and plasma chlorides in uranium nephritis in the dog, and of the protective action of sodium bicarbonate. J Exp Med. 1917;25(5):693-719.

11. Smith ES, Omerbašić D, Lechner SG, Anirudhan G, Lapatsina L, Lewin GR. The molecular basis of acid insensitivity in the African naked mole-rat. Science. 2011;334(6062):1557-60.

12. Edrey YH, Park TJ, Kang H, Biney A, Buffenstein R. Endocrine function and neurobiology of the longest-living rodent, the naked mole-rat. Exp Gerontol. 2011;46(2-3):116-23.

13. Liang S, Mele J, Wu Y, Buffenstein R, Hornsby PJ. Resistance to experimental tumorigenesis in cells of a long-lived mammal, the naked mole-rat (Heterocephalus glaber). Aging Cell. 2010;9(4):626-35.

14. Asdell SA, Doornenbal H, Joshi SR, Sperling GA. The effects of sex steroid hormones upon longevity in rats. J Reprod Fertil. 1967;14(1):113-20.

15. Suter P, Luetkemeier H, Zakova N, Christen P, Sachsse K, Hess R. Lifespan studies on male and female mice and rats under SPF-laboratory conditions. Arch Toxicol Suppl. 1979;(2):403-7.

16. Buffenstein R. The naked mole-rat: a new long-living model for human aging research. J Gerontol A Biol Sci Med Sci. 2005;60(11):1369-77.

17. O'connor TP, Lee A, Jarvis JU, Buffenstein R. Prolonged longevity in naked mole-rats: age-related changes in metabolism, body composition and gastrointestinal function. Comp Biochem Physiol, Part A Mol Integr Physiol. 2002;133(3):835-42.

18. Csiszar A, Labinskyy N, Orosz Z, Xiangmin Z, Buffenstein R, Ungvari Z. Vascular aging in the longest-living rodent, the naked mole rat. Am J Physiol Heart Circ Physiol. 2007;293(2):H919-27.

19. Edrey YH, Hanes M, Pinto M, Mele J, Buffenstein R. Successful aging and sustained good health in the naked mole rat: a long-lived mammalian model for biogerontology and biomedical research. ILAR J. 2011;52(1):41-53.

20. Lewis KN, Mele J, Hornsby PJ, Buffenstein R. Stress resistance in the naked mole-rat: the bare essentials - a mini-review. Gerontology. 2012;58(5):453-62.

21. Kim EB, Fang X, Fushan AA, et al. Genome sequencing reveals insights into physiology and longevity of the naked mole rat. Nature. 2011;479(7372):223-7.

22. Lewis KN, Andziak B, Yang T, Buffenstein R. The naked mole-rat response to oxidative stress: just deal with it. Antioxid Redox Signal. 2013;19(12):1388-99.

23. Peat R. *Protective CO2 and aging.* [Online]. Available: http://raypeat.com/articles/articles/co2.shtml. [February 15, 2017].

24. Shams I, Avivi A, Nevo E. Oxygen and carbon dioxide fluctuations in burrows of subterranean blind mole rats indicate tolerance to hypoxic-hypercapnic stresses. Comp Biochem Physiol, Part A Mol Integr Physiol. 2005;142(3):376-82.

25. Berkovits R, Boffa N, Deluca V. The effects of hypercapnic hypoxia on naked mole rat activity levels, memory, and social interaction. 2010. Available: https://macaulay.cuny.edu/eportfolios/newyorkcityonthebrain/files/2010/12/NMR-Poster.pdf [February 15, 2017].

26. Bahreini R, Currie RW. The Potential of Bee-Generated Carbon Dioxide for Control of Varroa Mite (Mesostigmata: Varroidae) in Indoor Overwintering Honey bee (Hymenoptera: Apidae) Colonies. J Econ Entomol. 2015;108(5):2153-67.

27. Remolina SC, Hughes KA. Evolution and mechanisms of long life and high fertility in queen honey bees. Age (Dordr). 2008;30(2-3):177-85.

28. Podlutsky AJ, Khritankov AM, Ovodov ND, Austad SN. A new field record for bat longevity. J Gerontol A Biol Sci Med Sci. 2005;60(11):1366-8.

29. Howarth FG, Stone FD. 1990. Elevated carbon dioxide levels in Bayliss Cave, Australia: implications for the evolution of obligate cave species. Pac Sci 44(3): 207-218.

30. Faeh D, Moser A, Panczak R, et al. Independent at heart: persistent association of altitude with ischaemic heart disease mortality after consideration of climate, topography and built environment. J Epidemiol Community Health. 2016;70(8):798-806.

31. Mortimer EA, Monson RR, Macmahon B. Reduction in mortality from coronary heart disease in men residing at high altitude. N Engl J Med. 1977;296(11):581-5.

32. Voors AW, Johnson WD. Altitude and arteriosclerotic heart disease mortality in white residents of 99 of the 100 largest cities in the United States. J Chronic Dis. 1979;32(1-2):157-62.

33. Burtscher M. Effects of living at higher altitudes on mortality: a narrative review. Aging Dis. 2014;5(4):274-80.

34. Faeh D, Gutzwiller F, Bopp M. Lower mortality from coronary heart disease and stroke at higher altitudes in Switzerland. Circulation. 2009;120(6):495-501.

35. Simeonov KP, Himmelstein DS. Lung cancer incidence decreases with elevation: evidence for oxygen as an inhaled carcinogen. PeerJ. 2015;3:e705.

36. Youk AO, Buchanich JM, Fryzek J, Cunningham M, Marsh GM. An ecological study of cancer mortality rates in high altitude counties of the United States. High Alt Med Biol. 2012;13(2):98-104.

37. Amsel J, Waterbor JW, Oler J, Rosenwaike I, Marshall K. Relationship of site-specific cancer mortality rates to altitude. Carcinogenesis. 1982;3(5):461-5.

38. Weinberg CR, Brown KG, Hoel DG. Altitude, radiation, and mortality from cancer and heart disease. Radiat Res. 1987;112(2):381-90.

39. Hart J. Cancer mortality in six lowest versus six highest elevation jurisdictions in the u.s. Dose Response. 2010;9(1):50-8.

40.	Klocke RA. Mechanism and kinetics of the Haldane effect in human erythrocytes. J Appl Physiol. 1973;35(5):673-81.

41.	Tripp KE, Peet MM, Pharr DM, Willits DH, Nelson PV. CO(2)-Enhanced Yield and Foliar Deformation among Tomato Genotypes in Elevated CO(2) Environments. Plant Physiol. 1991;96(3):713-9.

42.	Hinkleton PR, Joliffe PA. Effects of greenhouse co2 enrichment on the yield and photosynthetic physiology of tomato plants. Can J. Plant Sci. 1977;58:801-817.

43.	Srinivasa rao M, Manimanjari D, Vanaja M, et al. Impact of elevated CO_2 on tobacco caterpillar, Spodoptera litura on peanut, Arachis hypogea. J Insect Sci. 2012;12:103.

44.	Cheng W, Sakai H, Yagi K, Hasegawa T. Interactions of elevated [CO2] and night temperature on rice growth and yield. Agricultural and Forest Meteorology; vol.149, issue 1:51-58.

45.	Ghasemzadeh A, Jaafar HZ. Effect of CO(2) enrichment on synthesis of some primary and secondary metabolites in ginger (Zingiber officinale Roscoe). Int J Mol Sci. 2011;12(2):1101-14.

46.	Becker C, Kläring HP. CO_2 enrichment can produce high red leaf lettuce yield while increasing most flavonoid glycoside and some caffeic acid derivative concentrations. Food Chem. 2016;199:736-45.

47.	Idso SB, Kimball BA, Anderson MG, Mauney JR. Effects of atmospheric CO2 enrichment on plant growth: the interactive role of air temperature. Ag Eco and Envi. 1987; vol 20, issue 1:1-10.

48.	Zelikova TJ, Blumenthal DM, Williams DG, et al. Long-term exposure to elevated CO2 enhances plant community stability by suppressing dominant plant species in a mixed-grass prairie. Proc Natl Acad Sci USA. 2014;111(43):15456-61.

49.	Temperton VM, Grayston SJ, Jackson G, Barton CV, Millard P, Jarvis PG. Effects of elevated carbon dioxide concentration on growth and nitrogen fixation in Alnus glutinosa in a long-term field experiment. Tree Physiol. 2003;23(15):1051-9.

50.	Jach EM, Ceulemans R. Effects of elevated atmospheric co2 on growth and crown structure of scots pine (pinus sylvestris) seedlings after two years of exposure in the field. Tree Physiol. 1999;19(45):289-300.

51.	Bond WJ, Midgley GF. Carbon dioxide and the uneasy interactions of trees and savannah grasses. Philos Trans R Soc Lond, B, Biol Sci. 2012;367(1588):601-12.

52.	Campbell, C. D., Sage, R. F., Kocacinar, F. and Way, D. A. (2005), Estimation of the whole-plant CO_2 compensation point of tobacco *Nicotiana tabacum* L.). Global Change Biology, 11: 1956–1967.

53.	Escondido N. (2014). Cultivation clinic: co2 can increase yields 40%. High Times. [Online]. Available: http://hightimes.com/grow/cultivation-clinic-co2-can-increase-yields-40. [February 15, 2017].

54.	Holley WD, Goldsberry KL. Carbon dioxide increases growth of greenhouse roses. Colorado State University. 1961. Available: https://hortscans.ces.ncsu.edu/uploads/c/a/carbon_d_534d6d760c4ed.pdf [February 15, 2017].

55.	Singh SP, Singh P. Effect of CO2 concentration on algal growth: a review. Renewable and sustainable energy reviews. 2014; 38:172-179.

56.	Roberts DA, De nys R, Paul NA. The effect of CO2 on algal growth in industrial waste water for bioenergy and bioremediation applications. PLoS ONE. 2013;8(11):e81631.

57.	Ghasemzadeh A, Jaafar HZ, Rahmat A. Elevated carbon dioxide increases contents of flavonoids and phenolic compounds, and antioxidant activities in Malaysian young ginger (Zingiber officinale Roscoe.) varieties. Molecules. 2010;15(11):7907-22.

58. Stiling, P. and Cornelissen, T. How does elevated carbon dioxide (CO_2) affect plant–herbivore interactions? A field experiment and meta-analysis of CO_2-mediated changes on plant chemistry and herbivore performance. Global Change Biology, 13: 1823–1842.

59. Penuelas J, Estiarte M, Kimball BA, Idso SB, Pinter jr PJ, Wall GW, Garcia RL, Hansaker DJ, LaMorte RL, Hendrix DL. Variety of responses of plant phenolic concentration to CO2 enrichment. J Exper Bot. 1996;vol. 47, 302: 1463-1467.

60. Papitchaya T, Chen WT, Sripontan Y, Hwang SY. Elevated CO2 concentration promotes tomato plant growth but impairs Spodoptera litura performance. J zoo sci. 2015.

61. Coviella CE, Stipanovic RD, Trumble JT. Plant allocation to defensive compounds: interactions between elevated CO(2) and nitrogen in transgenic cotton plants. J Exp Bot. 2002;53(367):323-31.

62. Prior SA, Runion GB, Marble SC, Rogers HH, Gilliam CH, Torbert HA. A review of elevated atmospheric CO@ effects on plant growth and water relations: implications for horticulture. Hortscience. 2011;46(2).

63. Abdelgawad H, Farfan-vignolo ER, De vos D, Asard H. Elevated CO_2 mitigates drought and temperature-induced oxidative stress differently in grasses and legumes. Plant Sci. 2015;231:1-10.

64. Idso SB, Allen SG, Anderson MG, Kimball BA. Atmospheric CO2 enrichment enhances survival of Azolla at high temperatures. Env & Exp Bot. 1989; 29(3):337-341.

65. Abdelgawad H, Zinta G, Beemster GT, Janssens IA, Asard H. Future Climate CO2 Levels Mitigate Stress Impact on Plants: Increased Defense or Decreased Challenge?. Front Plant Sci. 2016;7:556.

66. Mhamdi A, Noctor G. High CO2 Primes Plant Biotic Stress Defences through Redox-Linked Pathways. Plant Physiol. 2016;172(2):929-942.

67. Hartwell jr AL, Baker JT, Boote KJ. The CO2 fertilization effects: higher carbohydrate production and retention as biomass and seed yield. Available: http://www.fao.org/docrep/w5183e/w5183e06.htm [February 15, 2017].

68. Reyes-fox M, Steltzer H, Trlica MJ, et al. Elevated CO2 further lengthens growing season under warming conditions. Nature. 2014;510(7504):259-62.

69. Choi HJ, Bae YS, Lee JS, Park MH, Kim GJ. Effects of carbon dioxide treatment and modified atmosphere packaging on the quality of long distance transporting "maehyang" strawberries. Ag Sci. 2016; 7:813-821.

70. Ramayya N, Niranjan K, Duncan E. Effects of modified atmosphere packaging on quality of 'Alphonso' Mangoes. J Food Sci Technol. 2012;49(6):721-8.

71. Almenar E, Hernández-muñoz P, Lagarón JM, Catalá R, Gavara R. Controlled atmosphere storage of wild strawberry fruit (Fragaria vesca L.). J Agric Food Chem. 2006;54(1):86-91.

72. Reilly S. The carbon dioxide requirements of anaerobic bacteria. J Med Microbiol. 1980;13(4):573-9.

73. Barrett, J. *CNN host links climate 'deniers' to genocidal mass murderers.* Daily Wire. [Online]. Available: http://www.dailywire.com/news/11152/cnn-correspondent-links-climate-deniers-genocidal-james-barrett. [February 15, 2017].

74. The Canadian Free Press. (2017). *Carbon tax not neutral.* Castanet. [Online]. Available: http://www.castanet.net/news/BC/189019/Carbon-tax-not-neutral. [February 15, 2017].

75. Essex C, McKitrick R, Andresen B. Does a global temperature exist? J. Non-equilibrium Thermo. 2006.

76. Gray, L. J., et al. (2010), Solar influences on climate, Rev. Geophys. 48, RG4001.

77. Camp, C. D., *and* K. K. Tung *(*2007*)*, Surface warming by the solar cycle as revealed by the composite mean difference projection, Geophys. Res. Lett., 34, *L14703*.

78. Schwartz SE. Heat capacity, time constant, and sensitivity of earth's climate system. J. Geo Res. 2007.

79. Tech-know-group. Dozens of unpublished scientific papers open for peer review.

80. Lu QB. Cosmic-ray-driven reaction and greenhouse effect of halogenated molecules: culprits for atmospheric ozone depletion and global climate change. Int. J. Mod. Phys. 2013;27:1350073.

81. Carter RM. Public misperceptions of human-caused climate change: the role of the media. 2006 testimony before the committee on Environment and Public Works. Available: https://www.epw.senate.gov/109th/Carter_Testimony.pdf [February 15, 2017].

82. Tsonis, A. A., K. Swanson, and S. Kravtsov (2007), A new dynamical mechanism for major climate shifts, Geophys. Res. Lett. 34, L13705.

83. Spencer RW. Satellite and climate model evidence against substantial manmade climate change (supercedes "has the climate sensitivity holy grail been found?") 2008.

84. Spencer RW. Global warming as a natural response to cloud changes associated with the pacific decadal oscillation (PDO). 2008.

85. Mackey R. Rhodes fairbridge and the idea that the solar system regulates the earth's climate. J. Ctl Res. 2007;50:955-968.

86. Shan LZ, Xian S. Multi-scale analysis of global temperature changes and trend of a drop in temperature in the next 20 years. Atmos. Phys. 2007; 95:115.

87. Manuel OK. Earth's heat source – the sun. Energy & Environment. 2009; 20:131-144.

88. Caruba, A. (2007). *The year the global warming hoax died.* Canada Free Press. [Online]. Available: http://canadafreepress.com/2007/caruba090307.htm. [February 15, 2017].

89. Schulte M-K. Scientific consensus on climate change? Energy & Environment. 2008; 19(2).

90. Al-Achi A, Meduri RT. An in vitro study of modulatory effects of sodium bicarbonate on human colon adenocarcinoma cell (caco-2). World J. Phar. & Phar. Sci. 2014;3(3):228-244.

91. Sircus, M. 2014. Sodium Bicarbonate: Nature's Unique First Aid Remedy. *Square One.* 224 pps.

92. Rofstad EK, Mathiesen B, Kindem K, Galappathi K. Acidic extracellular pH promotes experimental metastasis of human melanoma cells in athymic nude mice. Cancer Res. 2006;66(13):6699-707.

93. Robey IF, Baggett BK, Kirkpatrick ND, et al. Bicarbonate increases tumor pH and inhibits spontaneous metastases. Cancer Res. 2009;69(6):2260-8.

94. Estrella V, Chen T, Lloyd M, et al. Acidity generated by the tumor microenvironment drives local invasion. Cancer Res. 2013;73(5):1524-35.

95. Robey IF, Nesbit LA. Investigating mechanisms of alkalinization for reducing primary breast tumor invasion. Biomed Res Int. 2013;2013:485196.

96. Hoang BX, Tran DM, Tran HQ, et al. Dimethyl sulfoxide and sodium bicarbonate in the treatment of refractory cancer pain. J Pain Palliat Care Pharmacother. 2011;25(1):19-24.

97. Raghunand N, He X, Van sluis R, et al. Enhancement of chemotherapy by manipulation of tumour pH. Br J Cancer. 1999;80(7):1005-11.

98. Fassa, P. (2009). *Bicarbonate of soda used to cure stage four prostate cancer.* Natural News. [Online]. Available: http://www.naturalnews.com/027481_prostate_cancer_baking_soda.html. [February 15, 2017].

99. Loredana. seoleoINT. (2012). Breast cancer treatment with sodium bicarbonate. Available: https://www.youtube.com/watch?v=7fAK-56WCDg. [February 15, 2017].

100. Peterson R. seoleoINT. (2012). Dr. Simoncini – patient kidney cancer RCC. Available: https://www.youtube.com/watch?v=KGa3zhquQEk. [February 15, 2017].

101. Brunkhorst R. [Mineral and bone disorder in chronic kidney disease : Critical appraisal of pharmacotherapy]. Internist (Berl). 2014;55(3):334-9.

102. Wolinsky LE, Lott T. Effects of the inorganic salts sodium chloride, sodium bicarbonate, and magnesium sulfate upon the growth and motility of Treponema vincentii. J Periodontol. 1986;57(3):172-5.

103. Malik YS, Goyal SM. Virucidal efficacy of sodium bicarbonate on a food contact surface against feline calicivirus, a norovirus surrogate. Int J Food Microbiol. 2006;109(1-2):160-3.

104. Newbrun E. The use of sodium bicarbonate in oral hygiene products and practice. Compend Contin Educ Dent Suppl. 1997;18(21):S2-7.

105. Drake DR, Vargas K, Cardenzana A, Srikantha R. Enhanced bactericidal activity of Arm and Hammer Dental Care. Am J Dent. 1995;8(6):308-12.

106. Pinto L, Ippolito A, Baruzzi F. Control of spoiler Pseudomonas spp. on fresh cut vegetables by neutral electrolyzed water. Food Microbiol. 2015;50:102-8.

107. Miyasaki KT, Genco RJ, Wilson ME. Antimicrobial properties of hydrogen peroxide and sodium bicarbonate individually and in combination against selected oral, gram-negative, facultative bacteria. J Dent Res. 1986;65(9):1142-8.

108. Neavyn MJ, Boyer EW, Bird SB, Babu KM. Sodium acetate as a replacement for sodium bicarbonate in medical toxicology: a review. J Med Toxicol. 2013;9(3):250-4.

109. Bando H, Murao Y, Aoyagi U, Hirakawa A, Iwase M, Nakatani T. [Extreme hyperkalemia in a patient with a new glyphosate potassium herbicide poisoning: report of a case]. Chudoku Kenkyu. 2010;23(3):246-9.

110. Declerck MP, Bailey Y, Craig D, et al. Efficacy of Topical Treatments for Chrysaora chinensis Species: A Human Model in Comparison with an In Vitro Model. Wilderness Environ Med. 2016;27(1):25-38.

111. Ren A, Ren S, Jian X, Zhang Q. [The prevention and therapeutics effect of sodium bicarbonate with gastric lavage, atomization inhalation and intravenous injection on the patients with paraquat poisoning and pulmonary fibrosis induced by paraquat poisoning]. Zhonghua Lao Dong Wei Sheng Zhi Ye Bing Za Zhi. 2015;33(9):693-4.

112. Pierog J, Kane B, Kane K, Donovan JW. Management of isolated yew berry toxicity with sodium bicarbonate: a case report in treatment efficacy. J Med Toxicol. 2009;5(2):84-9.

113. Jang DH, Hoffman RS, Nelson LS. A case of near-fatal flecainide overdose in a neonate successfully treated with sodium bicarbonate. J Emerg Med. 2013;44(4):781-3.

114. Zhao B, Yang L, Xiao L, et al. [The influence of sodium bicarbonate combined with ulinastatin on cholinesterase activity for patients with acute phoxim pesticide poisoning]. Zhonghua Lao Dong Wei Sheng Zhi Ye Bing Za Zhi. 2016;34(1):53-5.

115. Stefanovic D, Antonijevic B, Bokonjic D, Stojiljkovic MP, Milovanovic ZA, Nedeljkovic M. Effect of sodium bicarbonate in rats acutely poisoned with dichlorvos. Basic Clin Pharmacol Toxicol. 2006;98(2):173-80.

116. García-padilla S, Duarte-vázquez MA, Gonzalez-romero KE, Caamaño Mdel C, Rosado JL. Effectiveness of intra-articular injections of sodium bicarbonate and calcium gluconate in the treatment of osteoarthritis of the knee: a randomized double-blind clinical trial. BMC Musculoskelet Disord. 2015;16:114.

117. Raphael KL. Approach to the Treatment of Chronic Metabolic Acidosis in CKD. Am J Kidney Dis. 2016;67(4):696-702.

118. Bakhru MR, Kumar A, Aneja A. A 58-year-old woman with mental status changes. Cleve Clin J Med. 2007;74(6):457-62.

119. De brito-ashurst I, Varagunam M, Raftery MJ, Yaqoob MM. Bicarbonate supplementation slows progression of CKD and improves nutritional status. J Am Soc Nephrol. 2009;20(9):2075-84.

120. Jeong J, Kwon SK, Kim HY. Effect of bicarbonate supplementation on renal function and nutritional indices in predialysis advanced chronic kidney disease. Electrolyte Blood Press. 2014;12(2):80-7.

121. Roumelioti ME, Ranpuria R, Hall M, et al. Abnormal nocturnal heart rate variability response among chronic kidney disease and dialysis patients during wakefulness and sleep. Nephrol Dial Transplant. 2010;25(11):3733-41.

122. Manley KJ. Will mouth wash solutions of water, salt, sodiumbicarbonate or citric acid improve upper gastrointestinal symptoms in chronic kidney disease. Nephrology (Carlton). 2017;22(3):213-219.

123. Ash A, Wilde PJ, Bradshaw DJ, King SP, Pratten JR. Structural modifications of the salivary conditioning film upon exposure to sodium bicarbonate: implications for oral lubrication and mouthfeel. Soft Matter. 2016;12(10):2794-801.

124. Ghassemi A, Hooper W, Vorwerk L, Domke T, Desciscio P, Nathoo S. Effectiveness of a new dentifrice with baking soda and peroxide in removing extrinsic stain and whitening teeth. J Clin Dent. 2012;23(3):86-91.

125. Charig A, Winston A, Flickinger M. Enamel mineralization by calcium-containing-bicarbonate toothpastes: assessment by various techniques. Compend Contin Educ Dent. 2004;25(9 Suppl 1):14-24.

126. Putt MS, Milleman KR, Ghassemi A, et al. Enhancement of plaque removal efficacy by tooth brushing with baking soda dentifrices: results of five clinical studies. J Clin Dent. 2008;19(4):111-9.

127. Ghassemi A, Vorwerk LM, Hooper WJ, Putt MS, Milleman KR. A four-week clinical study to evaluate and compare the effectiveness of a baking soda dentifrice and an antimicrobial dentifrice in reducing plaque. J Clin Dent. 2008;19(4):120-6.

128. Lomax A, Patel S, Wang N, Kakar K, Kakar A, Bosma ML. A randomized controlled trial evaluating the efficacy of a 67% sodium bicarbonate toothpaste on gingivitis. Int J Dent Hyg. 2016.

129. Messias DC, Turssi CP, Hara AT, Serra MC. Sodium bicarbonate solution as an anti-erosive agent against simulated endogenous erosion. Eur J Oral Sci. 2010;118(4):385-8.

130. Kashket S, Yaskell T. Effects of a high-bicarbonate dentifrice on intraoral demineralization. Compend Contin Educ Dent Suppl. 1997;18(21):S11-6.

131. Turssi CP, Vianna LM, Hara AT, Do amaral FL, França FM, Basting RT. Counteractive effect of antacid suspensions on intrinsic dental erosion. Eur J Oral Sci. 2012;120(4):349-52.

132. Alves Mdo S, Mantilla TF, Bridi EC, et al. Rinsing with antacid suspension reduces hydrochloric acid-induced erosion. Arch Oral Biol. 2016;61:66-70.

133. Kleber CJ, Putt MS, Milleman JL, Davidson KR, Proskin HM. An evaluation of sodium bicarbonate chewing gum in reducing dental plaque and gingivitis in conjunction with regular toothbrushing. Compend Contin Educ Dent. 2001;22(7A):4-12.

134. Kleber CJ, Davidson KR, Rhoades ML. An evaluation of sodium bicarbonate chewing gum as a supplement to toothbrushing for removal of dental plaque from children's teeth. Compend Contin Educ Dent. 2001;22(7A):36-42.

135. Sharma NC, Galustians JH, Qaqish JG. An evaluation of a commercial chewing gum in combination with normal toothbrushing for reducing dental plaque and gingivitis. Compend Contin Educ Dent. 2001;22(7A):13-7.

136. Ohmachi Y, Imamura T, Ikeda M, et al. Sodium bicarbonate protects uranium-induced acute nephrotoxicity through uranium-decorporation by urinary alkalinization in rats. J Toxicol Pathol. 2015;28(2):65-71.

137. Larson J, Park TJ. Extreme hypoxia tolerance of naked mole-rat brain. Neuroreport. 2009;20(18):1634-7.

138. Schoppen S, Sánchez-muniz FJ, Pérez-granados M, et al. Does bicarbonated mineral water rich in sodium change insulin sensitivity of postmenopausal women?. Nutr Hosp. 2007;22(5):538-44.

139. Reddy CM, Orti E. Insulin and sodium bicarbonate treatment in diabetic ketoacidosis in children. J Natl Med Assoc. 1977;69(5):355-7.

140. Yan T, Lapara TM, Novak PJ. The effect of varying levels of sodium bicarbonate on polychlorinated biphenyl dechlorination in Hudson River sediment cultures. Environ Microbiol. 2006;8(7):1288-98.

141. Neal C, Rowland P, Neal M, et al. Aluminium in UK rivers: a need for integrated research related to kinetic factors, colloidal transport, carbon and habitat. J Environ Monit. 2011;13(8):2153-64.

142. Phillips, E.J.P., Landa, E.R. & Lovley, D.R. Remediation of uranium contaminated soils with bicarbonate extraction and microbial U(VI) reduction. Journal of Industrial Microbiology (1995) 14: 203.

143. Popular Science. Recipe for PCB destruction: Add baking soda. August 1993;25.

144. Duncan MJ, Weldon A, Price MJ. The effect of sodium bicarbonate ingestion on back squat and bench press exercise to failure. J Strength Cond Res. 2014;28(5):1358-66.

145. Lindh AM, Peyrebrune MC, Ingham SA, Bailey DM, Folland JP. Sodium bicarbonate improves swimming performance. Int J Sports Med. 2008;29(6):519-23.

146. Siegler JC, Hirscher K. Sodium bicarbonate ingestion and boxing performance. J Strength Cond Res. 2010;24(1):103-8.

147. Miller P, Robinson AL, Sparks SA, Bridge CA, Bentley DJ, Mcnaughton LR. The Effects of Novel Ingestion of Sodium Bicarbonate on Repeated Sprint Ability. J Strength Cond Res. 2016;30(2):561-8.

148. Egger F, Meyer T, Such U, Hecksteden A. Effects of Sodium Bicarbonate on High-Intensity Endurance Performance in Cyclists: A Double-Blind, Randomized Cross-Over Trial. PLoS ONE. 2014;9(12):e114729.

149. Jallow DB, Hsia LC. Effect of sodium bicarbonate supplementation on carcass characteristics of lambs fed concentrate diets at different ambient temperature levels. Asian-australas J Anim Sci. 2014;27(8):1098-103.

150. Booth AJ, Naylor JM. Correction of metabolic acidosis in diarrheal calves by oral administration of electrolyte solutions with or without bicarbonate. J Am Vet Med Assoc. 1987;191(1):62-8.

151. Zhou W, Sui Z, Wang J, et al. Effects of sodium bicarbonate concentration on growth, photosynthesis, and carbonic anhydrase activity of macroalgae Gracilariopsis lemaneiformis, Gracilaria vermiculophylla, and Gracilaria chouae (Gracilariales, Rhodophyta). Photosyn Res. 2016;128(3):259-70.

152. Sarat chandra T, Deepak RS, Maneesh kumar M, et al. Evaluation of indigenous fresh water microalga Scenedesmus obtusus for feed and fuel applications: Effect of carbon dioxide, light and nutrient sources on growth and biochemical characteristics. Bioresour Technol. 2016;207:430-9.

153. Jiang MJ, Zhao JP, Jiao HC, Wang XJ, Zhang Q, Lin H. Dietary supplementation with sodium bicarbonate improves calcium absorption and eggshell quality of laying hens during peak production. Br Poult Sci. 2015;56(6):740-7.

154. Yuan Z, Zhao J, Chen Y, Yang Z, Cui W, Zheng Q. Regulating inflammation using acid-responsive electrospun fibrous scaffolds for skin scarless healing. Mediators Inflamm. 2014;2014:858045.

155. Faga A, Nicoletti G, Gregotti C, Finotti V, Nitto A, Gioglio L. Effects of thermal water on skin regeneration. Int J Mol Med. 2012;29(5):732-40.

156. Erzouki HK, Baum I, Goldberg SR, Schindler CW. Comparison of the effects of cocaine and its metabolites on cardiovascular function in anesthetized rats. J Cardiovasc Pharmacol. 1993;22(4):557-63.

157.   Miranda CH, Pazin-filho A. Crack cocaine-induced cardiac conduction abnormalities are reversed by sodium bicarbonate infusion. Case Rep Med. 2013;2013:396401.

158.   Kim J, Kim K, Park J, et al. Sodium bicarbonate administration during ongoing resuscitation is associated with increased return of spontaneous circulation. Am J Emerg Med. 2016;34(2):225-9.

159.   Paksu MS, Zengin H, Ilkaya F, et al. Can empirical hypertonic saline or sodium bicarbonate treatment prevent the development of cardiotoxicity during serious amitriptyline poisoning? Experimental research. Cardiovasc J Afr. 2015;26(3):134-9.

160.   Franco V. Wide complex tachycardia after bupropion overdose. Am J Emerg Med. 2015;33(10):1540.e3-5.

161.   Jang DH, Manini AF, Trueger NS, et al. Status epilepticus and wide-complex tachycardia secondary to diphenhydramine overdose. Clin Toxicol (Phila). 2010;48(9):945-8.

162.   Hodes D. Sodium bicarbonate and hyperventilation in treating an infant with severe overdose of tricyclic antidepressant. Br Med J (Clin Res Ed). 1984;288(6433):1800-1.

163.   Clement A, Raney JJ, Wasserman GS, Lowry JA. Chronic amitriptyline overdose in a child. Clin Toxicol (Phila). 2012;50(5):431-4.

164.   Toxqui L, Pérez-granados AM, Blanco-rojo R, Vaquero MP. A sodium-bicarbonated mineral water reduces gallbladder emptying and postprandial lipaemia: a randomised four-way crossover study. Eur J Nutr. 2012;51(5):607-14.

165.   Pérez-granados AM, Navas-carretero S, Schoppen S, Vaquero MP. Reduction in cardiovascular risk by sodium-bicarbonated mineral water in moderately hypercholesterolemic young adults. J Nutr Biochem. 2010;21(10):948-53.

166.   Riemann A, Wußling H, Loppnow H, Fu H, Reime S, Thews O. Acidosis differently modulates the inflammatory program in monocytes and macrophages. Biochim Biophys Acta. 2016;1862(1):72-81.

167.   Langfelder A, Okonji E, Deca D, Wei WC, Glitsch MD. Extracellular acidosis impairs P2Y receptor-mediated Ca(2+) signalling and migration of microglia. Cell Calcium. 2015;57(4):247-56.

168.   Shields EJ, Lam CJ, Cox AR, et al. Extreme Beta-Cell Deficiency in Pancreata of Dogs with Canine Diabetes. PLoS ONE. 2015;10(6):e0129809.

169.   Ori Y, Zingerman B, Bergman M, Bessler H, Salman H. The effect of sodium bicarbonate on cytokine secretion in CKD patients with metabolic acidosis. Biomed Pharmacother. 2015;71:98-101.

170.   Pilon-thomas S, Kodumudi KN, El-kenawi AE, et al. Neutralization of Tumor Acidity Improves Antitumor Responses to Immunotherapy. Cancer Res. 2016;76(6):1381-90.

171.   Singer RB, Deering RC, Clark JK. The acute effects in man of a rapid intravenous infusion of hypertonic sodium bicarbonate solution. II. Changes in respiration and output of carbon dioxide. J Clin Invest. 1956;35(2):245-53.

172.   Leibrock CB, Voelkl J, Kohlhofer U, Quintanilla-martinez L, Kuro-o M, Lang F. Bicarbonate-sensitive calcification and lifespan of klotho-deficient mice. Am J Physiol Renal Physiol. 2016;310(1):F102-8.

173.   Dakam W, Shang J, Agbor G, Oben J. Effects of sodium bicarbonate and albumin on the in vitro water-holding capacity and some physiological properties of Trigonella foenum graecum L. galactomannan in rats. J Med Food. 2007;10(1):169-74.

174.   Mallick S, Benson R, Rath GK. Radiation induced oral mucositis: a review of current literature on prevention and management. Eur Arch Otorhinolaryngol. 2016;273(9):2285-93.

175.   Liu Y, Wang DK, Chen LM. The physiology of bicarbonate transporters in mammalian reproduction. Biol Reprod. 2012;86(4):99.

176.   Quinn P, Cooke S. Equivalency of culture media for human in vitro fertilization formulated to have the same pH under an atmosphere containing 5% or 6% carbon dioxide. Fertil Steril. 2004;81(6):1502-6.

177.   Kurgan DM, Kokoruz MV, Kurgan MG, Novak VL. [The Dynamics of Immunological Results of Patients with T-Cell Skin Lymphomas and Psoriasis by The Therapy of Activation Mechanisms Sanogenesis Methods]. Lik Sprava. 2015;(3-4):31-8.

178.   Samsoen M. Sodium bicarbonate bath and psoriasis. First open study in a single center. 2007. Available: https://www.researchgate.net/publication/290279882_Sodium_bicarbonate_bath_and_psoriasis_First _open_study_in_a_single_center. [February 15, 2017].

179.   Verdolini R, Bugatti L, Filosa G, Mannello B, Lawlor F, Cerio RR. Old fashioned sodium bicarbonate baths for the treatment of psoriasis in the era of futuristic biologics: an old ally to be rescued. J Dermatolog Treat. 2005;16(1):26-30.

180.   Afsar B, Elsurer R. Association between serum bicarbonate and pH with depression, cognition and sleep quality in hemodialysis patients. Ren Fail. 2015;37(6):957-60.

181.   Disthabanchong S, Treeruttanawanich A. Oral sodium bicarbonate improves thyroid function in predialysis chronic kidney disease. Am J Nephrol. 2010;32(6):549-56.

182.   Brown JR, Block CA, Malenka DJ, O'Connor GT, Schoolwerth AC, Thompson CA. Sodium bicarbonate plus n-acetylcysteine prophylaxis : A meta-analysis. JACC. 2009;2(11):1116-1124.

183.   Merten GJ, Burgess WP, Rittase RA, Kennedy TP. Prevention of contrast-induced nephropathy with sodium bicarbonate: an evidence-based protocol. Crit Pathw Cardiol. 2004;3(3):138-43.

184.   Montalto AS, Bitto A, Irrera N, et al. CO2 pneumoperitoneum impact on early liver and lung cytokine expression in a rat model of abdominal sepsis. Surg Endosc. 2012;26(4):984-9.

185.   De smet HR, Bersten AD, Barr HA, Doyle IR. Hypercapnic acidosis modulates inflammation, lung mechanics, and edema in the isolated perfused lung. J Crit Care. 2007;22(4):305-13.

186.   Kimura D, Totapally BR, Raszynski A, Ramachandran C, Torbati D. The effects of CO2 on cytokine concentrations in endotoxin-stimulated human whole blood. Crit Care Med. 2008;36(10):2823-7.

187.   Gao W, Liu DD, Li D, Cui GX. Effect of Therapeutic Hypercapnia on Inflammatory Responses to One-lung Ventilation in Lobectomy Patients. Anesthesiology. 2015;122(6):1235-52.

188.   Cooker LA, Luneburg P, Holmes CJ, Jones S, Topley N. Interleukin-6 levels decrease in effluent from patients dialyzed with bicarbonate/lactate-based peritoneal dialysis solutions. Perit Dial Int. 2001;21 Suppl 3:S102-7.

189.   Takeshita K, Suzuki Y, Nishio K, et al. Hypercapnic acidosis attenuates endotoxin-induced nuclear factor-[kappa]B activation. Am J Respir Cell Mol Biol. 2003;29(1):124-32.

190.   Tawfik amin A, Shiraishi N, Ninomiya S, Tajima M, Inomata M, Kitano S. Activation of nuclear factor kappa B and induction of migration inhibitory factor in tumors by surgical stress of laparotomy versus carbon dioxide pneumoperitoneum: an animal experiment. Surg Endosc. 2010;24(3):578-83.

191.   Maurer M, Riesen W, Muser J, Hulter HN, Krapf R. Neutralization of Western diet inhibits bone resorption independently of K intake and reduces cortisol secretion in humans. Am J Physiol Renal Physiol. 2003;284(1):F32-40.

192.   Rojas vega S, Strüder HK, Wahrmann BV, Bloch W, Hollmann W. Bicarbonate reduces serum prolactin increase induced by exercise to exhaustion. Med Sci Sports Exerc. 2006;38(4):675-80.

193.   Strüder HK, Hollmann W, Donike M, Platen P, Weber K. Effect of O2 availability on neuroendocrine variables at rest and during exercise: O2 breathing increases plasma prolactin. Eur J Appl Physiol Occup Physiol. 1996;74(5):443-9.

194.   Capellini VK, Restini CB, Bendhack LM, Evora PR, Celotto AC. The effect of extracellular pH changes on intracellular pH and nitric oxide concentration in endothelial and smooth muscle cells from rat aorta. PLoS ONE. 2013;8(5):e62887.

195.   Pedoto A, Caruso JE, Nandi J, et al. Acidosis stimulates nitric oxide production and lung damage in rats. Am J Respir Crit Care Med. 1999;159(2):397-402.

196.   Sabatini S, Kurtzman NA. Bicarbonate therapy in severe metabolic acidosis. J Am Soc Nephrol. 2009;20(4):692-5.

197.   Malov IuS, Kulikov AN. [Bicarbonate deficiency and duodenal peptic ulcer]. Ter Arkh. 1998;70(2):28-32.

198. Haylor J, Toner JM, Jackson PR, Ramsay LE, Lote CJ. Is the urinary excretion of prostaglandin E in man dependent on urine pH?. Clin Sci. 1985;68(4):475-7.

199. Pepelko WE. The effect of cortisol upon lipolysis during cypercapnia and after beta-andrenergic blockade. Anat & Phys Pharmac. 1971. Available: http://oai.dtic.mil/oai/oai?verb=getRecord&metadataPrefix=html&identifier=AD0731124. [February 15, 2017].

200. Strider JW, Masterson CG, Durham PL. Treatment of mast cells with carbon dioxide suppresses degranulation via a novel mechanism involving repression of increased intracellular calcium levels. Allergy. 2011;66(3):341-50.

201. Soy FK, Ozbay C, Kulduk E, Dundar R, Yazıcı H, Sakarya EU. A new approach for cerumenolytic treatment in children: In vivo and in vitro study. Int J Pediatr Otorhinolaryngol. 2015;79(7):1096-100.

202. Sharma AP, Singh RN, Yang C, Sharma RK, Kapoor R, Filler G. Bicarbonate therapy improves growth in children with incomplete distal renal tubular acidosis. Pediatr Nephrol. 2009;24(8):1509-16.

203. Hess B. Metabolic syndrome, obesity and kidney stones. Arab J Urol. 2012;10(3):258-64.

204. Cicerello E, Merlo F, Maccatrozzo L. Urinary alkalization for the treatment of uric acid nephrolithiasis. Arch Ital Urol Androl. 2010;82(3):145-8.

205. Vivien P, Allannic H, Turpin J, Prunier P, Leborgne P, Loussouarn J. [A case of voluminous cystine lithiasis cured with high doses of sodium bicarbonate]. Therapie. 1971;26(1):121-7.

206. Stigliani M, Manniello MD, Zegarra-moran O, et al. Rheological Properties of Cystic Fibrosis Bronchial Secretion and in Vitro Drug Permeation Study: The Effect of Sodium Bicarbonate. J Aerosol Med Pulm Drug Deliv. 2016;29(4):337-45.

207. Piñero-zapata M, Cinesi-gómez C, Luna-maldonado A. [Mortality in patients with acute respiratory failure on chronic treatment with benzodiazepines]. Enferm Clin. 2013;23(3):89-95.

208. National Science Foundation. (2004). "Impact Of Earth's Rising Atmospheric Carbon Dioxide Found In World Oceans." ScienceDaily. [Online].Available: www.sciencedaily.com/releases/2004/07/040719092807.htm.[April 2,2017].

209. Poberezhskaya M. Media coverage of climate change in Russia: Governmental bias and climate science. Public understanding of science. 2014;24(1).

210. Shapiro JM. Special interests and the media: Theory and an application to climate change. J. Public Econ. 2016;144:91-108.

211. Abdo WF, Heunks LM. Oxygen-induced hypercapnia in COPD: myths and facts. Crit Care. 2012;16(5):323.

CHAPTER 10

UNRAVELING THE MYSTERIES OF CANCER

THE OFFICIAL POSITION of the cancer establishment is that "cancer is a genetic disease,"[1] whereby a specific set of gene mutations cause a single cell to turn irreversibly cancerous and multiply out-of-control, until enough of its mutant clones collectively form a tumor that strives to kill the host.

If this theory is correct, it means that cancer cells are like parasites that must be eradicated at all costs; even if patients are injured or nearly killed in the process. It also means that nothing in our environment or the way we live our lives have any bearing whatsoever on whether or not we develop cancer. And in this paradigm, since there's nothing we can do to prevent cancer from arising or stop it from progressing, if we happen to be one of the 'unlucky' ones who are diagnosed with the disease, we must depend on people more sophisticated than us for answers.

However, if cancer truly were a genetic disease then you'd think the vast sums of money spent on genetic cancer research over the past 50 years would have rendered us at least *some* progress.

It makes you wonder - *maybe researchers have been looking in the wrong place for answers*?

QUESTIONING THE GENETIC THEORY OF CANCER

In search of another paradigm that could adequately explain the underlying cause of cancer and why the war on cancer has been such a failure, I stumbled upon a series of fascinating studies whose conclusions completely contradicted the genetic theory of cancer. If cancer is a disease of genetic origin, then none of the following observations would have occurred.

CLONED MICE FROM TUMOR CELL DNA

Researchers from St. Jude Children's Research Hospital in Memphis, Tennessee, cloned a mouse using DNA derived from a mouse brain tumor cell in 2003. Published in the journal *Cancer Research*, the study found that the development of the cloned mouse occurred normally without cancer formation.[11]

FROG EGG TUMOR TRANSPLANTS

In 1969, a group of researchers transplanted frog tumor cells into frog eggs and found that despite the mutant cancer DNA contained within the transplanted tumor cells, from within the eggs emerged healthy, swimming tadpoles - demonstrating once again that mutated cancer DNA can direct normal development.[10]

CELL CYTOPLASM-SWAPPED 'CYBRIDS'

Since the 1970's, scientists have been experimenting with swapping normal cell cytoplasms (containing the energy-producing mitochondria, *not* DNA) with cancer cell cytoplasms and vice versa. They call the resultant cells 'cybrids.' When scientists transplanted normal cell cytoplasms into cancer cells (containing mutated DNA), the cancer cells transformed back into normal cells,[2-8] and when cancer cell cytoplasms were transplanted into normal cells (containing normal DNA), the cells turned into cancer cells.[9] These findings show that mutant cancer DNA doesn't cause cancer and that normal DNA doesn't prevent cancer; the cytoplasm seems to dictate carcinogenesis.

GENETIC THEORY UNLIKELY

Taken together, it appears that DNA has little (and perhaps nothing) to do with a cell becoming cancerous. Harry Rubin, Professor Emeritus of Cell and Developmental Biology from the University of California demonstrated in 2006 that cells can have hundreds of mutations and still behave normally within the organism.[12]

Another apparent flaw in the genetic theory is the claim that cancer cells are irreversible. There are hoards of studies in which scientists have observed cancer cells transform back into normal cells.[2-8,10,11,13-17,481-493,868] "...our data suggest quite strongly that nonmalignant tumor populations can be converted to a more malignant phenotype without additional mutations taking place and, conversely, malignant populations can be downregulated to a nontumorigenic phenotype," wrote researchers from Ohio State University in 1995.[17] But if cancer cells can revert back into normal cells, how can the cancer establishment justify carving out tumors, scorching patients with radiation and poisoning them with chemotherapy? They can't... and so their only option - if they wish to remain in business - is to pretend this evidence doesn't exist.

Despite the many experiments profoundly challenging the genetic theory of cancer, medical doctors are not presented these controversies in medical school and are instead taught the genetic theory as if it were fact, which is unfortunate because as the American Nobel Prize-winning virologist Peyton Rous said in 1959, "the somatic mutation theory acts like a tranquilizer on those who believe in it."[18]

What better way to resolve the controversies surrounding cancer's elusive origins than with the biggest and most comprehensive scientific investigation ever conducted on the genetics of cancer?

THE CANCER GENOME ATLAS PROJECT

In 2005, the National Cancer Institute launched a giant multi-national initiative called *The Cancer Genome Atlas Project* (TCGAP). The goal of the project was to expand human understanding of cancer genetics and to pinpoint a common sequence of genetic mutations that drive carcinogenesis so that new drugs targeting each mutation could be developed.[19] If there ever were a project that could finally either prove or disprove cancer as a genetic disease, this billion-dollar medical behemoth - spanning more than a decade - is it.[20] As you can imagine, the debut of the project spurred enormous excitement and hope among its many participants and supporters.

One of the greatest successes of the project, still underway, has been the accelerated speed at which scientists can fully sequence the genetic code of a cell. Each cell in our bodies is said to contain around 25,000 genes,[21] and using state-of-the-art technology scientists are now able to churn out the entire genomic sequence of cells with lightning speed. To date, TCGAP has compiled data from more than 10,000 tissue samples from over 30 types of cancer,[22] but to the surprise of many, the results have been vastly disappointing.

Looking at cancer cells from different people with the same type of tumor, scientists discovered the mutational signatures of cells were so immensely different that they appeared to occur completely at random.[23-25] Scientists also looked at the genomes of cells from within *the very same tumor*, but instead of finding a distinct series of mutations that could explain cancer initiation, every cell was found to have its own unique set of mutations.[26-30] Metastatic cancer cells were also analyzed, and researchers found their genetic defects were completely different than the genetic defects in cells of the original tumor.[29,31,32] Time and time again, the story was the same: not a single gene mutation - or any combination of mutations - was found to be absolutely responsible for initiating the disease.[27,33-37]

In 2010, researchers from the University of Washington called the results of the TCGA project 'sobering' and conceded, "it is becoming increasingly difficult to envision how it will be possible to develop a realistic number of targeted chemotherapies to be directed against a discrete panel of commonly mutated cancer genes."[26] Dr. David Agus, the University of California oncologist who treated Steve Jobs, suggested in a recent speech that cancer is simply too difficult to understand and that we should stop trying.[38]

The Cancer Genome Atlas Project - a fascinating milestone in the history of cancer research - has confirmed to us unequivocally that, above all - cancer is not a genetic disease. The 81-year-old "father of DNA" James Watson himself responded publically to these findings in 2013, recommending a shift in the focus of cancer research from genetics to metabolism.[39]

Although genetic defects are undeniably ubiquitous features of cancer cells of all types, they ultimately arise as downstream consequences of something else occurring first within cells.

THE PRIME CAUSE OF CANCER

If a scientific observation can be demonstrated repeatedly by many different people, then it's probably true. When it comes to the cause of genomic instability and genetic defects arising in cells, scientists have found that these events are consistently triggered by the same distinctive conditions inside cells: insufficient oxygen (hypoxia).[40-60] It's only after a cell is deprived of oxygen that genetic mutations begin to occur.

Insufficient oxygen, however, is not just the root cause of genomic instability; it's also the primary driver of tumor formation,[45,61-71] progression and metastasis;[48,51,52,72-80] or said differently, *the prime cause of cancer*. What's particularly striking is that German physiologist, medical doctor and Nobel Laureate, Dr. Otto Heinrich Warburg first discovered this almost 100 years ago, in 1923. In a presentation to other Nobel Laureates in 1966, Warburg stated,[96]

"The cause of cancer is no longer a mystery; we know it occurs whenever any cell is denied 60% of its oxygen requirements."

When a cell is deprived of oxygen, it responds by activating hypoxia-inducible factor-1alpha (HIF-1alpha),[67] which can be "found in high levels in malignant solid tumors, but not in normal tissues or slow-growing tumors."[81-89] HIF-1alpha then stimulates the release of vascular endothelial growth factor (VEGF) into the tumor microenvironment,[90-95] which signals cells in its proximity to grow (chapter 1).

Even more extraordinary than Dr. Warburg's discovery was a statement made in 1976 by the author of one of the most widely used medical textbooks in the world, *The Textbook of Medical Physiology*:

"All chronic pain, suffering and diseases are caused from a lack of oxygen at the cell level."
-Dr. Arthur C. Guyton

Suddenly, our quest to discover how to prevent and cure cancer, we've not only identified cancer's prime cause, but in doing so we've come face-to-face with the possibility that what cures cancer, cures all diseases. The fact that all three medicines reviewed in the preceding three chapters accelerate healing, enhance the immune system, protect the vital organs and are capable of treating a multitude of diseases and conditions validates considerably the idea that all diseases have a common origin. And if it is true, then cancer and all diseases are metabolic in nature, and remarkably, all are reversible and can be corrected by restoring the efficient use of oxygen.

CANCER CELL METABOLISM

The human body is comprised of an estimated 37.2 trillion cells,[97] all of which require energy to perform the vital functions that make our lives possible. So while we go about our days not thinking much about it, our cells are hard at work metabolizing the food we eat into the energy we use to breathe, move, eat, grow, exercise, regenerate and reproduce.

The metabolism of a healthy cell, put simply, involves a chemical reaction between glucose and oxygen in the 'power plants' of the cell, called mitochondria.[98] The end product of metabolism, often termed 'the energy currency of life,' is a high-energy molecule that provides energy to all our cells, called adenosine triphosphate (ATP).[99]

Without getting into all of the complex details, energy metabolism involves three basic steps – glycolysis, krebs cycle and oxidative phosphorylation.

Cancer Cell

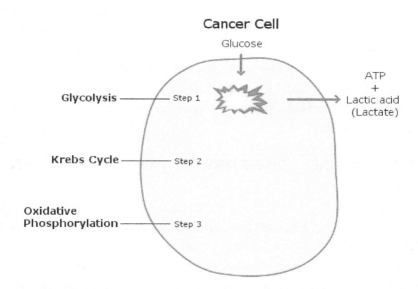

First, let's examine the defective metabolism of a cancer cell.

Whereas a normal cell produces energy using cellular respiration (all three steps; also known as mitochondrial respiration or oxidative metabolism),[100] a cancer cell uses glycolysis only, which ferments sugar and produces lactic acid as a byproduct.[101] This metabolic shift from cellular respiration to glycolysis occurs because – for reasons not yet established – the cell has lost its ability to use oxygen, and unlike the krebs cycle and oxidative phosphorylation, glycolysis doesn't require oxygen.[102] The moment a cell undergoes this metabolic shift, known as *the Warburg effect*,[98] is the moment it becomes a cancer cell.[109]

The production of lactic acid is normal during exercise when the oxygen supply is used up and not adequate to meet energy demands (anaerobic glycolysis),[103-108] but in cancer, lactic acid is produced even though oxygen is adequately present (aerobic glycolysis).

One of the downsides to using glycolysis for energy production is that it's highly inefficient and generates 15-times less ATP than cellular respiration.[110] This means that cancer cells must consume significantly more glucose in order to generate the same amount of energy[111-119] and consequently, they produce and release large amounts of lactic acid into the tumor microenvironment.[120-125]

Aside from the immunosuppressive[126] and carcinogenic effects[127,128] of lactic acid, large amounts of lactic acid also cause the breathing rate to increase, known as hyperventilation,[129-132] which quickly lowers the body's levels of carbon dioxide.[133-138]

THE EXTRAORDINARY DISCOVERY OF AN ELITE RUSSIAN SCIENTIST

While actively engaged in high-level research for the Russian military, space and sports programs at the First Medical Institute in Moscow, elite medical scientist Dr. Konstantin Pavlovich Buteyko (1923-2003) claimed to have made a discovery so vast that it would turn the whole of modern medicine on its head.[139]

Motivated by an intense interest in sophisticated medical diagnostics, Dr. Buteyko used state-of-the-art equipment and facilities to investigate the physiological and biochemical differences between healthy people and people with disease. After collecting empirical data from hundreds of patients, Dr. Buteyko made the extraordinary discovery that all people suffering from chronic diseases shared one thing in common: a lower than optimal level of carbon dioxide.

The medical norm of carbon dioxide concentration in the human body is around 5% (or 35-37mm Hg).[140,141] Dr. Buteyko found that people who had optimal levels of carbon dioxide never suffered from any chronic diseases and the greater the deficiency of carbon dioxide a person had, the worse their overall level of health.

Dr. Buteyko went on to develop a system of breathing called *The Buteyko Method*, which instructed patients to breathe shallower and less-frequently to raise their carbon dioxide levels and improve their health. Studies have confirmed that breathing less can normalize CO_2 deficiencies,[142,143] and statistics show that Buteyko's breathing method has helped more than 1,000 patients suffering from asthma, hypertension or stenocardia fully recover since 1967.[144] To date, eight clinical trials using

The Buteyko Method on human patients suffering from asthma have been conducted and in all studies, significant reductions in asthmatic symptoms and medication requirements by patients have been reported.[145-152]

Dr. Buteyko's radical discovery and his obsession with it lead him from being a privileged scientist within the soviet system to being cast a medical dissident. The medical establishment wanted nothing to do with his unconventional ideas and obstructed his progress to gain official acceptance at every turn.

"I was called a charlatan, a schizophrenic and a raving nutter, among other names," explained Dr. Buteyko. "They tried to poison me three times, and organised two car crashes. There were several attempts to put me in a psychiatric hospital. They physically destroyed my laboratory, which was unique throughout the world. And all of this because I had discovered a lever that patients could pull to be free from their piles of pills and complicated surgical procedures that were far from safe."[153]

The fact that Dr. Buteyko publically condemned the use of drug and surgical-based treatments - on the basis that most of them accelerated the loss of carbon dioxide and therefore worsened the health of patients - may have been why health authorities felt so threatened by him and went to such great lengths to suppress his discovery. Let's see if we can find any other evidence to substantiate Dr. Buteyko's finding that a deficiency of carbon dioxide occurs in all disease states.

Scientific experiments have determined that people with a wide variety of diseases are deficient in carbon dioxide, including heart disease,[154-162] diabetes,[163-167] asthma,[145,168-171] COPD,[172-174] sleep apnea,[175] cystic fibrosis,[176-182] bipolar disorder,[183] panic disorder,[184] epilepsy,[185] and of course, cancer.[186,187]

A CLOSER LOOK...

- In 2001, Ukranian medical doctor Sergey Paschenko measured the CO2 content in the exhaled breath of 120 women with metastasized breast cancer. Dr. Artour Rakhimov, who translated the study from Russian to English, reports, "The average value for end-tidal CO2 in these cancer patients was about 2.9%, while the official medical norm is about 5.3% that corresponds to 40 mm Hg at sea level."[187]

Interestingly, Dr. Rakhimov has graphed data on his website from a large list of studies showing that overall carbon dioxide levels in people worldwide have been in a steady, almost-linear decline since the 1920's.[188]

In 2015, an international team of scientists led by Dr. Darryl Leong of McMaster University in Hamilton, Ontario, analyzed the medical records of almost 140,000 people between the ages of 40 to 70 and discovered that hand grip strength was a strikingly accurate predictor of all-cause mortality; and even a more accurate predictor of heart disease than blood pressure.[189] A number of similar studies have authenticated the accuracy of grip strength as a predictor of all-cause mortality.[190-193]

With these findings in mind, a 2016 study from Winston-Salem State University in North Carolina found that over the past 30 years, the hand-grip strength of both men and women living in the US - particularly in younger people - has declined by 20% on average.[194] So while many people believe 'people are living longer than ever before,' given the decline of carbon dioxide levels and in grip strength in people over the past 100 years, it seems far more likely that the opposite is true.

Now that we've shown how CO2 deficiency can be caused and worsened by the lactic acid secreted from cancer cells, and provided substantial supporting evidence for Dr. Buteyko's groundbreaking discovery that all chronic disease is caused by a deficiency of carbon dioxide, you may be wondering: since both oxygen and carbon dioxide are deficient in sick people – *what is the relationship between oxygen and carbon dioxide?*

HEALTHY CELL METABOLISM

Unlike a cancer cell, which produces ATP and lactic acid through glycolytic metabolism, when a normal cell undergoes cellular respiration, in addition to ATP, it also generates carbon dioxide.

Normal Cell

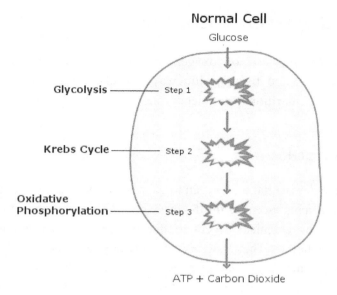

Glucose

Glycolysis — Step 1

Krebs Cycle — Step 2

Oxidative
Phosphorylation — Step 3

ATP + Carbon Dioxide

Dr. Buteyko has called carbon dioxide, "the main source of nutrition for any living matter on earth;" and its physiological effects are two-fold: First, CO_2 dilates blood vessels, increasing bloodflow.[133,195-197] Secondly, oxygen is transported through the bloodstream by red blood cells (hemoglobin), and the primary trigger for the release of oxygen from hemoglobin (*the Bohr effect*) is carbon dioxide.[198-200] In other words, without CO_2, oxygen cannot get into cells.

This has been confirmed by a number of studies looking at oxygen levels in various tissues following hyperventilation; CO_2 deficiency causes hypoxia in the brain,[201-212] heart,[213-217] liver,[218-220] kidneys,[214,220] spleen,[214] colon,[221] and indeed in all body tissues.[222,223]

So while lactic acid is constantly streaming from cancer cells - inhibiting oxygen use and cellular respiration - carbon dioxide is constantly streaming from healthy cells - promoting oxygen use and cellular respiration.

Let's take a closer look at what specifically can cause a cell to turn cancerous.

UNDERSTANDING METABOLIC DYSFUNCTION

Anything that inhibits the use of oxygen by cells is, by definition, carcinogenic - and there are two specific ways cellular oxygen can be inhibited: the first is a nutritional deficiency and the second is chemical toxicity.

1. NUTRITIONAL DEFICIENCY

While carbon dioxide is essential for oxygen to gain entry into cells, there are a number of other nutrients essential for the production of key enzymes that power the sequence of chemical reactions during the krebs cycle and oxidative phosphorylation. The B-series of vitamins are the primary nutrients that act as co-enzymes for cellular respiration, and include thiamine (B1), riboflavin (B2), niacinamide (B3), pantothenic acid (B5), pyridoxine (B6), biotin (B7) and folate (B9).[225]

Since respiration cannot occur without enzymes produced specifically by these nutrients, a deficiency in any one of them can inhibit the use of oxygen and turn a cell cancerous. And conversely, making these nutrients available to cancer cells can reverse cancer growth.

Foods with the greatest concentrations of B-vitamins include shellfish (clams, oysters, mussels), liver, caviar, octopus, crab, lobster, beef, lamb, fish, cheese and eggs.

Thiamine (Vitamin B1):

Thiamine is essential for a number of key metabolic enzymes[226] but the one we're going to focus on is called pyruvate dehydrogenase, which is critical because it links glycolysis to the krebs cycle.

Without thiamine and the pyruvate dehydrogenase enzyme made from it, a cell is forced to metabolize using glycolysis only.[227-229] Since glycolysis increases lactic acid, which lowers carbon dioxide - and since a deficiency of carbon dioxide can be seen in all disease states - we can expect to see a thiamine deficiency in many different diseases, including cancer.

234

Low levels of serum thiamine have been significantly associated with Parkinson's disease,[230,231] and administering thiamine to Parkinson's disease patients improves their brain function and overall condition.[231] Thiamine deficiency is also frequent in patients with heart disease, and administering thiamine to them improves their heart function.[232-234]

A number of studies have shown that a deficiency of thiamine is common in cancer patients and significantly associated with cancer progression,[237-243] and in 1970, Dr. Otto Warburg and his colleagues demonstrated they could induce cancer in normal cells specifically by depriving them of thiamine.[244]

The observation that thiamine can lower serum lactate concentrations[228,229,235,236] is evidence that cells are beginning to use oxygen more efficiently, and scientists from Westminster, California reported in 2013, "A very high dose of thiamine produces a growth-inhibitory effect in cancer."[237] Additionally, researchers from Kansas State University found that pyruvate dehydrogenase activation triggered apoptosis in cancer cells.[245]

Interestingly, breads, cereals and infant formula in the US and many other countries are fortified with thiamine,[246] so one could argue that people are getting enough dietary thiamine, except for one thing: most food manufacturers fortify foods with thiamine in the form of thiamine mononitrate,[247] which cancer patients have a difficult time absorbing[248] and converting[249] into the useable form found naturally in certain foods, like liver,[250] called thiamine pyrophosphate. The fact that growing tumor cells on rat liver tissue makes them revert back to healthy cells suggests that liver is an important food.[868]

Thiamine can also significantly protect the body from highly-toxic chemotherapy drugs, which illustrates just how powerful this one single nutrient can be - and how vital it is for a cell to undergo oxidative metabolism.[251-254] In one study, a patient went completely blind in both eyes following chemotherapy and after administering daily intravenous thiamine for just three days, their vision returned. "Symptomatic improvement with thiamine was rapid, with visual acuity improvement to 20/200 OU in three days."[255]

2. CHEMICAL TOXICITY

Environmental toxins can also turn cells cancerous by interfering with the production of these same critical respiratory enzymes; either by destroying the nutrients needed to make them or by accelerating their use in an attempt deal with the toxic insult, ultimately leading to a deficiency.[256,257]

Cytochrome c oxidase is an essential respiratory enzyme that interacts directly with oxygen[258] and catalyzes the very last step in the process of oxidative phosphorylation.[259,260] The nutrient needed to create this enzyme is copper[261-263] and its activity is amplified by thyroid hormone.[264]

Foods highest in copper include oysters, lobster, crab, squid, eggs, beef, lamb, fish, mushrooms and chocolate.

"Defects in cytochrome c oxidase expression induce a metabolic shift to glycolysis and carcinogenesis," wrote scientists from the University of Pennsylvania in 2015.[265] A deficiency of cytochrome c oxidase has also been implicated in tumor progression.[266]

A number of chemical toxins have been shown to inhibit cytochrome c oxidase activity; for example, chemotherapy,[267] cyanide,[268-270] carbon monoxide,[271,272] aluminum phosphide,[273] estrogen,[274] serotonin,[275] endotoxin,[276,277] aflatoxin B1,[278] UVB radiation,[279] X-ray radiation,[280,281] and most notably, unsaturated 'essential' fatty acids.[282]

A CLOSER LOOK...

- In 1951, researchers investigated the impact of the 'essential' unsaturated fatty acids (EFAs) on the respiratory enzyme cytochrome c oxidase. Results showed that EFAs strongly inhibited cytochrome c oxidase activity, and when rats were made *deficient* in the EFAs, both cytochrome c oxidase activity and cellular respiration were significantly higher than in normal rats.[282]

The fact that cigarette smoking inhibits cytochrome c oxidase activity and smoking cessation restores it[283] makes a good case for quitting.

Interestingly, light in the red (622-780nm wavelength) and near-infrared (700nm-1mm wavelength) spectrums is absorbed by cytochrome c oxidase and amplifies its activity.[284-302] This helps explain why cold and flu season occurs at the time of year with the least amount of sunlight, and provides a mechanism behind the incredible healing benefits of red and infrared light therapies; cognitive enhancement,[303-305] accelerated healing,[306] increased bone density,[307,308] increased testosterone,[309] reduced anxiety and depression,[310] reduced inflammation,[311] reduced acne,[312] pain relief,[314-318] and hair regrowth,[319] to name a few.

Dr. John Harvey Kellogg wrote in his book *Light Therapeutics:*

"Metabolism is unquestionably stimulated by the reflex action set out by the light rays impinging upon the nerve endings of the skin and retina… oxidation of living tissues is increased by the action of sunlight. In human beings as well as in animals, less carbon dioxide is emanated at night than during the same number of hours of daylight."

Nitric oxide is another toxin[320] that inhibits cytochrome c oxidase activity by binding directly to it.[321-323] Remarkably, red and infrared light is capable of unbinding nitric oxide from cytochrome c oxidase, allowing respiration and carbon dioxide production to resume.[324,325]

RETHINKING OUR FEARS SURROUNDING CANCER

Every day it seems we are inundated with the perception that cancer is some kind of biological terrorist that's entirely foreign to our bodies and trying to kill us - yet from what we've learned so far in this final chapter, it seems cancer is nothing more than a collection of cells not getting what they need to function properly. As Dr. Ray Peat has said, "The cancer business is based on something other than science or common sense."

The metabolic shift of cells to glycolysis that brands a cell cancerous - induced either by a nutrient deficiency or environmental toxin - causes free radical electrons to leak from the respiratory chain, which then react with unsaturated fats[342] and ultimately damage cells.[343-352] In other words, cancer cells are not just cells lacking nutrients; they're cells that have been injured.

German physician, anthropologist, pathologist, prehistorian, biologist, writer, editor, and politician Rudolph Virchow was the first to notice that tumors commonly form at sites of chronic injuries. So common do tumors grow from scars or old injuries that in 1862, Virchow suggested previous injuries were *a precondition* for tumor formation.[353] Swiss researchers acknowledged the "remarkable similarities between wound repair and cancer" in 2008,[354] and over the past 150 years, experiments have revealed there is virtually no difference between a wound and cancer.[355-364]

So when a doctor looks at a mammographic image and thinks he sees cancer, he's actually looking at a collection of injured cells that the body is trying to heal. A cancer doctor is trained to respond to injury by using treatments that cause further injury; and for that reason, far scarier than a diagnosis of cancer is what a doctor will try and do to you if he thinks you have it.

However, in contrast to a successfully healing wound, the healing process of a tumor is exaggerated and prolonged; an 'overhealing' as Sir Alexander Haddow put it.[354,365-367]

Chronic inflammation has been strongly associated with cancer development and progression[368-381] because an inflamed cell is an injured cell that has lost its ability to respire; it is swollen with water,[382] produces lactic acid,[383] and rapidly divides to try and replace itself with a fresh functioning cell[384-385] – the same archetypal characteristics as a cancer cell. Persistently injured and inflamed cells, like cells within a tumor, are evidence the body has been unable to properly repair the damage.

So what is preventing the body from completing the healing process in the case of a tumor? To answer that question, we look to the human embryo.

SCARLESS HEALING OF THE HUMAN EMBRYO

The opposite of a wound that won't heal is a wound that regenerates rapidly and without scarring. First observed in the 1970's, the embryos and fetus' of mice, rats, pigs, monkeys and humans have a remarkable capacity for healing; when wounded, they repair quickly, scarlessly and "with little or no inflammation," wrote Dr. Traci Wilgus at the University of Illinois in 2007.[386-402] Yet despite almost 50 years of investigation, researchers are still baffled by how this scarless healing occurs - admitting as recently as 2014, "the exact mechanisms of scarless fetal wound healing remain largely unknown."[386]

When investigators from the University of California transplanted adult sheepskin onto the backs of fetal lambs in 1995, they observed, "The adult-fetal interface healed without scar formation,"[403] suggesting that something within the embryonic/fetal environment is responsible for its regenerative capacity.

While arterial blood of a pregnant mother has an oxygen pressure of about 100 mm Hg, the blood that carries oxygen to the fetus through the umbilical vein is around 35 mm Hg.[404-406] This low-oxygen pressure allows the cells of the fetus to retain more carbon dioxide (*the Haldane effect*), which enhances cellular oxygenation and in turn cleans up the wound microenvironment and facilitates healing.[407]

Dr. Peat has mentioned another important factor involved in embryonic scarless healing: the uterus and placenta act as filters that let very little unsaturated fatty acids into the fetal environment; evidence of this can be seen in studies showing nearly all newborn babies are born deficient in the 'essential' fatty acids.[408-412]

"It is known that the child is virtually disease-free in the womb of the mother: only after the birth, do diatheses and all other abnormalities of metabolism appear," said Dr. Buteyko in a lecture at Moscow State University in 1969.[413] "After birth, during the first breaths," he continued, "there is a sudden increase in blood oxygenation and a sudden drop in CO2." This, according to Buteyko, is why babies have been traditionally tightly swaddled and sometimes even tightened to a wooden plate: "Folk wisdom understood, that this air, so poisonous for the newborn, requires gradual adaptation."

Interestingly, scientists studying the oral soft tissues of adult humans and pigs have discovered similarly rapid and scarless regenerative capacities;[414-417] "Wound healing in the oral mucosa proceeds faster than in skin and clinical observations have suggested that mucosal wounds rarely scar," wrote Canadian researchers from the University of British Columbia in 2009.[418]

Just as the mechanisms behind the flawless healing ability of the developing embryo and fetus remain a mystery in the published literature, scientists are perplexed by this one too. A group of researchers looking at cellular genetics of oral tissue made the following useful observation: "The striking difference between these tissues is transient and rapidly resolving inflammation in oral wounds compared with long-lasting inflammation in the skin wounds."[414]

In 1971, scientists from Boston, Massachusetts measured oxygen levels in the human mouth and found oxygen pressure was significantly reduced.[419] Just like the growing embryo in the womb, oral soft tissues accumulate increased carbon dioxide, stimulating oxidative metabolism and thus rapid, scarless regeneration.

STEM CELLS & THE HEALING PROCESS

If we define healing as the repair or replacement of defective cells with functioning ones, then the process has a lot to do with stem cells. Stem cells are like the body's rescue crew; anytime cells are injured they home to the injured tissue and either repair the damage or differentiate into the required cells and serve as replacements.[386,420-431]

Stem cell therapy - where doctors harvest stem cells from the bone marrow or fat tissue of patients and then administer it back to them – is portrayed by the media to be a highly-sophisticated medical innovation reserved for those who can afford the luxury. The irony is that the public is being sold something that is a normal part of the body's healing process. "It is well established that tissue repair depends on stem cells..." wrote researchers from the United Kingdom in 2012.[432]

The difference between a wound that heals, like the rapid and flawlessly healing embryo and adult oral soft tissues and a 'cancer' wound that's struggling to heal, is the extracellular conditions surrounding the wound when stem cells arrive.

240

STEM CELLS MEET THE TUMOR MICROENVIRONMENT

Interleukin-8,[433,434] vascular endothelial growth factor,[435] nerve growth factor,[436] hepatocyte growth factor,[437] nitric oxide[438,439] and estrogen[440,441] are some of the substances released by injured cells that signal the trafficking of stem cells to a wound.

Normally, the inbound stem cells would repopulate the tissues that have been damaged or lost, but since stem cells respond to the signals in their immediate environment,[442-445] abnormal substances within the tumor microenvironment send the wrong instructions and cause them to fail to complete the task. For example, the presence of toxic heavy metals like arsenic or cadmium in the tumor microenvironment will transform incoming stem cells into cancer cells.[446,447] Furthermore, all of the substances located within the tumor microenvironment of untreated cancer patients (chapter 6) also happen to promote carcinogenesis (chapter 1); so just as chemical carcinogens can induce metabolic dysfunction in arriving stem cells, the wide range of other stress and inflammatory substances in the tumor microenvironment also initiate aerobic glycolysis.[313,504,869-881]

"Cancer, the disease, is much more than a cellular defect. Most of the cells in a tumor are so defective that they are in the process of dying, and in that process they recruit replacement cells, which experience the same damaging conditions. The local and regional extracellular conditions, and the condition of the host, are just as central to the disease as the failing mitochondria."

- Dr. Raymond Peat

Although many people believe tumor growth occurs as a consequence of rapidly dividing tumor cells, Scottish researchers made a remarkable discovery in 1972 that revealed an entirely different process. Using electron microscopes in their laboratory at the University of Aberdeen, Andrew H. Wyllie and his colleagues found that the rate of cell death in tumors was enormous; and that cell division alone could only account for less than 5% of cells present in a growing tumor.[448-450]

What could account for the other 95% of cells in a tumor?

When conditions surrounding an injury are defective, incoming stem cells are immediately injured and recruit additional stem cells which also become injured. As this chronic influx of stem cells and high rate of cell death continues, cells - both living and dead - begin to accumulate within the injured region, forming what is commonly referred to as... a tumor. "Wounding recruits these cells from the follicle to the wound site,...giving rise to superficial BCC [basal cell carcinoma]-like tumors. These findings demonstrate that BCC-like tumors can originate from follicular stem cells and provide an explanation for the association between wounding and tumorigenesis," wrote scientists from the Cardiovascular Research Institute at the University of California in 2011.[451]

These fairly recent discoveries - that a constant flux of stem cells are responsible for tumor formation, growth and metastasis - have been confirmed so thoroughly[452-458] that even the cancer establishment has acknowledged them; except they've adapted them to fit in with their imaginary 'mutant boogeyman' theory of cancer, claiming that "cancer stem cells" are the true "villains" that need to be "eradicated" during cancer therapy. The fact that scientists would actually suggest killing the body's repair cells as a treatment for cancer exposes an astonishing lack of understanding about the disease.[459-474]

We've seen what happens to tumors when medicines like oranges, sodium bicarbonate and coconut oil work to normalize the tumor microenvironment (chapters 7-9). It's precisely these alterations that allow homing stem cells to repair damage and differentiate into healthy replacement cells, just as they do in a wounded embryo.

STEM CELLS MEET THE EMBRYONIC MICROENVIRONMENT

During the differentiation process of a stem cell into a specific cell type, some key metabolic changes take place: the number of mitochondria are increased, the cell begins consuming more oxygen and produces more energy as a result of the activation of the more efficient, aerobic metabolism.[475] "Cell differentiation is associated with an increase in mitochondrial content and activity and with a metabolic shift toward increased oxidative phosphorylation activity."[476]   In other words, an environment that signals cellular respiration is essential for successful stem cell differentiation.[477-479]

When a team of international scientists added embryonic stem cells to the blood serum of cancer patients, the cells transformed into cancer cells,[480] and conversely, experiments conducted as early as 1959 have demonstrated that implanting cancer cells into mouse, zebrafish and chicken embryos causes them to revert back into healthy, respiring cells.[481-492] "Indeed, our group and others have elucidated the unique ability of embryonic microenvironments to normalize aggressive melanoma cells toward a more benign melanocytic phenotype," wrote American scientists from Northwestern University's Feinberg School of Medicine in 2013.[493]

The high levels of carbon dioxide within a fetus or embryo - in addition to rapidly driving oxygen into cells and lowering virtually all of the stress and inflammatory factors within the wound microenvironment[908-925] – powerfully inhibit the generation of free radicals by keeping cells fully-oxidizing glucose for energy (preventing 'free radical' electron leakage from the transport chain) and also by preventing accidental free radical reactions from occurring within the blood; for example, involving unsaturated fats and heavy metals like iron.[494-501] "The results testify to the fact that CO2 is a powerful inhibitor of reactive oxygen species (ROS) generation by cells..."[502]   As a result of this incredibly nurturing CO2-rich embryonic environment, an embryo is able to withstand exposure to 10x more chemical toxins than an adult.[503]

After discovering that inflammation in fetal wound healing is minimal and resolves rapidly,[364,505] scientists looking more closely at the fetal/embryonic wound environment have observed decreased levels of pro-inflammatory cytokines interleukin-1,[386] interleukin-6,[505] interleukin-8,[506] tumor necrosis-factor alpha,[386] tumor growth factor beta[507] and prostaglandins.[508] Tumor growth factor beta (TGFb), which is absent in fetal wounds and abundant in tumor microenvironments, metabolically reprograms cells to shift to aerobic glycolysis (*the Warburg effect*).[509]

Most of the inflammatory mediators present in the 'defective' microenvironment of a tumor which are absent from the 'flawless-healing' fetal wound environment - interleukin-6, interleukin-8, tumor growth factor beta and prostaglandins - can all be induced by one single dietary constituent: unsaturated fat.[510-515]

CANCER AND THE IMMUNE SYSTEM

In 1909, German physician and scientist Paul Erhlich first proposed the existence of an immune 'surveillance' system in the body capable of eliminating transformed cells before they are clinically noticed.[535,536] Since then, it has been confirmed that this system does exist and scientists have been documenting a consistent association between a malfunctioning immune system and cancer development in both mice[537-542] and humans.[543-550] Epidemiological research has concluded, "Immune-suppressed populations experience higher rates of cancer than expected."[551]

In 1974, American immunologist Dr. George Friou stated the formation of cancer is not uncommon and cellular defects are overcome by a functional immune system before they develop into recognizable malignancies.[552] And in 2011, an Italian-American research team wrote, "Occult microscopic cancers are exceedingly common in the general population and are held in a dormant state by a balance between cell proliferation and cell death and also an intact host immune surveillance."[553]

Laughter has been shown to enhance the immune systems of cancer patients[554] and also decrease the risk of heart disease.[555]

Regular exercise of moderate intensity has been shown to boost the immune system[556,557] and reduce the risk of cancer,[558-561] while endurance or excessively intense exercise, both of which significantly elevate lactic acid production[562-564] and cause carbon dioxide loss through hyperventilation,[565] have been shown to impair immune function.[566-570]

For decades, vegetable oil (unsaturated fat) has been recognized as a drug that can knockout the immune system.[571-577] In fact, unsaturated fats are so potently immunosuppressive that they've been used specifically to disable the immune systems of kidney transplant patients to prevent their bodies from rejecting the foreign tissue.[578-580] One way unsaturated fats do this is by shrinking the thymus gland - an organ critical for immune function;[581] and they also directly kill white blood cells, which are the most important part of the immune system.[582]

THYROID HORMONE, CHOLESTEROL AND CANCER

Thyroid hormone is an essential component of cellular respiration; without it oxygen use and the production of carbon dioxide by cells cannot occur.[583-588] Thyroid hormone exerts two primary actions: First, it rapidly activates respiration,[661-666] which can be seen within minutes of a thyroid hormone injection, and secondly - within a few days of a thyroid injection - thyroid hormone stimulates the biogenesis of additional mitochondria within cells.[667-672]

Thyroid hormone is also used by the body to produce steroid hormones, which are some of the most powerful defenders against cancer and diseases in general. These hormones include pregnenolone, progesterone, DHEA and testosterone, which all seem to have similar anti-stress, anti-inflammation, anti-cancer effects mediated by the activation of oxidative metabolism.[589-602,673] The production of these hormones begins with thyroid hormone converting cholesterol into pregnenolone, and subsequently, pregnenolone can be converted into all of the other steroids. What's critical to understand is that without adequate cholesterol and thyroid hormone, none of these steroid hormones can be produced.

Impaired memory,[604,605] increased aggressive behavior and suicide,[606-608] and increased mortality from cardiovascular disease,[609-612] stroke and cancer,[613-616] are all consequences of not having enough cholesterol. The weight of evidence showing the detrimental effects of low cholesterol has recently become so titanic, that in 2015, the FDA completely reversed their position on cholesterol - a position held for over 50 years - officially removing the 'upper limit' on cholesterol consumption. In other words, there's no amount of dietary cholesterol you can consume that is bad for you.[603]

With this in mind, one of the primary ways the public has been sold on the 'essentiality' of unsaturated fat is that it potently inhibits LDL cholesterol synthesis.[617-620] "Diets rich in omega-3 fatty acids derived from fish oils lower the plasma concentrations of low density lipoproteins (LDL) and very low density lipoproteins in humans."[621] If cholesterol was unhealthy, then lowering it would be a good thing, but the research is exceptionally clear that inhibiting cholesterol synthesis by eating unsaturated fat (or in any other way, for example, statin drugs) will eventually lead to cancer and other degenerative diseases.

Anybody concerned about having high cholesterol should know that this situation has long been associated with a deficiency of thyroid (hypothyroidism).[622-648] "The thyroid hormone is required for using and eliminating cholesterol, so cholesterol is likely to be raised by anything which blocks the thyroid function," wrote Dr. Peat. Supplementation with a dessicated thyroid supplement (dry powdered thyroid gland pressed into a tablet) can be used to convert cholesterol into valuable hormones.

For decades, Dr. Peat has been saying that unsaturated fats, which include any oils that are liquid at room temperature, aside from olive oil (which contains about 11% unsaturated fat[650]), are potent inhibitors of thyroid function.[649]

Unsaturated oils obstruct thyroid hormone at every turn - including its secretion from the thyroid gland,[651] its transport through the blood,[652] its conversation in the liver,[653] its uptake by tissues[654] and its use inside cells.[655] This helps to explain why diets high in unsaturated 'essential' fatty acids promote weight gain and why animals made deficient in unsaturated fats are leaner and have higher metabolic rates, meaning they produce greater levels of energy and carbon dioxide as a result of increased oxidative metabolic activity.[656-660]

In summary: Thyroid hormone and the anti-aging steroid hormones it produces are essential for cellular respiration. Both thyroid hormone and cholesterol are essential for producing these hormones, and unsaturated fatty acids potently inhibit both thyroid hormone and cholesterol synthesis.

CO2, UNSATURATED FATS AND AGING

Since our lives begin in the womb with extraordinary health – characterized by optimal levels of carbon dioxide, and end with disease – characterized by a deficiency of carbon dioxide, it stands to reason that carbon dioxide gradually decreases with age. There's another very important thing that happens with age.

"We have conducted a systematic literature review of studies reporting the concentration of LA [Linoleic Acid/omega-6/unsaturated fat] in subcutaneous adipose tissue of US cohorts. Our results indicate that adipose tissue LA has increased by 136% over the last half century and that this increase is highly correlated with an increase in dietary LA intake over the same period of time," reported American researchers in 2015.[516]

It's no coincidence that as we age, decreasing levels of carbon dioxide are directly accompanied by an increased accumulation of unsaturated fatty acids in our tissues.[516-526]

Scientists have found that cytochrome c oxidase enzyme activity (and thus carbon dioxide production) in rats also declines with age,[527,528] while simultaneously cardiolipin, a major mitochondrial lipid that interacts directly with cytochrome c oxidase and plays a pivotal role in cellular respiration,[529-532] becomes increasingly unsaturated.[533] Feeding aged rats hydrogenated peanut oil (100% saturated fat) "completely restored" the respiratory enzyme activity in their muscles "to 80% of the value observed in muscles of young animals."[534]

In summary: Aging is a consequence of reduced levels of carbon dioxide in the body caused primarily by the increased accumulation of dietary unsaturated fatty acids in body tissues.

THE PRIMARY FUEL FOR A TUMOR

Discovered nearly 100 years ago by British medical scientist Philip Randle,[690] *the Randle effect* describes the observation that – similar to an "on" and "off" switch – having more glucose (sugar) than fat circulating in the blood will cause cells to metabolize sugar rather than fat, and reciprocally, having more fatty acids in the blood will cause cells to metabolize fat rather than sugar.[691]

While cancer cells do consume large amounts of sugar initially, once the bloodstream runs low on sugar (hypoglycemia), muscle will be catabolized into amino acids and fat mobilized from fat stores, which inhibit the use of glucose (*the Randle effect*) by cells - so tumor cells rely mostly on fat and protein for energy.[98,692-696]

The Randle effect also explains the metabolism of a person with diabetes. Like all diseases, excessive stress has mobilized fatty acids into the bloodstream, shutting off the body's ability to use glucose. This situation is so similar to what's happening in a person with cancer that the association between diabetes and cancer has been called 'a two-way street.'[697-704]

Aside from chronically elevated stress hormones, some of the adverse effects of fat and protein metabolism include: fat metabolism produces less carbon dioxide (per unit of oxygen consumed),[964-966] and protein metabolism results in the production of ammonia - "a highly toxic substance,"[705] which further promotes glycolysis and increases lactic acid production.[706-708]

Low blood sugar, caused by fasting, starvation, avoiding dietary carbohydrates and exercise (unless adequate sugar is consumed during exercise), stimulates the same stress metabolism as a person with cancer. This explains why most heart attacks occur in the early morning hours,[882] following an overnight 'fast' during sleep.

In 2017, researchers from the Barcelona Institute of Science and Technology in Spain investigated cancer cell metabolism and discovered that cancer metastasis relies on a single molecule whose function is to allow cells to absorb fat, called CD36. "The use of neutralizing antibodies to block CD36 causes almost complete inhibition of metastasis," they reported.[709] This study indicates that fat is *required* in order for cancer metastasis to occur. One year prior to this study, Spanish researchers also established a similarly remarkable finding: the ability of cancer cells to grow and proliferate is *exclusively dependent* on fat, which they called the "Achilles heel" of cancer.[710]

Animal experiments have determined that high fat diets of any kind will increase the frequency of cancer, but that it's the type of fat that determines the magnitude;[711-723] "Polyunsaturated vegetable oils enhance carcinogenesis more effectively than saturated fats;"[724] "In general, high dietary levels of unsaturated fats (e.g., corn oil, sunflower-seed oil) stimulate this tumorigenic process more than high levels of saturated fats (e.g., beef tallow, coconut oil)."[725]

Furthermore, the greater the degree of unsaturation, the more carcinogenic the fat is.[726-731]

A CLOSER LOOK...

- In 1998, Netherland researchers from the University of Amsterdam divided rats into three groups and fed them either - a low fat diet, a fish oil diet (omega-3), or a safflower oil diet (omega-6) - just three weeks before injecting colon cancer cells into their veins to induce tumors. "At 3 weeks after tumor transplantation, the fish oil diet and the safflower oil diet had induced, respectively, 10- and 4-fold more metastases (number) and over 1000- and 500-fold more metastases (size) than were found in the livers of rats on the low-fat diet."[729]

- In 1994, researchers from the University of Georgia compared the effects of feeding rats a high fat fish oil (omega-3) diet with a high fat corn oil (omega-6) diet. In the group of rats fed omega-3's - the most highly-unsaturated fat found in nature[730] – researchers found the largest increase in oxidative stress; "The omega-3 diet showed 675% increase in basal oxidation, a 2624% increase in auto-oxidation and a 4244% increase in iron-ascorbate catalyzed oxidation compared to the omega-6 diet in mammary tissue homogenates."[731]

In 1987, Dr. Leonard Sauer and his colleague looked at the effects of prolonged fasting on the growth of tumors in rats. The researchers found that tumor growth was increased in proportion to the availability of fat released from fat stores, substantiating the finding that tumor growth is dependent on fat.[732] **Here's the kicker:** no tumor growth occurred in the young rats - only in the adult rats - meaning the fats deemed essential for tumor growth were predominantly *unsaturated*. In other words, unsaturated fat is not only the primary fuel that drives tumor growth, but *a tumor cannot exist without it.*

When scientists from the University of Wisconsin fed rats a diet containing 5% corn oil for 6 months - 80% of the rats developed tumors. When they fed them hydrogenated coconut oil, containing 100% saturated fat, *no liver tumors developed*; "The feeding of the fatty acids of hydrogenated coconut oil lowered the incidence of hepatomas to zero."[733]

In rats chemically induced with pancreatic cancer, after 4 months, "Grossly visible tumors increased significantly in number as the EFA [essential fatty acid] content of the diet increased,"[734] and a number of studies have found that tumorigenesis could only be induced if a certain amount of unsaturated fat was included in the diet;[735-737] confirming what Dr. Peat has been stating boldly and repeatedly for decades:

"Cancer cannot exist unless there are unsaturated fatty acids in the diet."
- Dr. Raymond Peat

THE SELF-AMPLIFYING STRESS RESPONSE

In life-threatening situations, stress can save our lives by helping us physically escape danger; but in the modern world where stress is triggered more frequently, it can eventually result in disease and death.

During a stress response, stress hormones are released to break down muscle and fat tissues for emergency fuel, and depending on the composition of fats released into the bloodstream – which depends entirely on what foods we've chosen to eat in our lifetimes - two diametrically opposed reactions can occur.

Saturated Fat	When mostly saturated free fatty acids enter our bloodstream during stress, they will be oxidized for energy and at the same time inhibit additional stress hormones from being produced;[674-677] which quickly shuts off the stress response once the stressful situation is over.
Unsaturated Fat	When mostly unsaturated free fatty acids enter our bloodstream during stress, they will be oxidized for energy and at the same time – due to their toxicity - trigger the production of additional stress hormones,[678-684] which cause more unsaturated free fatty acids to be released, causing more stress hormones to be produced *in a vicious circle*.

"Various tumor cell-derived and contextual cues feed constantly this vicious circuitry sustaining inflammation and promoting proliferation, angiogenesis, invasion and eventually metastasis," wrote scientists from the University of Athens Medical School in 2013.[689]

If our tissues are comprised of mostly saturated fat, our stress response will be self-limiting, but if our tissues are comprised of mostly unsaturated fat, then our stress response will be self-amplifying; and when the self-amplifying stress response overwhelms the body's ability to deal with it - the stress will never be switched off; and cancer and diseases will emerge.

INTERRUPTING THE VICIOUS CYCLE OF STRESS

Anytime highly-reactive molecules like unsaturated free fatty acids are put into an environment rich in oxygen, the two will react - and the fat particles will be broken down into toxic fragments. And as the temperature of that oxygen-rich environment is increased, these reactions are enhanced; so between the toxic excess of oxygen in the air we breathe[738,739] and our relatively high body temperatures, the human body is a perfect setting for these oxidative reactions to occur.

One class of breakdown products (metabolites), which arise from oxidation of the unsaturated fat arachidonic acid (omega-6), that are heavily implicated in cancer growth and progression, are called prostaglandins.[740-748] Researchers studying dietary fat have suggested that prostaglandins might be the underlying reason why unsaturated fats promote tumor formation and saturated fats don't.[711]

Prostaglandins can also at least partly explain why feeding pigs diets containing unsaturated fat, which is common practice in convention pig farming, damages their lung function,[759] or why heart disease can be induced by eating unsaturated fat and prevented by adding cocoa butter (saturated fat) to the diet.[760]

The direct stimulation of cortisol[677-684] and estrogen[685-688] by unsaturated fatty acids as well as the prostaglandins produced from them are probably the three key factors sustaining the vicious cycle of stress and toxic tumor microenvironment that prevents stem cells from repairing a tumor wound.

Even if our tissues are brimming with unsaturated fatty acids, as long as they don't enter our bloodstream, none of these negative effects will occur, and therefore, finding ways to prevent unsaturated fatty acids from entering our bloodstream - so they can be safely detoxified from our tissues by the liver - is the paramount strategy for interrupting the vicious cycle of stress sustaining a tumor.

DIETARY CONSIDERATIONS

Since unsaturated fatty acids can enter the bloodstream either through exogenous (eating them) or from endogenous (released from tissues during stress) sources, the first step in healing a tumor (or preventing one) involves minimizing consumption of unsaturated fats or ideally, eliminating them from the diet entirely.

After inducing tumors in mice and amplifying their tumor size by feeding them high fat corn oil diets - researchers switched the mice to fat-free diets and after 20 weeks, tumors regressed in about half of the rats, and in some cases, completely disappeared.[761]

In the interest of cancer prevention, one strategy that Dr. Peat recommends for protecting the body when eating at a restaurant or a meal containing unsaturated fat, is supplemental vitamin E, which is probably based on evidence showing that vitamin E reduces lipid peroxidation caused by unsaturated fat,[762-764] meaning essentially that it saturates it.

Although consuming saturated fats like coconut oil can dilute the unsaturated fat content in the blood of a cancer patient and successfully interrupt the stress response (chapter 8), even coconut oil contains about 3% unsaturated fat, so a fat-free diet might be a better strategy. Hydrogenated coconut oil, however, would be a great medicine for cancer patients since it provides no inhibitory unsaturated fatty acids.

We've previously established that oranges, coconut oil and baking soda inhibit estrogen, cortisol and prostaglandins - suggesting they inhibit the movement of free fatty acids into the blood (lipolysis) - and there's one medicine in particular that can be used in conjunction with these foods to inhibit lipolysis probably more effectively than any other known substance.

CANCER MEDICINE

The enzyme responsible for the production of prostaglandins, which is highly expressed at sites of inflammation, like wounds and tumors,[741,743-746,765-770] is called COX-2 (cyclooxygenase-2).[771] "Cyclooxygenase-2 is frequently overexpressed in many cancers and is functionally involved in the pathogenesis of tumours. Therefore, it represents an important target for pharmaceutical intervention," wrote Swiss researchers from the Institute of Cell Biology in Zurich.[354]

Drugs that inhibit the COX-2 enzyme have been shown to significantly prevent cancer, including a 40-50% reduction in the incidence of colorectal cancer in people taking COX-2 inhibitors (which was directly attributed to decreased prostaglandins[742,772-774]) and reduce the growth of existing tumors, in both animals and in humans.[742,744,775-782] And since prostaglandins are one of the mechanisms by which unsaturated fats knockout the immune system,[783-788] anything that inhibits COX-2 will also stimulate the immune system.[785]

Interestingly, all drugs classified as COX-2 inhibitors, for example, acetaminophen, ibuprofen, etc., have been shown to be extremely toxic and increase the risk of heart disease, except one.

ASPIRIN

Comprised of acetic acid (found in vinegar) and salicylic acid (found in willow bark, fruit and vegetables[789]), aspirin (acetylsalicylic acid) is a safe and inexpensive drug that can effectively inhibit the enzyme COX-2.

Ancient Egyptians used willow bark extract thousands of years ago to help mothers cope with the pain of childbirth,[790] and this same medicine is being widely used today for the same and many other purposes.

In 2016, after analyzing the available scientific evidence, the U.S. Preventive Services Task Force officially began recommending daily low-dose aspirin for people aged 50 to 69 to prevent heart disease, stroke and cancer.[791] Even the Acting Director of the U.S. National Cancer Institute Dr.

Douglas Lowy publically endorsed the use of daily low-dose aspirin as a cancer preventive,[792] which can reduce the cancer death rate by 30%, heart disease by 22% and stroke by 17% and save 900,000 lives over the next 20 years, according to a 2016 study from the University of California.[793] A 2016 systematic review concluded aspirin was as effective as screening for preventing colon cancer incidence and mortality; meaning daily low-dose aspirin can completely replace an annual colonoscopy.[794]

Aspirin works in part by inhibiting the COX-2 enzyme that converts unsaturated fatty acids into prostaglandins – but aspirin is far more than just a COX-2 inhibitor. Aspirin directly inhibits the release of free fatty acids into the bloodstream (lipolysis)[795-797] and it also inhibits the enzyme responsible for the synthesis of cortisol.[798] So while aspirin prevents the production of prostaglandins, it's also inhibiting cortisol production and lipolysis, which cuts off the direct estrogenic, anti-thyroid and immunosuppressive effects of unsaturated fatty acids.

When you eliminate toxic unsaturated fats from the equation with medicines like aspirin, the vicious cycle of stress seen in cancer is shut off, damaged cells are repaired, mitochondrial respiration is restored,[799] carbon dioxide levels rise and amazing things begin to take place.

Aspirin can reduce pain,[800] prevent cataracts,[801,802] protect the brain from glutamate[803] and nitric oxide toxicity,[804] prevent neurodegenerative diseases like Alzheimer's, Parkinson's and Huntington's diseases,[805] improve insulin sensitivity in diabetics,[798] enhance brain function,[806] alleviate depression,[807] chelate toxic heavy metal iron,[808] prevent damage from ionizing radiation,[809,810] prevent miscarriage,[811] improve fertility,[812] extend the lifespan of nematodes by up to 23%;[813,814] of mice by 10%;[815] and of yeast by almost 400%; in fact, the active ingredient in aspirin was found to be more effective at extending lifespans than over 10,000 other plant extracts tested.[816]

Highlights of the anti-cancer effects of aspirin in vitro and in animal studies include stopping the growth of endometrial tumors,[817] triggering apoptosis in gastric cancer cells,[818] preventing lung tumor formation[819] and shrinking fibrosarcoma tumors by 30%.[820]

A groundbreaking study by scientists at the University of Kansas Medical Center in 2015 administered the human-equivalent dose of a single 325mg aspirin tablet to mice with breast tumors and found that aspirin not only prevented tumor growth, but it actually 'reprogrammed' stem cells to begin differentiating and repairing the damage, instead of becoming injured and maintaining tumor mass.[821]

Human breast cancer patients were treated with aspirin in a study from the Bose Institute in Kolkata, India in 2010, and researchers found that aspirin completely stopped tumor growth in 80% of patients. [822] At doses as low as 100mg/day, aspirin can halt the growth of non-metastatic human pancreatic and colon cancer cells, and at doses between 3-12 grams/day it can halt the growth of metastatic cancer cells.[823]

Aspirin's effects on the tumor microenvironment are significant and include reductions in free radicals,[824,825] tumor necrosis factor-alpha,[826,827] interleukin-1,[828] interleukin-4,[829,830] interleukin-6,[831-833] interleukin-8,[834-836] interleukin-13,[837] nuclear factor kappa-b,[828] cortisol,[798,838,839] adrenaline,[840-843] high mobility group box 1 protein,[844,845] vascular endothelial growth factor,[846] epidermal growth factor,[847,848] nitric oxide,[849-852] lactic acid,[853-855] estrogen[856-858] and serotonin.[841,859,860]

ASPIRIN SAFETY

Mainstream medicine seems devoted to bashing aspirin in the media; claiming it is a dangerous drug with lethal side effects like bleeding in the stomach or brain. But like every statement we hear in the media, our first response is to exert a healthy skepticism until we've investigated the subject for ourselves. So let's take a look at some evidence and decide if the concerns surrounding aspirin use are warranted.

An extensive 2015 review looking at the safety of aspirin use in patients with aneurisms declared, "Aspirin has been found to be a safe in patients harboring cerebral aneurysms." The researchers also cited a number of clinical studies in which aspirin was demonstrated to *decrease* the overall chances of rupture/brain bleeding in patients with aneurisms.[861]

Lebanese researchers examined mortality of patients admitted to hospital for gastrointestinal bleeding in 2015 and found, "being on aspirin was protective against in-hospital mortality, rebleeding, and predictive of a shorter hospital stay."[862]

Another well-established benefit of aspirin is that repeated doses actually protect the stomach from damage caused by strong irritants.[866] In

1995, Polish researchers from the Jagiellonian University School of Medicine found that administering human-equivalent doses of 1.5 grams of aspirin to rats for 5 days enhanced their resistance to stomach irritation; "Gastric adaptation to ASA enhances the mucosal resistance to injury by strong irritants..." they concluded. [867]

So how is it possible that aspirin can both prevent stomach and brain bleeding while simultaneously causing it? The doses used may have a lot to do with it. Dr. Peat has mentioned that in animal experiments where aspirin was found to produce stomach ulcers/bleeding, enormous single human-equivalent doses of anywhere between 10 and 100 aspirin tablets have been used;[864] basically these studies were designed to produce ulcers. So for all practical purposes, typical doses used by people will not even come close to having these effects and the evidence seems to substantiate this.

In 2000, researchers from the United Kingdom investigated the effects of low-dose asprin on the formation of ulcers or stomach damage. Results showed that low-doses of aspirin caused no increase in intestinal permeability, ulcers or stomach damage; "Aspirin caused no inflammation or ulcers." However, when the researchers tested aspirin use in combination with the highly-toxic drug dinitrophenol, they found that stomach ulcers did form.[865]

Since people often take multiple other drugs together with aspirin, it makes you wonder if reports of stomach bleeding have been caused by other medications being used at the same time as aspirin, and yet aspirin has taken the blame. Contrary to rumors that aspirin can cause deadly stomach bleeding, a 2016 review and meta-analysis by an international team of researchers found *no evidence* of aspirin ever causing fatal stomach bleeding.[863]

From my own experience, I've read about and experimented with dozens of different supplements, nutrients and drugs over the past decade and nothing has even come close to being as helpful for me as aspirin; I feel it has completely turned my health around, which began when I upped my dose from 1 to 3 tablets (about 1 gram) per day. For the past 8 months, I've been taking between 3-5 grams of aspirin daily and it's allowed me to keep my energy levels high and stress levels low enough to sit, stand and think while writing this book at an intense pace for usually 8 to 12 hours a day. While I did notice slight irritation when I first increased my dose of aspirin, I've certainly never experienced any stomach bleeding from it; in fact, my stomach seemed to adapt rather quickly and I no longer have any issues at all.

It seems the fears being pushed by the media regarding aspirin use are vastly overstated and that the decreased risk of heart attack, stroke, cancer and the many other benefits aspirin delivers greatly outweigh any minor risk that may exist. The fact that aspirin is unpatented, costs next to nothing, and has the potential to completely replace everything the cancer industry has to offer and most of what the drug industry has to offer might have a lot to do with the deliberate falsehoods and scare tactics being endorsed in the media.

When purchasing aspirin, be sure to read the ingredients list as many companies have been adding harmful chemicals to their tablets. The best options seem to be either pure aspirin (acetylsalicylic acid) powder or a number brands offer tablets containing only aspirin and either cornstarch or cellulose. Buy these, boycott the rest, and drug companies can either clean up their asprin products or go out of business.

CARBOHYDRATES AND CANCER

It's interesting that for the past half century our society has vilified saturated fat and now that evidence has overwhelmingly shown that saturated fat doesn't 'clog your arteries' or have any negative impact on human health, government food recommendations have switched to vilifying sugar. Everyone knows sugar makes you fat, right?

Here's an inconvenient truth: In 2011, Australian researchers compared sugar consumption and obesity rates in Australia, the UK and USA, and found that between the years 1980-2003, Australian obesity rates increased 3-fold while sugar consumption decreased by 23%.[883]

Coconut oil stimulates weight loss by diluting the content of unsaturated fatty acids in the blood, which is marked by a boost in thyroid function and increased thermogenesis. Therefore, the higher your metabolic rate (the more your cells are respiring/the more carbon dioxide in your body), the leaner and less obese you will be. It is probable that dietary consumption of unsaturated fat - a major metabolic inhibitor that can be incredibly difficult to avoid eating - is the main culprit behind the increased obesity seen in Australians during this study period.

Since stress hormones are elevated primarily to replenish glucose stores in the blood, ingesting sugar is one of the quickest and most effective ways to turn off stress. A 1987 study published in *Life Sciences* examined the effects of different diets on hormonal production in men who ate either high carbohydrate diets (20% fat, 10% protein, 70% carbs) or low carbohydrate diets (20% fat, 44% protein 35% carbs). The results showed, "Testosterone concentrations in seven normal men were consistently higher after ten days on a high carbohydrate diet" and "cortisol concentrations were consistently lower during the high carbohydrate diet." [884] Another study came to similar conclusions: Two groups of men were asked to perform three consecutive days of intensive exercise training while consuming different diets - one consumed a diet containing 60% carbohydrates and the other 30% carbohydrates. Blood samples revealed that the men who ate low-carbohydrate diets had higher cortisol levels and lower testosterone levels compared to the men who ate high-carbohydrate diets.[885] In both studies, carbohydrates had an androgenic and stress-reducing effect.

One useful way of looking at metabolism is that we have two options – the stress metabolism or the health metabolism. Which one we spend the most of our time in is a choice we make everyday, primarily by the food we eat: either we eat sugar – yes, even plain white sugar - or in its absence, our body will elevate stress hormones and begin tearing itself apart in order to make sugar.

The fact that the body is willing to destroy itself to make glucose when it is lacking reveals how critical dietary consumption of sugar actually is. "Glucose metabolism in mitochondria through oxidative phosphorylation (OXPHOS) for generation of adenosine triphosphate (ATP) is vital for cell function," wrote scientists in 2015.[224]

In cancer, since sugar metabolism is switched off by the presence of free fatty acids in the bloodstream (*the Randle effect*), inhibiting lipolysis using medicines like aspirin will effectively switch cells back to metabolizing sugar. This, in combination with a diet containing adequate protein and high in carbohydrates, particularly from fruit, like oranges, will elevate the body's supply of carbon dioxide, supporting a high metabolic rate and a disease-free organism.

There are a number of advanced healing technologies that can also be used as strategies for disease prevention, treatment, athletic performance enhancement and life extension.

CARBOGEN

In the 1940's, fire trucks, police rescue crews and paramedics all across the United States were equipped with devices called 'H-H Inhalators,' which created a healing mixture of oxygen and carbon dioxide - called carbogen - that was administered to patients during emergencies.[886] The common practice of using carbogen by emergency response crews was spurred by the early 19th century work of Yale professor Dr. Yandell Henderson and his colleagues, whose pioneering research on carbogen uncovered some of the many virtues of the therapeutic inhalation of carbon dioxide.

The administration of pure oxygen to patients during emergency situations, which is standard practice today, actually lowers carbon dioxide levels (*the Haldane effect*), which constricts blood vessels[887,888] and ironically, reduces tissue oxygenation[201-223] and the overall health status of patients.[889,890] In a 2010 study published in the British Medical Journal, patients with COPD receiving high-flow oxygen had significantly increased rates of mortality compared to the titrated oxygen group.[891] A 2016 study published in the Journal of the American Medical Association found that giving less oxygen to patients in intensive care units reduced mortality.[887] And animals administered 100% oxygen for just 1 hour had markedly worsened neurological outcomes than a control group of animals. Interestingly, the animals administered the excess of oxygen had increased oxidation of brain lipids (unsaturated fats) and increased neuronal cell death.[892]

In 1921, Dr. Henderson and his colleagues found that administering 8% carbon dioxide in air to patients after major surgical interventions facilitated a rapid return to consciousness and elimination of anesthetic.[893] "The cutaneous circulation improved. The skin changed in color and temperature, from blue- gray and cold to pink and warm. The volume of the pulse, previously thready, rapidly became full; and arterial pressure was restored to normal... Nausea and vomiting were either greatly reduced or entirely absent and after the inhalation the patient dropped off to sleep," wrote Henderson.[886]

Carbogen can stimulate the breathing of babies in hospitals at birth, and also the breathing of patients with respiratory failure following severe alcohol intoxication, drowning, electric shock; it can even reverse a deep coma caused by severe carbon monoxide poisoning.[894-897]

"Experience has demonstrated that the return of natural breathing is considerably aided and accelerated by the administration oxygen and carbon dioxide from an inhalator, while artificial respiration is being applied."
- Dr. Yandell Henderson

In dogs experimentally induced with pneumonia, their lungs were cleared and their pneumonia cured by putting them in closed chambers containing about 8% carbon dioxide in air for 12 to 24 hours, according to a study published in the *Archives of Internal Medicine* in 1930.[898] By 1932, these findings were widely adopted by the medical community and treatment of pneumonia in humans with carbogen had become common practice; "Many cases of pneumonia have now been treated with inhalation of CO2 in O2," wrote Dr. Henderson.[899]

Carbogen has clearly proven itself a highly-effective aid during emergency situations and in hospital settings and therefore, it's of high priority that rescue crews and hospitals worldwide are re-equipped with H-H Inhalators and the use of carbogen be permanently reinstated.

In addition to helping people in emergency situations, carbogen inhalation therapy has also been shown to potently suppress seizures in epileptic patients[940] and significantly improve recovery rates in patients with sudden hearing loss.[941] It has also been tested on people with cancer.

CARBON DIOXIDE THERAPY

Carbon dioxide is a potent anti-inflammatory substance[901-907] that reverses cancer growth by rapidly oxygenating cells and lowering carcinogenic substances within the extracellular matrix of tumors, including interleukin-1,[908] interleukin-1b,[909] interleukin-6,[908] interleukin-8,[908] nuclear factor-kappa b, [910,911] tumor necrosis-factor alpha,[912] nitric oxide,[913-915] free radicals,[916] cortisol,[917] prolactin,[918,919] lactic acid,[920-922] prostaglandins,[923,924] and histamine,[925] which in turn allows incoming stem cells to differentiate into healthy, replacement cells and complete the healing process.

When carbon dioxide levels are increased therapeutically, tumors shrink,[326-328,900] and cancer metastasis - the number one cause of cancer mortality[329-336] – is prevented.[75-77,337-341] There are a number of ways this can be accomplished.

CARBON DIOXIDE INJECTIONS

Japanese researchers experimented with carbon dioxide as a treatment for cancer in 2012 by directly injecting it into rat skin tumors at Kobe University School of Medicine. Published in the journal *PLOS one*, carbon dioxide injections were found to enrich cytochrome c oxidase activity, multiply the number of mitochondria in cells, trigger apoptosis in tumor cells and significantly reduce tumor volumes.[926] In 2014, researchers from the same university injected carbon dioxide into another type of skin tumor - squamous cell carcinoma - and found that it triggered cancer cell apoptosis and reduced the expression of hypoxia inducible factor 1-alpha (HIF-1α),[337] signifying tumor cells began receiving adequate oxygen.

CARBON DIOXIDE BATHS

The benefits of bathing in naturally carbonated springs or baths infused with carbon dioxide have long been known in Europe[337] and this type of therapy (balneotherapy) has been in use therapeutically since the Middle Ages.[927] Interestingly, carbon dioxide is readily absorbed through the skin; 100 times more powerfully than water.[934]

261

In 1997, German researchers from the University of Freiburg compared the effects of soaking the lower legs of people in either fresh water or in carbon dioxide enriched water (1200mg CO2 per kg water). While legs immersed in fresh water were found to have no increase in circulation and little increase in oxygen use, researchers discovered that circulation in legs immersed in carbon dioxide enriched water was enhanced by 300% and oxygen pressure within tissues was increased by 10%.[928] A number of other studies have confirmed that CO2-enriched baths significantly increase blood circulation and enhance cellular oxygenation.[929-933]

Slovakian researchers tested the effects of a series of 20 carbon dioxide baths on patients and assessed their health after the first, 10th and 20th sessions. Results confirmed that although the effects of the first bath were the most pronounced, "a series of carbon dioxide baths had a gradually improving effect."[935]

423 patients with high blood pressure were given a 4-week course of carbon dioxide baths to determine the effects on blood pressure in 1989. Patients were randomly assigned to baths containing either high or low concentrations of carbon dioxide and the results showed, "A significant fall in blood pressure, both at rest and during exercise was observed in both groups during the course of treatment."[936]

Japanese scientists tested the effects of carbon dioxide baths on the athletic performance of swimmers. Results showed that swimmers who underwent carbon dioxide baths prior to swimming had improved muscle performance, increased endurance and accumulated lower levels of lactic acid during their swim.[937]

For those looking to utilize carbon dioxide baths at home, it's useful to know that the CO2-enriched bathwater used in many of these studies was generated by adding products containing sodium bicarbonate and an acid to water; commonly known as *bath bombs*.

CARBOGEN INHALATION THERAPY

Scientists experimenting with the use of carbogen on cancer patients have confirmed its effectiveness for improving tumor oxygenation;[942-949] "This study confirms that breathing 2% CO2 and 98% O2 is well tolerated and effective in increasing tumour oxygenation."[950] In normal rats and in rats with implanted brain tumors, inhalation of 5% carbogen was found to increase brain tissue oxygenation by "at least 100%,"[951] and cancer patients administered 4 minutes of 100% oxygen, followed by 10 minutes of room air, and then 4 minutes of 5% carbogen had improved tumor oxygenation *by an average of 21-times.*[952]

Most of these studies were testing carbogen to see if it could improve the 'effectiveness' of either radiotherapy or chemotherapy, so there are no reports of the fate of a tumor following carbogen administration on its own - but by now we're well aware of what happens when carbon dioxide meets a tumor and its environment.

CAPNOMETRY

In recent years, the revival of Warburg's finding that cancer cells produce lactic acid as a result of aerobic glycolysis has inspired some doctors to begin measuring blood levels of lactic acid as a way of diagnosing cancer.[938]

Since healthy cells produce carbon dioxide and malfunctioning cells produce lactic acid - a person who is healthy will have high levels of carbon dioxide and low levels of lactic acid, while a person who is ill will have low levels of carbon dioxide and high levels of lactic acid; and therefore, blood levels of lactic acid and carbon dioxide are the two most accurate indicators of overall health.

As it turns out, the concentration of carbon dioxide present in the exhaled breath, which can be measured using a device called a capnometer, is an accurate way of determining arterial levels of carbon dioxide in the body[939] and can therefore be used by anyone, at home, to determine their overall level of health and as an assessment tool during disease treatment.

HEALTH RISING

If there is a creator of man and all of nature, and there seems to be no shortage of evidence for this, then it appears our creator has a plan. Prior to 1800, the concentrations of carbon dioxide in Earth's air were said to have been 280ppm[953] and in 2015, measurements revealed that the rising CO2 levels had officially surpassed the 400ppm (0.04%) mark. Remarkably, carbon dioxide concentrations in our air are not just rising - they're rising *exponentially.*[954-957]

And if that news wasn't good enough - the toxic, excessive levels of oxygen in our air have simultaneously been in exponential decline; 0.1% (1000ppm) over the past 100 years, according to a 2016 study by researchers from Princeton University.[958] Oxygen levels in all of the world's oceans are dropping at an even faster rate; a 2015 study published in nature found that oceanic oxygen levels have declined more than 2% since 1960.[959]

For those still uncomfortable with the idea that reduced oxygen is something beneficial for life - remember that less oxygen in our air means more carbon dioxide in our bodies, which drives oxygen into cells. Here are a few more fascinating examples to further illustrate this effect.

In the 1980's, Russian researchers transplanted tumors into rats and then took them to high altitudes to see the effects of hypoxia (reduced oxygen) on their recovery. These studies showed that hypoxic high-altitude environments inhibited tumor growth;[960] "It was shown in rat experiments that high-altitude hypoxia inhibits the growth of transplantable tumors..."[961] Furthermore, some of the rats in these studies were given chemotherapy, and not only did high-altitude hypoxia help them recover, but it significantly diminished the toxicity of the chemotherapy drugs.[960,961]

In 2011, scientists from Harvard Medical School studied the effects of hypoxia on tumor progression in vivo. After transplanting lung tumors into rats and then putting them in environments containing 10% oxygen for 14 days, researchers found that tumor growth and cancer metastasis were both significantly suppressed.[962]

While the beneficial effects of exponentially increasing carbon dioxide levels and exponentially decreasing oxygen levels in our environment are certainly being felt and make for a promising future, like the naked mole rat, frogs, bats, bees and many other living creatures, I think it's time we begin focusing our attention on how to optimize our environment even further. Identifying the ideal concentration of these two gases in air might be a good starting point.

THE END OF ALL DISEASE

Current carbon dioxide levels in sea level air are currently only 0.04% and oxygen levels are 21%;[963] an environment that Dr. Buteyko once called 'poisonous in its composition;' containing 10-times more oxygen and 250-times less carbon dioxide than what our bodies need. "...the cells of animals and humans need about 7% CO2 and only 2% O2 in the surrounding environment. This is the way our cells live: cells of the heart, brain, and kidneys," explained Dr. Buteyko.[413]

	Oxygen	Carbon Dioxide
Current Concentration	21%	0.04%
Target Concentration	2%	7%

Once the most efficient methods of achieving these environmental modifications have been realized and implemented, human beings, animals and nature will be virtually immune to the harmful effects of all environmental contaminants, and the day will soon follow when humankind witnesses an end to all suffering and disease.

Until then, that the people now have the understanding needed to heal themselves, independent of doctors and systems of healthcare, means they are free.

REFERENCES

1. Canadian Cancer Society. What is Cancer? [Online]. Available: https://www.cancer.gov/about-cancer/understanding/what-is-cancer. [March 1st, 2017].

2. Shay JW, Werbin H. Cytoplasmic suppression of tumorigenicity in reconstructed mouse cells. Cancer Res. 1988;48(4):830-3.

3. Israel BA, Schaeffer WI. Cytoplasmic suppression of malignancy. In Vitro Cell Dev Biol. 1987;23(9):627-32.

4. Howell AN, Sager R. Tumorigenicity and its suppression in cybrids of mouse and Chinese hamster cell lines. Proc Natl Acad Sci USA. 1978;75(5):2358-62.

5. Shay JW, Liu YN, Werbin H. Cytoplasmic suppression of tumor progression in reconstituted cells. Somat Cell Mol Genet. 1988;14(4):345-50.

6. Giguère L, Morais R. On suppression of tumorigenicity in hybrid and cybrid mouse cells. Somatic Cell Genet. 1981;7(4):457-71.

7. Koura M, Isaka H, Yoshida MC, Tosu M, Sekiguchi T. Suppression of tumorigenicity in interspecific reconstituted cells and cybrids. Gan. 1982;73(4):574-80.

8. Shay JW, Lorkowski G, Clark MA. Suppression of tumorigenicity in cybrids. J Supramol Struct Cell Biochem. 1981;16(1):75-82.

9. Israel BA, Schaeffer WI. Cytoplasmic mediation of malignancy. In Vitro Cell Dev Biol. 1988;24(5):487-90.

10. Mckinnell RG, Deggins BA, Labat DD. Transplantation of pluripotential nuclei from triploid frog tumors. Science. 1969;165(3891):394-6.

11. Li L, Connelly MC, Wetmore C, Curran T, Morgan JI. Mouse embryos cloned from brain tumors. Cancer Res. 2003;63(11):2733-6.

12. Rubin H. What keeps cells in tissues behaving normally in the face of myriad mutations?. Bioessays. 2006;28(5):515-24.

13. Nikolaou N, Green CJ, Gunn PJ, Hodson L, Tomlinson JW. Optimizing human hepatocyte models for metabolic phenotype and function: effects of treatment with dimethyl sulfoxide (DMSO). Physiol Rep. 2016;4(21).

14. Weaver VM, Petersen OW, Wang F, et al. Reversion of the malignant phenotype of human breast cells in three-dimensional culture and in vivo by integrin blocking antibodies. J Cell Biol. 1997;137(1):231-45.

15. Brinster RL. The effect of cells transferred into the mouse blastocyst on subsequent development. J Exp Med. 1974;140(4):1049-56.

16. Mintz B, Illmensee K. Normal genetically mosaic mice produced from malignant teratocarcinoma cells. Proc Natl Acad Sci USA. 1975;72(9):3585-9.

17. Milo GE, Shuler CF, Lee H, Casto BC. A conundrum in molecular toxicology: molecular and biological changes during neoplastic transformation of human cells. Cell Biol Toxicol. 1995;11(6):329-45.

18. Rous P. Surmise and fact on the nature of cancer. Nature. 1959;183(4672):1357-61.

19. Tomczak K, Czerwińska P, Wiznerowicz M. The Cancer Genome Atlas (TCGA): an immeasurable source of knowledge. Contemp Oncol (Pozn). 2015;19(1A):A68-77.

20. Kaiser J. Genomics. Billion-dollar cancer mapping project steps forward. Science. 2008;321(5885):26-7.

21. Poethig RS. Life with 25,000 genes. Genome Res. 2001;11(3):313-6.

22. Lee JS. Exploring cancer genomic data from the cancer genome atlas project. BMB Rep. 2016;49(11):607-611.

23. Greenman C, Stephens P, Smith R, et al. Patterns of somatic mutation in human cancer genomes. Nature. 2007;446(7132):153-8.

24. Loeb LA. A mutator phenotype in cancer. Cancer Res. 2001;61(8):3230-9.

25. Parsons DW, Jones S, Zhang X, et al. An integrated genomic analysis of human glioblastoma multiforme. Science. 2008;321(5897):1807-12.

26. Salk JJ, Fox EJ, Loeb LA. Mutational heterogeneity in human cancers: origin and consequences. Annu Rev Pathol. 2010;5:51-75.

27. Gibbs WW. Untangling the roots of cancer. Sci Am. 2003;289(1):56-65.

28. Steeg PS. Heterogeneity of drug target expression among metastatic lesions: lessons from a breast cancer autopsy program. Clin Cancer Res. 2008;14(12):3643-5.

29. Wu JM, Fackler MJ, Halushka MK, et al. Heterogeneity of breast cancer metastases: comparison of therapeutic target expression and promoter methylation between primary tumors and their multifocal metastases. Clin Cancer Res. 2008;14(7):1938-46.

30. Gabor miklos GL. The human cancer genome project--one more misstep in the war on cancer. Nat Biotechnol. 2005;23(5):535-7.

31. Stoecklein NH, Hosch SB, Bezler M, et al. Direct genetic analysis of single disseminated cancer cells for prediction of outcome and therapy selection in esophageal cancer. Cancer Cell. 2008;13(5):441-53.

32. The patterns and dynamics of genomic instability in metastatic pancreatic cancer. Nature. 2010;467(7319):1109.

33. Seyfried TN, Shelton LM. Cancer as a metabolic disease. Nutr Metab (Lond). 2010;7:7.

34. The cancer genome. Nature. 2009;458(7239):719.

35. Mandinova A, Lee SW. The p53 pathway as a target in cancer therapeutics: obstacles and promise. Sci Transl Med. 2011;3(64):64rv1.

36. Gravendeel LA, Kouwenhoven MC, Gevaert O, et al. Intrinsic gene expression profiles of gliomas are a better predictor of survival than histology. Cancer Res. 2009;69(23):9065-72.

37. Dang L, White DW, Gross S, et al. Cancer-associated IDH1 mutations produce 2-hydroxyglutarate. Nature. 2009;462(7274):739-44.

38. Agus, D. [TED]. (2010). David Agus: A New Strategy in the War Against Cancer. Available: https://www.youtube.com/watch?v=IRxgDMSp9Gs.[March 1, 2017].

39. Begley, S. (2013). DNA pioneer James Watson takes aim at "cancer establishments". [Online]. Available: http://www.reuters.com/article/us-usa-cancer-watson-idUSBRE90805N20130109.[March 1, 2017].

40. Luoto KR, Kumareswaran R, Bristow RG. Tumor hypoxia as a driving force in genetic instability. Genome Integr. 2013;4(1):5.

41. Kumareswaran R, Ludkovski O, Meng A, Sykes J, Pintilie M, Bristow RG. Chronic hypoxia compromises repair of DNA double-strand breaks to drive genetic instability. J Cell Sci. 2012;125(Pt 1):189-99.

42. Taiakina D, Dal pra A, Bristow RG. Intratumoral hypoxia as the genesis of genetic instability and clinical prognosis in prostate cancer. Adv Exp Med Biol. 2014;772:189-204.

43. Scanlon SE, Glazer PM. Multifaceted control of DNA repair pathways by the hypoxic tumor microenvironment. DNA Repair (Amst). 2015;32:180-9.

44. Chan N, Koch CJ, Bristow RG. Tumor hypoxia as a modifier of DNA strand break and cross-link repair. Curr Mol Med. 2009;9(4):401-10.

45. Chan N, Ali M, Mccallum GP, et al. Hypoxia provokes base excision repair changes and a repair-deficient, mutator phenotype in colorectal cancer cells. Mol Cancer Res. 2014;12(10):1407-15.

46. Meng AX, Jalali F, Cuddihy A, et al. Hypoxia down-regulates DNA double strand break repair gene expression in prostate cancer cells. Radiother Oncol. 2005;76(2):168-76.

47. Bristow RG, Hill RP. Hypoxia and metabolism. Hypoxia, DNA repair and genetic instability. Nat Rev Cancer. 2008;8(3):180-92.

48. Chan N, Bristow RG. "Contextual" synthetic lethality and/or loss of heterozygosity: tumor hypoxia and modification of DNA repair. Clin Cancer Res. 2010;16(18):4553-60.

49. Bindra RS, Crosby ME, Glazer PM. Regulation of DNA repair in hypoxic cancer cells. Cancer Metastasis Rev. 2007;26(2):249-60.

50. Bindra RS, Schaffer PJ, Meng A, et al. Down-regulation of Rad51 and decreased homologous recombination in hypoxic cancer cells. Mol Cell Biol. 2004;24(19):8504-18.

51. Bindra RS, Schaffer PJ, Meng A, et al. Alterations in DNA repair gene expression under hypoxia: elucidating the mechanisms of hypoxia-induced genetic instability. Ann N Y Acad Sci. 2005;1059:184-95.

52. Chan N, Pires IM, Bencokova Z, et al. Contextual synthetic lethality of cancer cell kill based on the tumor microenvironment. Cancer Res. 2010;70(20):8045-54.

53. Chan N, Milosevic M, Bristow RG. Tumor hypoxia, DNA repair and prostate cancer progression: new targets and new therapies. Future Oncol. 2007;3(3):329-41.

54. Bindra RS, Glazer PM. Genetic instability and the tumor microenvironment: towards the concept of microenvironment-induced mutagenesis. Mutat Res. 2005;569(1-2):75-85.

55. Wigerup C, Påhlman S, Bexell D. Therapeutic targeting of hypoxia and hypoxia-inducible factors in cancer. Pharmacol Ther. 2016;164:152-69.

56. Glazer PM, Hegan DC, Lu Y, Czochor J, Scanlon SE. Hypoxia and DNA repair. Yale J Biol Med. 2013;86(4):443-51.

57. Yoo YG, Hayashi M, Christensen J, Huang LE. An essential role of the HIF-1alpha-c-Myc axis in malignant progression. Ann N Y Acad Sci. 2009;1177:198-204.

58. Nowell PC. The clonal evolution of tumor cell populations. Science. 1976;194(4260):23-8.

59. Kaiser J. Combining targeted drugs to stop resistant tumors. Science. 2011;331(6024):1542-5.

60. Sonnenschein C, Soto AM. Somatic mutation theory of carcinogenesis: why it should be dropped and replaced. Mol Carcinog. 2000;29(4):205-11.

61. Ryan HE, Lo J, Johnson RS. HIF-1 alpha is required for solid tumor formation and embryonic vascularization. EMBO J. 1998;17(11):3005-15.

62. Ryan HE, Poloni M, Mcnulty W, et al. Hypoxia-inducible factor-1alpha is a positive factor in solid tumor growth. Cancer Res. 2000;60(15):4010-5.

63. Acker T, Plate KH. A role for hypoxia and hypoxia-inducible transcription factors in tumor physiology. J Mol Med. 2002;80(9):562-75.

64. Harris AL. Hypoxia--a key regulatory factor in tumour growth. Nat Rev Cancer. 2002;2(1):38-47.

65. Pullamsetti SS, Banat GA, Schmall A, et al. Phosphodiesterase-4 promotes proliferation and angiogenesis of lung cancer by crosstalk with HIF. Oncogene. 2013;32(9):1121-34.

66. Thienpont B, Steinbacher J, Zhao H, et al. Tumour hypoxia causes DNA hypermethylation by reducing TET activity. Nature. 2016;537(7618):63-68.

67. Dayan F, Mazure NM, Brahimi-horn MC, Pouysségur J. A dialogue between the hypoxia-inducible factor and the tumor microenvironment. Cancer Microenviron. 2008;1(1):53-68.

68. Ayyasamy V, Owens KM, Desouki MM, et al. Cellular model of Warburg effect identifies tumor promoting function of UCP2 in breast cancer and its suppression by genipin. PLoS ONE. 2011;6(9):e24792.

69. Seoane M, Mosquera-miguel A, Gonzalez T, Fraga M, Salas A, Costoya JA. The mitochondrial genome is a "genetic sanctuary" during the oncogenic process. PLoS ONE. 2011;6(8):e23327.

70. The Metabolism of Tumors. JAMA Otolaryngol Head Neck Surg. 2015;141(5):428.

71. Roskelley RC, Mayer N, Horwitt BN, Salter WT. STUDIES IN CANCER. VII. ENZYME DEFICIENCY IN HUMAN AND EXPERIMENTAL CANCER. J Clin Invest. 1943;22(5):743-51.

72. Brizel DM, Scully SP, Harrelson JM, et al. Tumor oxygenation predicts for the likelihood of distant metastases in human soft tissue sarcoma. Cancer Res. 1996;56(5):941-3.

73. Kunz M, Ibrahim SM. Molecular responses to hypoxia in tumor cells. Mol Cancer. 2003;2:23.

74. De jaeger K, Kavanagh MC, Hill RP. Relationship of hypoxia to metastatic ability in rodent tumours. Br J Cancer. 2001;84(9):1280-5.

75. Denko NC, Fontana LA, Hudson KM, et al. Investigating hypoxic tumor physiology through gene expression patterns. Oncogene. 2003;22(37):5907-14.

76. Semenza GL. Hypoxia-inducible factors: mediators of cancer progression and targets for cancer therapy. Trends Pharmacol Sci. 2012;33(4):207-14.

77. Burroughs SK, Kaluz S, Wang D, Wang K, Van meir EG, Wang B. Hypoxia inducible factor pathway inhibitors as anticancer therapeutics. Future Med Chem. 2013;5(5):553-72.

78. Onnis B, Rapisarda A, Melillo G. Development of HIF-1 inhibitors for cancer therapy. J Cell Mol Med. 2009;13(9A):2780-6.

79. Xia Y, Choi HK, Lee K. Recent advances in hypoxia-inducible factor (HIF)-1 inhibitors. Eur J Med Chem. 2012;49:24-40.

80. Melillo G. Inhibiting hypoxia-inducible factor 1 for cancer therapy. Mol Cancer Res. 2006;4(9):601-5.

81. Marín-hernández A, Gallardo-pérez JC, Ralph SJ, Rodríguez-enríquez S, Moreno-sánchez R. HIF-1alpha modulates energy metabolism in cancer cells by inducing over-expression of specific glycolytic isoforms. Mini Rev Med Chem. 2009;9(9):1084-101.

82. Porporato PE, Dhup S, Dadhich RK, Copetti T, Sonveaux P. Anticancer targets in the glycolytic metabolism of tumors: a comprehensive review. Front Pharmacol. 2011;2:49.

83. Guzy RD, Schumacker PT. Oxygen sensing by mitochondria at complex III: the paradox of increased reactive oxygen species during hypoxia. Exp Physiol. 2006;91(5):807-19.

84. Favier J, Brière JJ, Burnichon N, et al. The Warburg effect is genetically determined in inherited pheochromocytomas. PLoS ONE. 2009;4(9):e7094.

85. Semenza GL. HIF-1 mediates the Warburg effect in clear cell renal carcinoma. J Bioenerg Biomembr. 2007;39(3):231-4.

86. Dang CV, Semenza GL. Oncogenic alterations of metabolism. Trends Biochem Sci. 1999;24(2):68-72.

87. Denko NC. Hypoxia, HIF1 and glucose metabolism in the solid tumour. Nat Rev Cancer. 2008;8(9):705-13.

88. Vander heiden MG, Cantley LC, Thompson CB. Understanding the Warburg effect: the metabolic requirements of cell proliferation. Science. 2009;324(5930):1029-33.

89. Semenza GL. Oxygen-dependent regulation of mitochondrial respiration by hypoxia-inducible factor 1. Biochem J. 2007;405(1):1-9.

90. Fang J, Yan L, Shing Y, Moses MA. HIF-1alpha-mediated up-regulation of vascular endothelial growth factor, independent of basic fibroblast growth factor, is important in the switch to the angiogenic phenotype during early tumorigenesis. Cancer Res. 2001;61(15):5731-5.

91. Tsuzuki Y, Fukumura D, Oosthuyse B, Koike C, Carmeliet P, Jain RK. Vascular endothelial growth factor (VEGF) modulation by targeting hypoxia-inducible factor-1alpha--> hypoxia response element--> VEGF cascade differentially regulates vascular response and growth rate in tumors. Cancer Res. 2000;60(22):6248-52.

92. Mazure NM, Brahimi-horn MC, Pouysségur J. Protein kinases and the hypoxia-inducible factor-1, two switches in angiogenesis. Curr Pharm Des. 2003;9(7):531-41.

93. Vandenbunder B. [Hypoxia and tumors: does HIF-1 transcription factor favor tumor growth or hypoxia?]. Bull Cancer. 1998;85(10):843-5.

94. Büchler P, Reber HA, Büchler M, et al. Hypoxia-inducible factor 1 regulates vascular endothelial growth factor expression in human pancreatic cancer. Pancreas. 2003;26(1):56-64.

95. Choi KS, Bae MK, Jeong JW, Moon HE, Kim KW. Hypoxia-induced angiogenesis during carcinogenesis. J Biochem Mol Biol. 2003;36(1):120-7.

96. Francis, R. 2011. Never Fear Cancer Again: How to Prevent and Reverse Cancer. HCI. 384ps.

97. Bianconi E, Piovesan A, Facchin F, et al. An estimation of the number of cells in the human body. Ann Hum Biol. 2013;40(6):463-71.

98. Jang M, Kim SS, Lee J. Cancer cell metabolism: implications for therapeutic targets. Exp Mol Med. 2013;45:e45.

99. Jurtshuk, P Jr. 1996. Medical Microbiology: 4th Edition. The University of Texas Medical Branch at Galveston.

100. Zheng J. Energy metabolism of cancer: Glycolysis versus oxidative phosphorylation (Review). Oncol Lett. 2012;4(6):1151-1157.

101. Rogatzki MJ, Ferguson BS, Goodwin ML, Gladden LB. Lactate is always the end product of glycolysis. Front Neurosci. 2015;9:22.

102. Carpenter KLH, Jalloh I, Hutchinson JP. Glycolysis and the significant of lactate in traumatic brain injury. Front. Neuro. 2015.

103. Sahlin K, Katz A, Henriksson J. Redox state and lactate accumulation in human skeletal muscle during dynamic exercise. Biochem J. 1987;245(2):551-6.

104. Katz A, Sahlin K. Regulation of lactic acid production during exercise. J Appl Physiol. 1988;65(2):509-18.

105. Sahlin K. Muscle energetics during explosive activities and potential effects of nutrition and training. Sports Med. 2014;44 Suppl 2:S167-73.

106. Ishii H, Nishida Y. Effect of Lactate Accumulation during Exercise-induced Muscle Fatigue on the Sensorimotor Cortex. J Phys Ther Sci. 2013;25(12):1637-42.

107. Ghosh AK. Anaerobic threshold: its concept and role in endurance sport. Malays J Med Sci. 2004;11(1):24-36.

108. Faude O, Kindermann W, Meyer T. Lactate threshold concepts: how valid are they?. Sports Med. 2009;39(6):469-90.

109. Warburg O. Uber den Stoffwechsel der Hefe.pp252-254.

110. Alberts B, Johnson A, Lewis J, et al. 2002. Molecular Biology of the Cell: 4th Edition. New York. Garland Science.

111. Archetti M. Evolutionary dynamics of the Warburg effect: glycolysis as a collective action problem among cancer cells. J Theor Biol. 2014;341:1-8.

112. Phan LM, Yeung SC, Lee MH. Cancer metabolic reprogramming: importance, main features, and potentials for precise targeted anti-cancer therapies. Cancer Biol Med. 2014;11(1):1-19.

113. Chen X, Qian Y, Wu S. The Warburg effect: evolving interpretations of an established concept. Free Radic Biol Med. 2015;79:253-63.

114. Ganapathy-kanniappan S, Geschwind JF. Tumor glycolysis as a target for cancer therapy: progress and prospects. Mol Cancer. 2013;12:152.

115. Gatenby RA, Gillies RJ. Why do cancers have high aerobic glycolysis?. Nat Rev Cancer. 2004;4(11):891-9.

116. Gatenby RA, Gawlinski ET. The glycolytic phenotype in carcinogenesis and tumor invasion: insights through mathematical models. Cancer Res. 2003;63(14):3847-54.

117. Lincet H, Icard P. How do glycolytic enzymes favour cancer cell proliferation by nonmetabolic functions?. Oncogene. 2015;34(29):3751-9.

118. Masson N, Ratcliffe PJ. Hypoxia signaling pathways in cancer metabolism: the importance of co-selecting interconnected physiological pathways. Cancer Metab. 2014;2(1):3.

119. Poliakov E, Managadze D, Rogozin IB. Generalized portrait of cancer metabolic pathways inferred from a list of genes overexpressed in cancer. Genet Res Int. 2014;2014:646193.

120. Lipid metabolic reprogramming in cancer cells. Oncogenesis. 2016;5(1):e189.

121. Dart A. Tumour metabolism: Lactic acid: not just a waste product?. Nat Rev Cancer. 2016;16(11):676-677.

122. Annibaldi A, Widmann C. Glucose metabolism in cancer cells. Curr Opin Clin Nutr Metab Care. 2010;13(4):466-70.

123. Cantor JR, Sabatini DM. Cancer cell metabolism: one hallmark, many faces. Cancer Discov. 2012;2(10):881-98.

124. Ward PS, Thompson CB. Metabolic reprogramming: a cancer hallmark even warburg did not anticipate. Cancer Cell. 2012;21(3):297-308.

125. Phan LM, Yeung SC, Lee MH. Cancer metabolic reprogramming: importance, main features, and potentials for precise targeted anti-cancer therapies. Cancer Biol Med. 2014;11(1):1-19.

126. Fischer K, Hoffmann P, Voelkl S, et al. Inhibitory effect of tumor cell-derived lactic acid on human T cells. Blood. 2007;109(9):3812-9.

127. Mothersill C, Seymour CB, Moriarty M. Lactate-mediated changes in growth morphology and transformation frequency of irradiated C3H 10T1/2 cells. Cell Biol Int Rep. 1983;7(11):971-80.

128. San-millán I, Brooks GA. Reexamining cancer metabolism: lactate production for carcinogenesis could be the purpose and explanation of the Warburg Effect. Carcinogenesis. 2016.

129. Olsson M, Ho HP, Annerbrink K, Thylefors J, Eriksson E. Respiratory responses to intravenous infusion of sodium lactate in male and female Wistar rats. Neuropsychopharmacology. 2002;27(1):85-91.

130. Liebowitz MR, Gorman JM, Fyer AJ, et al. Lactate provocation of panic attacks. II. Biochemical and physiological findings. Arch Gen Psychiatry. 1985;42(7):709-19.

131. Gorman JM, Cohen BS, Liebowitz MR, Fyer AJ, Ross D, Davies SO, Klein DF. Blood Gas Changes and Hypophosphatemia in Lactate-Induced Panic. Arch Gen Psychiatry. 1986;43(11):1067-1071.

132. Jack M. Gorman, Raymond R. Goetz, Judy Uy, Donald Ross, Jose Martinez, Abby J. Fyer, Michael R. Liebowitz, Donald F. Klein. Hyperventilation occurs during lactate-induced panic. Journal of Anxiety Disorders, Volume 2, Issue 3, Pages 193-202.

133. Raichle ME, Plum F. Hyperventilation and cerebral blood flow. Stroke. 1972;3(5):566-75.

134. Naschitz JE, Mussafia-priselac R, Peck ER, et al. Hyperventilation and amplified blood pressure response: is there a link?. J Hum Hypertens. 2005;19(5):381-7.

135. Hayashi K, Fujikawa M, Sawa T. Hyperventilation-induced hypocapnia changes the pattern of electroencephalographic bicoherence growth during sevoflurane anaesthesia. Br J Anaesth. 2008;101(5):666-72.

136. Chin LM, Leigh RJ, Heigenhauser GJ, Rossiter HB, Paterson DH, Kowalchuk JM. Hyperventilation-induced hypocapnic alkalosis slows the adaptation of pulmonary O_2 uptake during the transition to moderate-intensity exercise. J Physiol (Lond). 2007;583(Pt 1):351-64.

137. Meuret AE, Ritz T. Hyperventilation in panic disorder and asthma: empirical evidence and clinical strategies. Int J Psychophysiol. 2010;78(1):68-79.

138. Ter avest E, Patist FM, Ter maaten JC, Nijsten MW. Elevated lactate during psychogenic hyperventilation. Emerg Med J. 2011;28(4):269-73.

139. Learn Buteyko. (2011). Learn Buteyko Presentation Part 1. Available: https://www.youtube.com/watch?v=h-WvOFfgmZs.[March 1, 2017].

140. Puybasset L, Stewart T, Rouby JJ, et al. Inhaled nitric oxide reverses the increase in pulmonary vascular resistance induced by permissive hypercapnia in patients with acute respiratory distress syndrome. Anesthesiology. 1994;80(6):1254-67.

141. Lam AM, Artru AA. Autoregulation of cerebral blood flow in response to adenosine-induced hypotension in dogs. J Neurosurg Anesthesiol. 1992;4(2):120-7.

142. Buteyko KP & Shurgal SI, Functional diagnostic of coronary disease. In: Surgical treatment of the coronary disease (in Russian), Moscow, 1965: p. 117-118.

143. Sinichenko VV, Leschenko GY, Melekhin VD, Emotional-volitional training in complex treatment of patients with rheumatoid arthritis (in Russian), Therap Arch 1990, 62: p. 58-61.

144. Breathing Retraining Center. History of the Buteyko Breathing Technique. [Online]. Available: http://www.breathingretrainingcenter.com/history-of-buteyko.php.[March 1, 2017].

145. Bowler SD, Green A, Mitchell CA. Buteyko breathing techniques in asthma: a blinded randomised controlled trial. Med J Aust. 1998;169(11-12):575-8.

146. Mchugh P, Aitcheson F, Duncan B, Houghton F. Buteyko Breathing Technique for asthma: an effective intervention. N Z Med J. 2003;116(1187):U710.

147. Cooper S, Oborne J, Newton S, et al. Effect of two breathing exercises (Buteyko and pranayama) in asthma: a randomised controlled trial. Thorax. 2003;58(8):674-9.

148. Mchugh P, Duncan B, Houghton F. Buteyko breathing technique and asthma in children: a case series. N Z Med J. 2006;119(1234):U1988.

149. Cowie RL, Conley DP, Underwood MF, Reader PG. A randomised controlled trial of the Buteyko technique as an adjunct to conventional management of asthma. Respir Med. 2008;102(5):726-32.

150. Hassan ZM, Riad NM, Ahmed FH. Effect of Buteyko breathing technique on patients with bronchial asthma. 2012;61(4):235-241.

CANCER CURED

151. Ravinder N, Bhaduri SN, Ajita M. A study of the effects of Buteyko Breathing Technique on Asthmatic Patients. Ind. J. Phys. & Occ. Ther. 2012;6(4):224-228.

152. Adelola OA, Oosthuizen JC, Oosthuiven JC, Fenton JE. Role of Buteyko breathing technique in asthmatics with nasal symptoms. Clin Otolaryngol. 2013;38(2):190-1.

153. Altukhov, S. (2009). 150 Diseases of Deep Breathing. Doctor Buteyko's Discovery Trilogy. [Online]. Available: http://www.doctorbuteykodiscoverytrilogy.com/150-diseases-of-deep-breathing.php.[March 1, 2017].

154. Matsumoto A, Itoh H, Eto Y, et al. End-tidal CO2 pressure decreases during exercise in cardiac patients: association with severity of heart failure and cardiac output reserve. J Am Coll Cardiol. 2000;36(1):242-9.

155. Dimopoulou I, Tsintzas OK, Alivizatos PA, Tzelepis GE. Pattern of breathing during progressive exercise in chronic heart failure. Int J Cardiol. 2001;81(2-3):117-21.

156. Johnson BD, Beck KC, Olson LJ, et al. Ventilatory constraints during exercise in patients with chronic heart failure. Chest. 2000;117(2):321-32.

157. Fanfulla F, Mortara A, Maestri R, et al. The development of hyperventilation in patients with chronic heart failure and Cheyne-Strokes respiration: a possible role of chronic hypoxia. Chest. 1998;114(4):1083-90.

158. Clark AL, Volterrani M, Swan JW, Coats AJ. The increased ventilatory response to exercise in chronic heart failure: relation to pulmonary pathology. Heart. 1997;77(2):138-46.

159. Banning AP, Lewis NP, Northridge DB, Elborn JS, Hendersen AH. Perfusion/ventilation mismatch during exercise in chronic heart failure: an investigation of circulatory determinants. Br Heart J. 1995;74(1):27-33.

160. Clark AL, Chua TP, Coats AJ. Anatomical dead space, ventilatory pattern, and exercise capacity in chronic heart failure. Br Heart J. 1995;74(4):377-80.

161. Buller NP, Poole-wilson PA. Mechanism of the increased ventilatory response to exercise in patients with chronic heart failure. Br Heart J. 1990;63(5):281-3.

162. Elborn JS, Riley M, Stanford CF, Nicholls DP. The effects of flosequinan on submaximal exercise in patients with chronic cardiac failure. Br J Clin Pharmacol. 1990;29(5):519-24.

163. Bottini P, Dottorini ML, Cristina cordoni M, Casucci G, Tantucci C. Sleep-disordered breathing in nonobese diabetic subjects with autonomic neuropathy. Eur Respir J. 2003;22(4):654-60.

164. Tantucci C, Bottini P, Fiorani C, et al. Cerebrovascular reactivity and hypercapnic respiratory drive in diabetic autonomic neuropathy. J Appl Physiol. 2001;90(3):889-96.

165. Mancini M, Filippelli M, Seghieri G, et al. Respiratory muscle function and hypoxic ventilatory control in patients with type I diabetes. Chest. 1999;115(6):1553-62.

166. Tantucci C, Scionti L, Bottini P, et al. Influence of autonomic neuropathy of different severities on the hypercapnic drive to breathing in diabetic patients. Chest. 1997;112(1):145-53.

167. Tantucci C, Bottini P, Dottorini ML, et al. Ventilatory response to exercise in diabetic subjects with autonomic neuropathy. J Appl Physiol. 1996;81(5):1978-86.

168. Chalupa DC, Morrow PE, Oberdörster G, Utell MJ, Frampton MW. Ultrafine particle deposition in subjects with asthma. Environ Health Perspect. 2004;112(8):879-82.

169. Johnson BD, Scanlon PD, Beck KC. Regulation of ventilatory capacity during exercise in asthmatics. J Appl Physiol. 1995;79(3):892-901.

170. Kassabian J, Miller KD, Lavietes MH. Respiratory center output and ventilatory timing in patients with acute airway (asthma) and alveolar (pneumonia) disease. Chest. 1982;81(5):536-43.

171. Mcfadden ER, Lyons HA. Arterial-blood gas tension in asthma. N Engl J Med. 1968;278(19):1027-32.

172. Palange P, Valli G, Onorati P, et al. Effect of heliox on lung dynamic hyperinflation, dyspnea, and exercise endurance capacity in COPD patients. J Appl Physiol. 2004;97(5):1637-42.

173. Sinderby C, Spahija J, Beck J, et al. Diaphragm activation during exercise in chronic obstructive pulmonary disease. Am J Respir Crit Care Med. 2001;163(7):1637-41.

174. Stulbarg MS, Winn WR, Kellett LE. Bilateral carotid body resection for the relief of dyspnea in severe chronic obstructive pulmonary disease. Physiologic and clinical observations in three patients. Chest. 1989;95(5):1123-8.

175. Radwan L, Maszczyk Z, Koziorowski A, et al. Control of breathing in obstructive sleep apnoea and in patients with the overlap syndrome. Eur Respir J. 1995;8(4):542-5.

176. Fauroux B, Nicot F, Boelle PY, et al. Mechanical limitation during CO2 rebreathing in young patients with cystic fibrosis. Respir Physiol Neurobiol. 2006;153(3):217-25.

177. Browning IB, D'alonzo GE, Tobin MJ. Importance of respiratory rate as an indicator of respiratory dysfunction in patients with cystic fibrosis. Chest. 1990;97(6):1317-21.

178. Ward SA, Tomezsko JL, Holsclaw DS, Paolone AM. Energy expenditure and substrate utilization in adults with cystic fibrosis and diabetes mellitus. Am J Clin Nutr. 1999;69(5):913-9.

179. Dodd JD, Barry SC, Barry RB, Gallagher CG, Skehan SJ, Masterson JB. Thin-section CT in patients with cystic fibrosis: correlation with peak exercise capacity and body mass index. Radiology. 2006;240(1):236-45.

180. Mckone EF, Barry SC, Fitzgerald MX, Gallagher CG. Role of arterial hypoxemia and pulmonary mechanics in exercise limitation in adults with cystic fibrosis. J Appl Physiol. 2005;99(3):1012-8.

181. Bell SC, Saunders MJ, Elborn JS, Shale DJ. Resting energy expenditure and oxygen cost of breathing in patients with cystic fibrosis. Thorax. 1996;51(2):126-31.

182. Tepper RS, Skatrud JB, Dempsey JA. Ventilation and oxygenation changes during sleep in cystic fibrosis. Chest. 1983;84(4):388-93.

183. Mackinnon DF, Craighead B, Hoehn-saric R. Carbon dioxide provocation of anxiety and respiratory response in bipolar disorder. J Affect Disord. 2007;99(1-3):45-9.

184. Pain MC, Biddle N, Tiller JW. Panic disorder, the ventilatory response to carbon dioxide and respiratory variables. Psychosom Med. 1988;50(5):541-8.

185. Esquivel E, Chaussain M, Plouin P, Ponsot G, Arthuis M. Physical exercise and voluntary hyperventilation in childhood absence epilepsy. Electroencephalogr Clin Neurophysiol. 1991;79(2):127-32.

186. Travers J, Dudgeon DJ, Amjadi K, et al. Mechanisms of exertional dyspnea in patients with cancer. J Appl Physiol. 2008;104(1):57-66.

187. Paschenko SN. Study of application of the shallow breathing method in combined treatment of breast cancer. Oncology. 2001;3(1):77-78.

188. Rakhimov, A. References for Table (Minute Ventilation in Normal Subjects). [Online]. Available: http://www.normalbreathing.com/refer-table-normals.php.[March 1, 2017].

189. Leong DP, Teo KK, Rangarajan S, et al. Prognostic value of grip strength: findings from the Prospective Urban Rural Epidemiology (PURE) study. Lancet. 2015;386(9990):266-73.

190. Vogt BP, Borges MCC, de Goes CR, Costa J, Caramori T. Handgrip strength is an independent predictor of all-cause mortality in maintenance dialysis patients. Clinical Nutrition. 2016;35(6):1429-1433.

191. Rantanen T, Volpato S, Ferrucci L, Heikkinen E, Fried LP, Guralnik JM. Handgrip strength and cause-specific and total mortality in older disabled women: exploring the mechanism. J Am Geriatr Soc. 2003;51(5):636-41.

192. Rantanen T, Harris T, Leveille SG, et al. Muscle strength and body mass index as long-term predictors of mortality in initially healthy men. J Gerontol A Biol Sci Med Sci. 2000;55(3):M168-73.

193. Metter EJ, Talbot LA, Schrager M, Conwit R. Skeletal muscle strength as a predictor of all-cause mortality in healthy men. J Gerontol A Biol Sci Med Sci. 2002;57(10):B359-65.

194. Fain E, Weatherford C. Comparative study of millennials' (age 20-34 years) grip and lateral pinch with the norms. J Hand Ther. 2016;29(4):483-488.

195. Raichle ME, Posner JB, Plum F. Cerebral blood flow during and after hyperventilation. Arch Neurol. 1970;23(5):394-403.

196. Alterations in Cerebral Blood Flow and Oxygen Consumption during Prolonged Hypocarbia. Pediatric Research. 1986;20(2):147.

197. Voors AW, Johnson WD. Altitude and arteriosclerotic heart disease mortality in white residents of 99 of the 100 largest cities in the united states. J Clin. Epid. 1979;32(1-2):157-162.

198. Poyart CF, Bursaux E. [Current conception of the Bohr effect]. Poumon Coeur. 1975;31(4):173-7.

199. Tyuma I. The Bohr effect and the Haldane effect in human hemoglobin. Jpn J Physiol. 1984;34(2):205-16.

200. Kilmartin JV. The Bohr effect of human hemoglobin. Trends in Bio. Sci. 1977;2(11):247-249.

201. Brown EB, Physiological effects of hyperventilation 1953, Physiol Rev 33:445-471.

202. Kennealy JA, McLennan JE, Loudon RG, McLaurin RL, Hyperventilation-induced cerebral hypoxia, Am Rev Respir Dis 1980, 122: p. 407-412.

203. Wilson DF, Pastuszko A, Digiacomo JE, Pawlowski M, Schneiderman R, Delivoria-papadopoulos M. Effect of hyperventilation on oxygenation of the brain cortex of newborn piglets. J Appl Physiol. 1991;70(6):2691-6.

204. Liem KD, Kollee LA, Hopman JC, De Haan AF, Oeseburg B, The influence of arterial carbon dioxide on cerebral oxygenation and hemodynamics during ECMO in normoxaemic and hypoxaemic piglets, Acta Anaesthesiolica Scandanavica Supplement, 1995; 107: p.157-164.

205. Lum LC, Hyperventilation: The Tip and the Iceberg, Journal of Psychosomatic Research, 1975, Vol. 19, pp. 375-383.

206. Lum LC, Hyperventilation and Anxiety State, Journal of the Royal Society of Medicine, 1981 (74) 1-4.

207. Macey PM, Woo MA, Harper RM, Hyperoxic brain effects are normalized by addition of CO2, PLoS Medicine, 2007 May; 4(5): p. e173.

208. Litchfield PM, A brief overview of the chemistry of respiration and the breathing heart wave, California Biofeedback, 2003 Spring, 19(1).

209. Santiago T V & Edelman NH, Brain blood flow and control of breathing, in Handbook of Physiology, Sect ion 3: The respiratory system, vol. II, ed. by AP Fishman. American Physiological Society, Betheda, Maryland, 1986, p. 163-179.

210. Skippen P, Seear M, Poskitt K, et al. Effect of hyperventilation on regional cerebral blood flow in head-injured children. Crit Care Med 1997, 25: p. 1402-1409.

211. Starling E & Lovatt EC, Principles of human physiology, 14th ed., 1968, Lea & Febiger, Philadelphia.

212. Tsuda Y, Kimura K, Yoneda S, Hartmann A, Etani H, Hashikawa K, Kamada T, Effect of hypocapnia on cerebral oxygen metabolism and blood flow in ischemic cerebrovascular disorders, Eur Neurol. 1987; 27(3): p.155-163.

213. Foex P, Ryder WA, Effect of CO2 on the systemic and coronary circulations and on coronary sinus blood gas tensions, Bulletin of European Physiopathology and Respirology, 1979 Jul-Aug; 15(4): p.625-638.

214. Karlsson T, St jernström EL, St jernström H, Norlén K, Wiklund L, Central and regional blood flow during hyperventilation. An experimental study in the pig, Act a Anaesthesiol Scand. 1994 Feb; 38(2): p.180-186.

215. Okazaki K, Hashimoto K, Okutsu Y, Okumura F, Effect of arterial carbon dioxide tension on regional myocardial tissue oxygen tension in the dog [Article in Japanese], Masui, 1991 Nov; 40(11): p. 1620-1624.

216. Okazaki K, Hashimoto K, Okutsu Y, Okumura F, Effect of carbon dioxide (hypocapnia and hypercapnia) on regional myocardial tissue oxygen tension in dogs with coronary stenosis [Article in Japanese], Masui, 1992 Feb; 41(2): p. 221-224.

217. Wexels JC, Myhre ES, Mjos OD, Effects of carbon dioxide and pH on myocardial blood-flow and metabolism in the dog, Clin Physiol. 1985 Dec; 5(6): p.575-588.

218. Fujita Y, Sakai T, Ohsumi A, Takaori M, Effects of hypocapnia and hypercapnia on splanchnic circulation and hepatic function in the beagle, Anesthesia and Analgesia, 1989 Aug; 69(2): p. 152-157.

219. Hughes RL, Mathie RT, Fitch W, Campbell D, Liver blood flow and oxygen consumption during hypocapnia and IPPV in the greyhound, Journal of Applied Physiology, 1979 Aug; 47(2): p. 290-295.

220. Okazaki K, Okutsu Y, Fukunaga A, Effect of carbon dioxide (hypocapnia and hypercapnia) on tissue blood flow and oxygenation of liver, kidneys and skeletal muscle in the dog, Masui, 1989 Apr, 38 (4): p. 457-464.

221. Guzman JA, Kruse JA. Gut mucosal-arterial PCO2 gradient as an indicator of splanchnic perfusion during systemic hypo- and hypercapnia, Crit Care Med 1999; 27: p. 2760-2765.

222. Laffey JG & Kavanagh BP, Hypocapnia, New England Journal of Medicine 2002, 347(1) 43-53.

223. Nunn JF. Applied respiratory physiology, 1987, 3rd ed. London: Butterworths.

224. Zhang S, Yang C, Yang Z, et al. Homeostasis of redox status derived from glucose metabolic pathway could be the key to understanding the Warburg effect. Am J Cancer Res. 2015;5(3):928-44.

225. Zastre JA, Sweet RL, Hanberry BS, Ye S. Linking vitamin B1 with cancer cell metabolism. Cancer Metab. 2013;1(1):16.

226. Raschke M, Bürkle L, Müller N, et al. Vitamin B1 biosynthesis in plants requires the essential iron sulfur cluster protein, THIC. Proc Natl Acad Sci USA. 2007;104(49):19637-42.

227. Naito E, Ito M, Yokota I, Saijo T, Ogawa Y, Kuroda Y. Diagnosis and molecular analysis of three male patients with thiamine-responsive pyruvate dehydrogenase complex deficiency. J Neurol Sci. 2002;201(1-2):33-7.

228. Naito E, Ito M, Yokota I, et al. Thiamine-responsive pyruvate dehydrogenase deficiency in two patients caused by a point mutation (F205L and L216F) within the thiamine pyrophosphate binding region. Biochim Biophys Acta. 2002;1588(1):79-84.

229. Lee EH, Ahn MS, Hwang JS, Ryu KH, Kim SJ, Kim SH. A Korean female patient with thiamine-responsive pyruvate dehydrogenase complex deficiency due to a novel point mutation (Y161C)in the PDHA1 gene. J Korean Med Sci. 2006;21(5):800-4.

230. Lu'o'ng Kv, Nguyên LT. Thiamine and Parkinson's disease. J Neurol Sci. 2012;316(1-2):1-8.

231. Luong KV, Nguyễn LT. The beneficial role of thiamine in Parkinson disease. CNS Neurosci Ther. 2013;19(7):461-8.

232. Dinicolantonio JJ, Niazi AK, Lavie CJ, O'keefe JH, Ventura HO. Thiamine supplementation for the treatment of heart failure: a review of the literature. Congest Heart Fail. 2013;19(4):214-22.

233. Dinicolantonio JJ, Lavie CJ, Niazi AK, O'keefe JH, Hu T. Effects of thiamine on cardiac function in patients with systolic heart failure: systematic review and metaanalysis of randomized, double-blind, placebo-controlled trials. Ochsner J. 2013;13(4):495-9.

234. Seligmann H, Halkin H, Rauchfleisch S, et al. Thiamine deficiency in patients with congestive heart failure receiving long-term furosemide therapy: a pilot study. Am J Med. 1991;91(2):151-5.

235. Rouzet P, Rubie H, Robert A, et al. [Severe hyperlactacidemia in 2 children treated for malignant tumors. Role of vitamin B1]. Arch Fr Pediatr. 1991;48(6):423-6.

236. Rovelli A, Bonomi M, Murano A, Locasciulli A, Uderzo C. Severe lactic acidosis due to thiamine deficiency after bone marrow transplantation in a child with acute monocytic leukemia. Haematologica. 1990;75(6):579-81.

237. Lu'o'ng KV, Nguyễn LT. The role of thiamine in cancer: possible genetic and cellular signaling mechanisms. Cancer Genomics Proteomics. 2013;10(4):169-85.

238. Van zaanen HC, Van der lelie J. Thiamine deficiency in hematologic malignant tumors. Cancer. 1992;69(7):1710-3.

239. Trebukhina RV, Ostrovsky YM, Shapot VS, Mikhaltsevich GN, Tumanov VN. Turnover of [14C]thiamin and activities of thiamin pyrophosphate-dependent enzymes in tissues of mice with Ehrlich ascites carcinoma. Nutr Cancer. 1984;6(4):260-73.

240. Bartley JC, Mcgrath H, Abraham S. Glucose and acetate utilization by hyperplastic, alveolar nodule outgrowths and adenocarcinomas of mouse mammary gland. Cancer Res. 1971;31(5):527-37.

241. Basu TK, Dickerson JW, Raven RW, Williams DC. The thiamine status of patients with cancer as determined by the red cell transketolase activity. Int J Vitam Nutr Res. 1974;44(1):53-8.

242. Seligmann H, Levi R, Konijn AM, Prokocimer M. Thiamine deficiency in patients with B-chronic lymphocytic leukaemia: a pilot study. Postgrad Med J. 2001;77(911):582-5.

243. Kaul L, Heshmat MY, Kovi J, et al. The role of diet in prostate cancer. Nutr Cancer. 1987;9(2-3):123-8.

244. Warburg O, Geissler AW, Lorenz S. [Genesis of tumor metabolism by vitamin B1 deficiency (thiamine deficiency)]. Z Naturforsch B. 1970;25(3):332-3.

245. Roche TE, Hiromasa Y. Pyruvate dehydrogenase kinase regulatory mechanisms and inhibition in treating diabetes, heart ischemia, and cancer. Cell Mol Life Sci. 2007;64(7-8):830-49.

246. Bettendorff L. Thiamin. In: Erdman JW, Macdonald IA, Zeisel SH, eds. Present Knowledge in Nutrition. 10th ed. Washington, DC: Wiley-Blackwell; 2012:261-79.

247. Said HM. Thiamin. In: Coates PM, Betz JM, Blackman MR, et al., eds. Encyclopedia of Dietary Supplements. 2nd ed. London and New York: Informa Healthcare; 2010:748-53.

248. De reuck JL, Sieben GJ, Sieben-praet MR, Ngendahayo P, De coster WJ, Vander eecken HM. Wernicke's encephalopathy in patients with tumors of the lymphoid-hemopoietic systems. Arch Neurol. 1980;37(6):338-41.

249. Basu TK, Dickerson JW. The thiamin status of early cancer patients with particular reference to those with breast and bronchial carcinomas. Oncology. 1976;33(5-6):250-2.

250. Goethart G. The thiamine pyrophosphate content of centrifugally-prepared fractions of rat liver homogenate; the influence of a thiamine-deficient diet. Biochim Biophys Acta. 1952;8(4):479-80.

251. Turan MI, Siltelioglu turan I, Mammadov R, Altınkaynak K, Kisaoglu A. The effect of thiamine and thiamine pyrophosphate on oxidative liver damage induced in rats with cisplatin. Biomed Res Int. 2013;2013:783809.

252. Turan MI, Cayir A, Cetin N, Suleyman H, Siltelioglu turan I, Tan H. An investigation of the effect of thiamine pyrophosphate on cisplatin-induced oxidative stress and DNA damage in rat brain tissue compared with thiamine: thiamine and thiamine pyrophosphate effects on cisplatin neurotoxicity. Hum Exp Toxicol. 2014;33(1):14-21.

253. Moore DH, Fowler WC, Crumpler LS. 5-Fluorouracil neurotoxicity. Gynecol Oncol. 1990;36(1):152-4.

254. Turan MI, Cetin N, Turan IS, Suleyman H. Effects of Thiamine and Thiamine Pyrophosphate on Oxidative Stress by Methotrexate in the Rat Brain. Latin Am. J. Pharm. 2013;32(2):203-207.

255. Zeng KL, Kuruvilla S, Sanatani M, Louie AV. Bilateral Blindness Following Chemoradiation for Locally Advanced Oropharyngeal Carcinoma. Cureus. 2015;7(10):e352.

256. Basu TK, Aksoy M, Dickerson JW. Effects of 5-fluorouracil on the thiamin status of adult female rats. Chemotherapy. 1979;25(2):70-6.

257. Gonzalez MJ, Miranda massari JR, Duconge J, et al. The bio-energetic theory of carcinogenesis. Med Hypotheses. 2012;79(4):433-9.

258. Yonetani T, Kidder GW. Studies on Cytochrome Oxidase. J Bio Chem. 1963;238(1).

259. Li Y, Park JS, Deng JH, Bai Y. Cytochrome c oxidase subunit IV is essential for assembly and respiratory function of the enzyme complex. J Bioenerg Biomembr. 2006;38(5-6):283-91.

260. Herrmann PC, Herrmann EC. Oxygen metabolism and a potential role for cytochrome c oxidase in the Warburg effect. J Bioenerg Biomembr. 2007;39(3):247-50.

261. Ekici S, Turkarslan S, Pawlik G, et al. Intracytoplasmic copper homeostasis controls cytochrome c oxidase production. MBio. 2014;5(1):e01055-13.

262. Kako K, Takehara A, Arai H, et al. A selective requirement for copper-dependent activation of cytochrome c oxidase by Cox17p. Biochem Biophys Res Commun. 2004;324(4):1379-85.

263. Nair PM, Mason HS. Reconstitution of cytochrome C oxidase from a copper-depleted enzyme and Cu. J Biol Chem. 1967;242(7):1406-15.

264. Stevens RJ, Nishio ML, Hood DA. Effect of hypothyroidism on the expression of cytochrome c and cytochrome c oxidase in heart and muscle during development. Mol Cell Biochem. 1995;143(2):119-27.

265. Dong DW, Srinivasan S, Guha M, Avadhani NG. Defects in cytochrome c oxidase expression induce a metabolic shift to glycolysis and carcinogenesis. Genom Data. 2015;6:99-107.

266. Srinivasan S, Guha M, Dong DW, et al. Disruption of cytochrome c oxidase function induces the Warburg effect and metabolic reprogramming. Oncogene. 2016;35(12):1585-95.

267. Hasinoff BB, Davey JP, O'brien PJ. The Adriamycin (doxorubicin)-induced inactivation of cytochrome c oxidase depends on the presence of iron or copper. Xenobiotica. 1989;19(2):231-41.

268. Stannard JN, Horecker BL. The in vitro inhibition of cytochrome oxidase by azide and cyanide. J Biol. Chem. 1948;172:599-608.

269. Wilson MT, Antonini G, Malatesta F, Sarti P, Brunori M. Probing the oxygen binding site of cytochrome c oxidase by cyanide. J Bio Chem.1994;269(39):24114-24119.

270. Jensen P, Wilson MT, Aasa R, Malmström BG. Cyanide inhibition of cytochrome c oxidase. A rapid-freeze e.p.r. investigation. Biochem J. 1984;224(3):829-37.

271. Miró O, Casademont J, Barrientos A, Urbano-márquez A, Cardellach F. Mitochondrial cytochrome c oxidase inhibition during acute carbon monoxide poisoning. Pharmacol Toxicol. 1998;82(4):199-202.

272. Alonso JR, Cardellach F, López S, Casademont J, Miró O. Carbon monoxide specifically inhibits cytochrome c oxidase of human mitochondrial respiratory chain. Pharmacol Toxicol. 2003;93(3):142-6.

273. Singh S, Bhalla A, Verma SK, Kaur A, Gill K. Cytochrome-c oxidase inhibition in 26 aluminum phosphide poisoned patients. Clin Toxicol (Phila). 2006;44(2):155-8.

274. Kotwicka M, Skibinska I, Jendraszak M, Jedrzejczak P. 17β-estradiol modifies human spermatozoa mitochondrial function in vitro. Reprod Biol Endocrinol. 2016;14(1):50.

275. Harvey AT, Preskorn SH. Cytochrome P450 enzymes: interpretation of their interactions with selective serotonin reuptake inhibitors. Part II. J Clin Psychopharmacol. 1996;16(5):345-55.

276. Levy RJ, Vijayasarathy C, Raj NR, Avadhani NG, Deutschman CS. Competitive and noncompetitive inhibition of myocardial cytochrome C oxidase in sepsis. Shock. 2004;21(2):110-4.

277. Nagai N, Ito Y. Dysfunction in cytochrome c oxidase caused by excessive nitric oxide in human lens epithelial cells stimulated with interferon-γ and lipopolysaccharide. Curr Eye Res. 2012;37(10):889-97.

278. Mohapatra NK, Roberts JF. In vitro effect of aflatoxin B1 on rat liver macrophages (Kuffer cells). Toxicol Lett. 1985;29(2-3):177-81.

279. Oriowo O, Sivak J, Bols N. UVB-Radiation attenuation of cytochrome c oxidase enzyme in ocular lens-uv cataract implication. Am. Acad. Opt. 2003.

280. Warburg O. On the origin of cancer cells. Science. 1956;123(3191):309-14.

281. Zhong J, Rajaram N, Brizel DM, et al. Radiation induces aerobic glycolysis through reactive oxygen species. Radiother Oncol. 2013;106(3):390-6.

282. Kunkel, H. O., and Williams, J. N., Jr., J. Biol. Chem., 189, 755 (1951).

283. Cardellach F, Alonso JR, López S, Casademont J, Miró O. Effect of smoking cessation on mitochondrial respiratory chain function. J Toxicol Clin Toxicol. 2003;41(3):223-8.

284. Hamblin MR. Mechanisms of Low Level Light Therapy. Photobiology. Harvard Medical School.

285. Karu T, Tiphlova O, Esenaliev R, Letokhov V. Two different mechanisms of low-intensity laser photobiological effects on Escherichia coli. J Photochem Photobiol B, Biol. 1994;24(3):155-61.

286. Morimoto Y, Arai T, Kikuchi M, Nakajima S, Nakamura H. Effect of low-intensity argon laser irradiation on mitochondrial respiration. Lasers Surg Med. 1994;15(2):191-9.

287. Passarella S, Ostuni A, Atlante A, Quagliariello E. Increase in the ADP/ATP exchange in rat liver mitochondria irradiated in vitro by helium-neon laser. Biochem Biophys Res Commun. 1988;156(2):978-86.

288. Greco M, Guida G, Perlino E, Marra E, Quagliariello E. Increase in RNA and protein synthesis by mitochondria irradiated with helium-neon laser. Biochem Biophys Res Commun. 1989;163(3):1428-34.

289. Karu T, Pyatibrat L, Kalendo G. Irradiation with He-Ne laser increases ATP level in cells cultivated in vitro. J Photochem Photobiol B, Biol. 1995;27(3):219-23.

290. Pastore D, Di martino C, Bosco G, Passarella S. Stimulation of ATP synthesis via oxidative phosphorylation in wheat mitochondria irradiated with helium-neon laser. Biochem Mol Biol Int. 1996;39(1):149-57.

291. Pastore D, Greco M, Passarella S. Specific helium-neon laser sensitivity of the purified cytochrome c oxidase. Int J Radiat Biol. 2000;76(6):863-70.

292. Karu T. Primary and secondary mechanisms of action of visible to near-IR radiation on cells. J Photochem Photobiol B, Biol. 1999;49(1):1-17.

293. Eells JT, Henry MM, Summerfelt P, et al. Therapeutic photobiomodulation for methanol-induced retinal toxicity. Proc Natl Acad Sci USA. 2003;100(6):3439-44.

294. Karu TI, Pyatibrat LV, Ryabykh TP. Melatonin modulates the action of near infrared radiation on cell adhesion. J Pineal Res. 2003;34(3):167-72.

295. Karu TI, Pyatibrat LV, Kalendo GS. Photobiological modulation of cell attachment via cytochrome c oxidase. Photochem Photobiol Sci. 2004;3(2):211-6.

296. Eells JT, Wong-riley MT, Verhoeve J, et al. Mitochondrial signal transduction in accelerated wound and retinal healing by near-infrared light therapy. Mitochondrion. 2004;4(5-6):559-67.

297. Karu TI, Pyatibrat LV, Afanasyeva NI. Cellular effects of low power laser therapy can be mediated by nitric oxide. Lasers Surg Med. 2005;36(4):307-14.

298. Karu TI, Pyatibrat LV, Kolyakov SF, Afanasyeva NI. Absorption measurements of a cell monolayer relevant to phototherapy: reduction of cytochrome c oxidase under near IR radiation. J Photochem Photobiol B, Biol. 2005;81(2):98-106.

299. Karu TI, Kolyakov SF. Exact action spectra for cellular responses relevant to phototherapy. Photomed Laser Surg. 2005;23(4):355-61.

300. Wong-riley MT, Liang HL, Eells JT, et al. Photobiomodulation directly benefits primary neurons functionally inactivated by toxins: role of cytochrome c oxidase. J Biol Chem. 2005;280(6):4761-71.

301. Yeager RL, Franzosa JA, Millsap DS, et al. Survivorship and mortality implications of developmental 670-nm phototherapy: dioxin co-exposure. Photomed Laser Surg. 2006;24(1):29-32.

302. Liang HL, Whelan HT, Eells JT, et al. Photobiomodulation partially rescues visual cortical neurons from cyanide-induced apoptosis. Neuroscience. 2006;139(2):639-49.

303. Gonzalez-lima F, Barrett DW. Augmentation of cognitive brain functions with transcranial lasers. Front Syst Neurosci. 2014;8:36.

304. Hwang J, Castelli DM, Gonzalez-lima F. Cognitive enhancement by transcranial laser stimulation and acute aerobic exercise. Lasers Med Sci. 2016;31(6):1151-60.

305. Barrett DW, Gonzalez-lima F. Transcranial infrared laser stimulation produces beneficial cognitive and emotional effects in humans. Neuroscience. 2013;230:13-23.

306. Hopkins JT, Mcloda TA, Seegmiller JG, David baxter G. Low-Level Laser Therapy Facilitates Superficial Wound Healing in Humans: A Triple-Blind, Sham-Controlled Study. J Athl Train. 2004;39(3):223-229.

307. De souza merli LA, De medeiros VP, Toma L, et al. The low level laser therapy effect on the remodeling of bone extracellular matrix. Photochem Photobiol. 2012;88(5):1293-301.

308. Saad A, El yamany M, Abbas O, Yehia M. Possible role of low level laser therapy on bone turnover in ovariectomized rats. Endocr Regul. 2010;44(4):155-63.

309. Ahn JC, Kim YH, Rhee CK. The effects of low level laser therapy (LLLT) on the testis in elevating serum testosterone level in rats. Biomed Res. 2013;24(1):28-32.

310. Schiffer F, Johnston AL, Ravichandran C, et al. Psychological benefits 2 and 4 weeks after a single treatment with near infrared light to the forehead: a pilot study of 10 patients with major depression and anxiety. Behav Brain Funct. 2009;5:46.

311. Gomes LE, Dalmarco EM, André ES. The brain-derived neurotrophic factor, nerve growth factor, neurotrophin-3, and induced nitric oxide synthase expressions after low-level laser therapy in an axonotmesis experimental model. Photomed Laser Surg. 2012;30(11):642-7.

312. Aziz-jalali MH, Tabaie SM, Djavid GE. Comparison of Red and Infrared Low-level Laser Therapy in the Treatment of Acne Vulgaris. Indian J Dermatol. 2012;57(2):128-30.

313. Shi DY, Xie FZ, Zhai C, Stern JS, Liu Y, Liu SL. The role of cellular oxidative stress in regulating glycolysis energy metabolism in hepatoma cells. Mol Cancer. 2009;8:32.

314. Bjordal JM, Johnson MI, Iversen V, Aimbire F, Lopes-martins RA. Low-level laser therapy in acute pain: a systematic review of possible mechanisms of action and clinical effects in randomized placebo-controlled trials. Photomed Laser Surg. 2006;24(2):158-68.

315. Falaki F, Nejat AH, Dalirsani Z. The Effect of Low-level Laser Therapy on Trigeminal Neuralgia: A Review of Literature. J Dent Res Dent Clin Dent Prospects. 2014;8(1):1-5.

316. Sumen A, Sarsan A, Alkan H, Yildiz N, Ardic F. Efficacy of low level laser therapy and intramuscular electrical stimulation on myofascial pain syndrome. J Back Musculoskelet Rehabil. 2015;28(1):153-8.

317. Yousefi-nooraie R, Schonstein E, Heidari K, et al. Low level laser therapy for nonspecific low-back pain. Cochrane Database Syst Rev. 2008;(2):CD005107.

318. Chow RT, Johnson MI, Lopes-martins RA, Bjordal JM. Efficacy of low-level laser therapy in the management of neck pain: a systematic review and meta-analysis of randomised placebo or active-treatment controlled trials. Lancet. 2009;374(9705):1897-908.

319. Avci P, Gupta GK, Clark J, Wikonkal N, Hamblin MR. Low-level laser (light) therapy (LLLT) for treatment of hair loss. Lasers Surg Med. 2014;46(2):144-51.

320. Barry Weinberger, Debra L. Laskin, Diane E. Heck, Jeffrey D. Laskin; The Toxicology of Inhaled Nitric Oxide. Toxicol Sci 2001; 59 (1): 5-16.

321. Brown GC, Cooper CE. Nanomolar concentrations of nitric oxide reversibly inhibit synaptosomal respiration by competing with oxygen at cytochrome oxidase. FEBS Lett. 1994;356(2-3):295-8.

322. Bolaños JP, Peuchen S, Heales SJ, Land JM, Clark JB. Nitric oxide-mediated inhibition of the mitochondrial respiratory chain in cultured astrocytes. J Neurochem. 1994;63(3):910-6.

323. Cleeter MW, Cooper JM, Darley-usmar VM, Moncada S, Schapira AH. Reversible inhibition of cytochrome c oxidase, the terminal enzyme of the mitochondrial respiratory chain, by nitric oxide. Implications for neurodegenerative diseases. FEBS Lett. 1994;345(1):50-4.

324. Brown GC, Borutaite V. Nitric oxide, cytochrome c and mitochondria. Biochem Soc Symp. 1999;66:17-25.

325. Hamblin M. The role of nitric oxide in low level light therapy. 2008;6846.

326. Ristow M, Cuezva JM. Oxidative phosphorylation and cancer: the ongoing Warburg hypothesis. 2008;1-18.

327. Gogvadze V, Orrenius S, Zhivotovsky B. Mitochondria in cancer cells: what is so special about them?. Trends Cell Biol. 2008;18(4):165-73.

328. Cuezva JM, Ortega AD, Willers I, Sánchez-cenizo L, Aldea M, Sánchez-aragó M. The tumor suppressor function of mitochondria: translation into the clinics. Biochim Biophys Acta. 2009;1792(12):1145-58.

329. Chambers AF, Groom AC, Macdonald IC. Dissemination and growth of cancer cells in metastatic sites. Nat Rev Cancer. 2002;2(8):563-72.

330. Poste G, Fidler IJ. The pathogenesis of cancer metastasis. Nature. 1980;283(5743):139-46.

331. Chaffer CL, Weinberg RA. A perspective on cancer cell metastasis. Science. 2011;331(6024):1559-64.

332. Welch DR. Do we need to redefine a cancer metastasis and staging definitions?. Breast Dis. 2006;26:3-12.

333. Lazebnik Y. What are the hallmarks of cancer?. Nat Rev Cancer. 2010;10(4):232-3.

334. Tarin D. Comparisons of metastases in different organs: biological and clinical implications. Clin Cancer Res. 2008;14(7):1923-5.

335. Bacac M, Stamenkovic I. Metastatic cancer cell. Annu Rev Pathol. 2008;3:221-47.

336. Hanahan D, Weinberg RA. The hallmarks of cancer. Cell. 2000;100(1):57-70.

337. Takeda D, Hasegawa T, Ueha T, et al. Transcutaneous carbon dioxide induces mitochondrial apoptosis and suppresses metastasis of oral squamous cell carcinoma in vivo. PLoS ONE. 2014;9(7):e100530.

338. Kamarajugadda S, Stemboroski L, Cai Q, et al. Glucose oxidation modulates anoikis and tumor metastasis. Mol Cell Biol. 2012;32(10):1893-907.

339. Lu J, Tan M, Cai Q. The Warburg effect in tumor progression: mitochondrial oxidative metabolism as an anti-metastasis mechanism. Cancer Lett. 2015;356(2 Pt A):156-64.

340. Liu W, Beck BH, Vaidya KS, et al. Metastasis suppressor KISS1 seems to reverse the Warburg effect by enhancing mitochondrial biogenesis. Cancer Res. 2014;74(3):954-63.

341. Ristow M. Oxidative metabolism in cancer growth. Curr Opin Clin Nutr Metab Care. 2006;9(4):339-45.

342. Addabbo F, Montagnani M, Goligorsky MS. Mitochondria and reactive oxygen species. Hypertension. 2009;53(6):885-92.

343. Naviaux RK. Oxidative shielding or oxidative stress?. J Pharmacol Exp Ther. 2012;342(3):608-18.

344. Brand MD, Affourtit C, Esteves TC, et al. Mitochondrial superoxide: production, biological effects, and activation of uncoupling proteins. Free Radic Biol Med. 2004;37(6):755-67.

345. Korshunov SS, Skulachev VP, Starkov AA. High protonic potential actuates a mechanism of production of reactive oxygen species in mitochondria. FEBS Lett. 1997;416(1):15-8.

346. Srinivasan S, Avadhani NG. Cytochrome c oxidase dysfunction in oxidative stress. Free Radic Biol Med. 2012;53(6):1252-63.

347. Turrens JF. Mitochondrial formation of reactive oxygen species. J Physiol (Lond). 2003;552(Pt 2):335-44.

348. John AP. Dysfunctional mitochondria, not oxygen insufficiency, cause cancer cells to produce inordinate amounts of lactic acid: the impact of this on the treatment of cancer. Med Hypotheses. 2001;57(4):429-31.

349. Srinivasan S, Avadhani NG. Cytochrome c oxidase dysfunction in oxidative stress. Free Radic Biol Med. 2012;53(6):1252-63.

350. Pinheiro CH, Silveira LR, Nachbar RT, Vitzel KF, Curi R. Regulation of glycolysis and expression of glucose metabolism-related genes by reactive oxygen species in contracting skeletal muscle cells. Free Radic Biol Med. 2010;48(7):953-60.

351. Sullivan LB, Chandel NS. Mitochondrial reactive oxygen species and cancer. Cancer Metab. 2014;2:17.

352. Szatrowski TP, Nathan CF. Production of large amounts of hydrogen peroxide by human tumor cells. Cancer Res. 1991;51(3):794-8.

353. Virchow, R. Virchow, R. Aetiologie der neoplastischen Geschwulste/Pathogenie der neoplastischen Geschwulste. (Verlag von August Hirschwald, Berlin, Germany, 1863.

354. Schäfer M, Werner S. Cancer as an overhealing wound: an old hypothesis revisited. Nat Rev Mol Cell Biol. 2008;9(8):628-38.

355. Mokbel K, Price RK, Carpenter R. Radial Scars and Breast Cancer. NEJM. 1999;341:210.

356. Sloane JP, Mayers MM. Carcinoma and atypical hyperplasia in radial scars and complex sclerosing lesions: importance of lesion size and patient age. Histopathology. 1993;23(3):225-31.

357. Frouge C, Tristant H, Guinebretière JM, et al. Mammographic lesions suggestive of radial scars: microscopic findings in 40 cases. Radiology. 1995;195(3):623-5.

358. Meng X, Riordan NH. Cancer is a functional repair tissue. Med Hypotheses. 2006;66(3):486-90.

359. Morgan C, Shah ZA, Hamilton R, et al. The radial scar of the breast diagnosed at core needle biopsy. Proc (Bayl Univ Med Cent). 2012;25(1):3-5.

360. Kennedy M, Masterson AV, Kerin M, Flanagan F. Pathology and clinical relevance of radial scars: a review. J Clin Pathol. 2003;56(10):721-4.

361. Nassar A, Conners AL, Celik B, Jenkins SM, Smith CY, Hieken TJ. Radial scar/complex sclerosing lesions: a clinicopathologic correlation study from a single institution. Ann Diagn Pathol. 2015;19(1):24-8.

362. Lv M, Zhu X, Zhong S, et al. Radial scars and subsequent breast cancer risk: a meta-analysis. PLoS ONE. 2014;9(7):e102503.

363. Dunham LJ. Cancer in man at site of prior benign lesion of skin or mucous membrane: a review. Cancer Res. 1972;32(7):1359-74.

364. Ennis WJ, Sui A, Bartholomew A. Stem Cells and Healing: Impact on Inflammation. Adv Wound Care (New Rochelle). 2013;2(7):369-378.

365. Dvorak HF. Tumors: wounds that do not heal. Similarities between tumor stroma generation and wound healing. N Engl J Med. 1986;315(26):1650-9.

366. Meng X, Zhong J, Liu S, Murray M, Gonzalez-angulo AM. A new hypothesis for the cancer mechanism. Cancer Metastasis Rev. 2012;31(1-2):247-68.

367. Haddow A. Molecular repair, wound healing, and carcinogenesis: tumor production a possible overhealing?. Adv Cancer Res. 1972;16:181-234.

368. Coussens LM, Werb Z. Inflammation and cancer. Nature. 2002;420(6917):860-7.

369. Rakoff-nahoum S. Why cancer and inflammation?. Yale J Biol Med. 2006;79(3-4):123-30.

370. Bonomi M, Patsias A, Posner M, Sikora A. The role of inflammation in head and neck cancer. Adv Exp Med Biol. 2014;816:107-27.

371. Borrello MG, Degl'innocenti D, Pierotti MA. Inflammation and cancer: the oncogene-driven connection. Cancer Lett. 2008;267(2):262-70.

372. Allavena P, Garlanda C, Borrello MG, Sica A, Mantovani A. Pathways connecting inflammation and cancer. Curr Opin Genet Dev. 2008;18(1):3-10.

373. Kundu JK, Surh YJ. Inflammation: gearing the journey to cancer. Mutat Res. 2008;659(1-2):15-30.

374. Mantovani A. Molecular pathways linking inflammation and cancer. Curr Mol Med. 2010;10(4):369-73.

375. Dobrovolskaia MA, Kozlov SV. Inflammation and cancer: when NF-kappaB amalgamates the perilous partnership. Curr Cancer Drug Targets. 2005;5(5):325-44.

376. Keibel A, Singh V, Sharma MC. Inflammation, microenvironment, and the immune system in cancer progression. Curr Pharm Des. 2009;15(17):1949-55.

377. Shacter E, Weitzman SA. Chronic inflammation and cancer. Oncology (Williston Park, NY). 2002;16(2):217-26, 229.

378. Colotta F, Allavena P, Sica A, Garlanda C, Mantovani A. Cancer-related inflammation, the seventh hallmark of cancer: links to genetic instability. Carcinogenesis. 2009;30(7):1073-81.

379.   Mantovani A, Sica A. Macrophages, innate immunity and cancer: balance, tolerance, and diversity. Curr Opin Immunol. 2010;22(2):231-7.

380.   Hanahan D, Weinberg RA. Hallmarks of Cancer: The Next Generation. Cell. 2011;144(5):646-674.

381.   Karin M. Nuclear factor-kappaB in cancer development and progression. Nature. 2006;441(7092):431-6.

382.   Zhejiang University. Ischemic and Hypoxic Injury. [Online]. Available: http://jpck.zju.edu.cn/jcyxjp/files/ge/03/MT/0365.pdf. [March 30, 2017].

383.   Haas R, Smith J, Rocher-ros V, et al. Lactate Regulates Metabolic and Pro-inflammatory Circuits in Control of T Cell Migration and Effector Functions. PLoS Biol. 2015;13(7):e1002202.

384.   Kiraly O, Gong G, Olipitz W, Muthupalani S, Engelward BP. Inflammation-induced cell proliferation potentiates DNA damage-induced mutations in vivo. PLoS Genet. 2015;11(2):e1004901.

385.   Boschetti G, Kanjarawi R, Bardel E, et al. Gut Inflammation in Mice Triggers Proliferation and Function of Mucosal Foxp3+ Regulatory T Cells but Impairs Their Conversion from CD4+ T Cells. J Crohns Colitis. 2017;11(1):105-117.

386.   Larson BJ, Longaker MT, Lorenz HP. Scarless fetal wound healing: a basic science review. Plast Reconstr Surg. 2010;126(4):1172-80.

387.   Wilgus TA. Regenerative healing in fetal skin: a review of the literature. Ostomy Wound Manage. 2007;53(6):16-31.

388.   Colwell AS, Longaker MT, Lorenz HP. Mammalian fetal organ regeneration. Adv Biochem Eng Biotechnol. 2005;93:83-100.

389.   Mackool RJ, Gittes GK, Longaker MT. Scarless healing. The fetal wound. Clin Plast Surg. 1998;25(3):357-65.

390.   Lorenz HP, Adzick NS. Scarless skin wound repair in the fetus. West J Med. 1993;159(3):350-5.

391.   Bullard KM, Longaker MT, Lorenz HP. Fetal wound healing: current biology. World J Surg. 2003;27(1):54-61.

392.   Rolfe KJ, Grobbelaar AO. A review of fetal scarless healing. ISRN Dermatol. 2012;2012:698034.

393.   Lo DD, Zimmermann AS, Nauta A, Longaker MT, Lorenz HP. Scarless fetal skin wound healing update. Birth Defects Res C Embryo Today. 2012;96(3):237-47.

394.   Dang C, Ting K, Soo C, Longaker MT, Lorenz HP. Fetal wound healing current perspectives. Clin Plast Surg. 2003;30(1):13-23.

395.   Bleacher JC, Adolph VR, Dillon PW, Krummel TM. Fetal tissue repair and wound healing. Dermatol Clin. 1993;11(4):677-83.

396.   Stelnicki EJ, Chin GS, Gittes GK, Longaker MT. Fetal wound repair: where do we go from here?. Semin Pediatr Surg. 1999;8(3):124-30.

397.   Kathju S, Gallo PH, Satish L. Scarless integumentary wound healing in the mammalian fetus: molecular basis and therapeutic implications. Birth Defects Res C Embryo Today. 2012;96(3):223-36.

398.   Ferguson MW, O'kane S. Scar-free healing: from embryonic mechanisms to adult therapeutic intervention. Philos Trans R Soc Lond, B, Biol Sci. 2004;359(1445):839-50.

399.   Jun Q, Ji-hong Z. Mechanism of scarless healing of embryonic skin. J Clin. Rehab. Tiss. Eng. Res. 2005;9(22):228-230.

400.   Lee YS, Wysocki A, Warburton D, Tuan TL. Wound healing in development. Birth Defects Res C Embryo Today. 2012;96(3):213-22.

401. Samuels P, Tan AK. Fetal scarless wound healing. J Otolaryngol. 1999;28(5):296-302.

402. Yates CC, Hebda P, Wells A. Skin wound healing and scarring: fetal wounds and regenerative restitution. Birth Defects Res C Embryo Today. 2012;96(4):325-33.

403. Sullivan KM, Meuli M, Macgillivray TE, Adzick NS. An adult-fetal skin interface heals without scar formation in sheep. Surgery. 1995;118(1):82-6.

404. Resnik, R, Creasy, RK. Lockwood, CJ, Moore, T, Greene MF. 2013. Creasy and Resnik's Maternal-Fetal Medicine: Principles and Practise. Elsevier Canada: 7th Edition. 1320 pps.

405. Rodesch F, Simon P, Donner C, Jauniaux E. Oxygen measurements in endometrial and trophoblastic tissues during early pregnancy. Obstet Gynecol. 1992;80(2):283-5.

406. Jauniaux E, Gulbis B, Burton GJ. The human first trimester gestational sac limits rather than facilitates oxygen transfer to the foetus--a review. Placenta. 2003;24 Suppl A:S86-93.

407. Kloth LC. Electrical stimulation for wound healing: a review of evidence from in vitro studies, animal experiments, and clinical trials. Int J Low Extrem Wounds. 2005;4(1):23-44.

408. Al MD, Hornstra G, Van der schouw YT, Bulstra-ramakers MT, Huisjes HJ. Biochemical EFA status of mothers and their neonates after normal pregnancy. Early Hum Dev. 1990;24(3):239-48.

409. Otto SJ, Houwelingen AC, Antal M, et al. Maternal and neonatal essential fatty acid status in phospholipids: an international comparative study. Eur J Clin Nutr. 1997;51(4):232-42.

410. Hornstra G, Van houwelingen AC, Simonis M, Gerrard JM. Fatty acid composition of umbilical arteries and veins: possible implications for the fetal EFA-status. Lipids. 1989;24(6):511-7.

411. Rump P, Mensink RP, Kester AD, Hornstra G. Essential fatty acid composition of plasma phospholipids and birth weight: a study in term neonates. Am J Clin Nutr. 2001;73(4):797-806.

412. Hornstra G, Al MD, Van houwelingen AC, Foreman-van drongelen MM. Essential fatty acids in pregnancy and early human development. Eur J Obstet Gynecol Reprod Biol. 1995;61(1):57-62.

413. Rakhimov, A. 1969. Dr. Buteyko Lecture in the Moscow State University on 9 December 1969. Available: http://www.normalbreathing.com/book-lecture.php.[March 1, 2017].

414. Larjava H, Wiebe C, Gallant-behm C, Hart DA, Heino J, Häkkinen L. Exploring scarless healing of oral soft tissues. J Can Dent Assoc. 2011;77:b18.

415. Harrison JW. Healing of surgical wounds in oral mucoperiosteal tissues. J Endod. 1991;17(8):401-8.

416. Glim JE, Van egmond M, Niessen FB, Everts V, Beelen RH. Detrimental dermal wound healing: what can we learn from the oral mucosa?. Wound Repair Regen. 2013;21(5):648-60.

417. Mak K, Manji A, Gallant-behm C, et al. Scarless healing of oral mucosa is characterized by faster resolution of inflammation and control of myofibroblast action compared to skin wounds in the red Duroc pig model. J Dermatol Sci. 2009;56(3):168-80.

418. Wong JW, Gallant-behm C, Wiebe C, et al. Wound healing in oral mucosa results in reduced scar formation as compared with skin: evidence from the red Duroc pig model and humans. Wound Repair Regen. 2009;17(5):717-29.

419. Eskow RN, Loesche WJ. Oxygen tensions in the human oral cavity. Arch Oral Biol. 1971;16(9):1127-8.

420. Kørbling M, Estrov Z. Adult stem cells for tissue repair - a new therapeutic concept?. N Engl J Med. 2003;349(6):570-82.

421. Hennessy B, Körbling M, Estrov Z. Circulating stem cells and tissue repair. Panminerva Med. 2004;46(1):1-11.

422. Mizuno H. Adipose-derived stem cells for tissue repair and regeneration: ten years of research and a literature review. J Nippon Med Sch. 2009;76(2):56-66.

423. Hu MS, Rennert RC, Mcardle A, et al. The Role of Stem Cells During Scarless Skin Wound Healing. Adv Wound Care (New Rochelle). 2014;3(4):304-314.

424. Roubelakis MG, Trohatou O, Roubelakis A, et al. Platelet-rich plasma (PRP) promotes fetal mesenchymal stem/stromal cell migration and wound healing process. Stem Cell Rev. 2014;10(3):417-28.

425. Taghavi S, George JC. Homing of stem cells to ischemic myocardium. Am J Transl Res. 2013;5(4):404-11.

426. Pytlík R, Rentsch C, Soukup T, et al. Efficacy and safety of human mesenchymal stromal cells in healing of critical-size bone defects in immunodeficient rats. Physiol Res. 2016.

427. Covacu R, Brundin L. Endogenous spinal cord stem cells in multiple sclerosis and its animal model. J Neuroimmunol. 2016.

428. Collins JN, Collins JJ. Tissue Degeneration following Loss of Schistosoma mansoni cbp1 Is Associated with Increased Stem Cell Proliferation and Parasite Death In Vivo. PLoS Pathog. 2016;12(11):e1005963.

429. Cheng CW, Adams GB, Perin L, et al. Prolonged fasting reduces IGF-1/PKA to promote hematopoietic-stem-cell-based regeneration and reverse immunosuppression. Cell Stem Cell. 2014;14(6):810-23.

430. Wagers AJ, Christensen JL, Weissman IL. Cell fate determination from stem cells. Gene Ther. 2002;9(10):606-12.

431. Hardy D, Besnard A, Latil M, et al. Comparative Study of Injury Models for Studying Muscle Regeneration in Mice. PLoS ONE. 2016;11(1):e0147198.

432. Arwert EN, Hoste E, Watt FM. Epithelial stem cells, wound healing and cancer. Nat Rev Cancer. 2012;12(3):170-80.

433. Laterveer L, Lindley IJ, Hamilton MS, Willemze R, Fibbe WE. Interleukin-8 induces rapid mobilization of hematopoietic stem cells with radioprotective capacity and long-term myelolymphoid repopulating ability. Blood. 1995;85(8):2269-75.

434. Laterveer L, Lindley IJ, Heemskerk DP, et al. Rapid mobilization of hematopoietic progenitor cells in rhesus monkeys by a single intravenous injection of interleukin-8. Blood. 1996;87(2):781-8.

435. Westenbrink BD, Lipsic E, Van der meer P, et al. Erythropoietin improves cardiac function through endothelial progenitor cell and vascular endothelial growth factor mediated neovascularization. Eur Heart J. 2007;28(16):2018-27.

436. Meloni M, Caporali A, Graiani G, et al. Nerve growth factor promotes cardiac repair following myocardial infarction. Circ Res. 2010;106(7):1275-84.

437. Rota M, Padin-iruegas ME, Misao Y, et al. Local activation or implantation of cardiac progenitor cells rescues scarred infarcted myocardium improving cardiac function. Circ Res. 2008;103(1):107-16.

438. Ii M, Nishimura H, Iwakura A, et al. Endothelial progenitor cells are rapidly recruited to myocardium and mediate protective effect of ischemic preconditioning via "imported" nitric oxide synthase activity. Circulation. 2005;111(9):1114-20.

439. Taghavi S, George JC. Homing of stem cells to ischemic myocardium. Am J Transl Res. 2013;5(4):404-11.

440. Ruifrok WP, De boer RA, Iwakura A, et al. Estradiol-induced, endothelial progenitor cell-mediated neovascularization in male mice with hind-limb ischemia. Vasc Med. 2009;14(1):29-36.

441. Iwakura A, Shastry S, Luedemann C, et al. Estradiol enhances recovery after myocardial infarction by augmenting incorporation of bone marrow-derived endothelial progenitor cells into sites of

ischemia-induced neovascularization via endothelial nitric oxide synthase-mediated activation of matrix metalloproteinase-9. Circulation. 2006;113(12):1605-14.

442. Bergsland M, Covacu R, Perez estrada C, Svensson M, Brundin L. Nitric oxide-induced neuronal to glial lineage fate-change depends on NRSF/REST function in neural progenitor cells. Stem Cells. 2014;32(9):2539-49.

443. Drummond-barbosa D. Stem cells, their niches and the systemic environment: an aging network. Genetics. 2008;180(4):1787-97.

444. Towns CR, Jones DG. Stem cells, embryos, and the environment: a context for both science and ethics. J Med Ethics. 2004;30(4):410-3.

445. Gattazzo F, Urciuolo A, Bonaldo P. Extracellular matrix: a dynamic microenvironment for stem cell niche. Biochim Biophys Acta. 2014;1840(8):2506-19.

446. Tokar EJ, Diwan BA, Waalkes MP. Arsenic exposure transforms human epithelial stem/progenitor cells into a cancer stem-like phenotype. Environ Health Perspect. 2010;118(1):108-15.

447. Xu Y, Tokar EJ, Person RJ, Orihuela RG, Ngalame NN, Waalkes MP. Recruitment of normal stem cells to an oncogenic phenotype by noncontiguous carcinogen-transformed epithelia depends on the transforming carcinogen. Environ Health Perspect. 2013;121(8):944-50.

448. Lowe SW, Lin AW. Apoptosis in cancer. Carcinogenesis. 2000;21(3):485-95.

449. Wyllie AH, Kerr JF, Currie AR. Cell death: the significance of apoptosis. Int Rev Cytol. 1980;68:251-306.

450. Kerr JF, Wyllie AH, Currie AR. Apoptosis: a basic biological phenomenon with wide-ranging implications in tissue kinetics. Br J Cancer. 1972;26(4):239-57.

451. Wong SY, Reiter JF. Wounding mobilizes hair follicle stem cells to form tumors. Proc Natl Acad Sci USA. 2011;108(10):4093-8.

452. Houghton J, Stoicov C, Nomura S, et al. Gastric cancer originating from bone marrow-derived cells. Science. 2004;306(5701):1568-71.

453. Kasper M, Jaks V, Are A, et al. Wounding enhances epidermal tumorigenesis by recruiting hair follicle keratinocytes. Proc Natl Acad Sci USA. 2011;108(10):4099-104.

454. Grachtchouk M, Pero J, Yang SH, et al. Basal cell carcinomas in mice arise from hair follicle stem cells and multiple epithelial progenitor populations. J Clin Invest. 2011;121(5):1768-81.

455. Donovan J. Review of the hair follicle origin hypothesis for basal cell carcinoma. Dermatol Surg. 2009;35(9):1311-23.

456. Hutchin ME, Kariapper MS, Grachtchouk M, et al. Sustained Hedgehog signaling is required for basal cell carcinoma proliferation and survival: conditional skin tumorigenesis recapitulates the hair growth cycle. Genes Dev. 2005;19(2):214-23.

457. Gupta S, Takebe N, Lorusso P. Targeting the Hedgehog pathway in cancer. Ther Adv Med Oncol. 2010;2(4):237-50.

458. Catalano V, Turdo A, Di franco S, Dieli F, Todaro M, Stassi G. Tumor and its microenvironment: a synergistic interplay. Semin Cancer Biol. 2013;23(6 Pt B):522-32.

459. Hong M, Tan HY, Li S, et al. Cancer Stem Cells: The Potential Targets of Chinese Medicines and Their Active Compounds. Int J Mol Sci. 2016;17(6).

460. Dragu DL, Necula LG, Bleotu C, Diaconu CC, Chivu-economescu M. Therapies targeting cancer stem cells: Current trends and future challenges. World J Stem Cells. 2015;7(9):1185-201.

461. Baek SJ, Ishii H, Tamari K, et al. Cancer stem cells: The potential of carbon ion beam radiation and new radiosensitizers (Review). Oncol Rep. 2015;34(5):2233-7.

462.   Hong IS, Lee HY, Nam JS. Cancer stem cells: the 'Achilles heel' of chemo-resistant tumors. Recent Pat Anticancer Drug Discov. 2015;10(1):2-22.

463.   Vochem R, Einenkel J, Horn LC, Ruschpler P. [Importance of the tumor stem cell hypothesis for understanding ovarian cancer]. Pathologe. 2014;35(4):361-70.

464.   Chhabra R. Cervical cancer stem cells: opportunities and challenges. J Cancer Res Clin Oncol. 2015;141(11):1889-97.

465.   Ahmed N, Abubaker K, Findlay JK. Ovarian cancer stem cells: Molecular concepts and relevance as therapeutic targets. Mol Aspects Med. 2014;39:110-25.

466.   Ahmed N, Abubaker K, Findlay J, Quinn M. Cancerous ovarian stem cells: obscure targets for therapy but relevant to chemoresistance. J Cell Biochem. 2013;114(1):21-34.

467.   Bar JK, Grelewski P, Lis-nawara A, Drobnikowska K. [The role of cancer stem cells in progressive growth and resistance of ovarian cancer: true or fiction?]. Postepy Hig Med Dosw (Online). 2015;69:1077-86.

468.   Chen K, Huang YH, Chen JL. Understanding and targeting cancer stem cells: therapeutic implications and challenges. Acta Pharmacol Sin. 2013;34(6):732-40.

469.   Ogawa K, Yoshioka Y, Isohashi F, Seo Y, Yoshida K, Yamazaki H. Radiotherapy targeting cancer stem cells: current views and future perspectives. Anticancer Res. 2013;33(3):747-54.

470.   Zhang Q, Feng Y, Kennedy D. Multidrug-resistant cancer cells and cancer stem cells hijack cellular systems to circumvent systemic therapies, can natural products reverse this?. Cell Mol Life Sci. 2017;74(5):777-801.

471.   Chen LS, Wang AX, Dong B, Pu KF, Yuan LH, Zhu YM. A new prospect in cancer therapy: targeting cancer stem cells to eradicate cancer. Chin J Cancer. 2012;31(12):564-72.

472.   Hu Y, Fu L. Targeting cancer stem cells: a new therapy to cure cancer patients. Am J Cancer Res. 2012;2(3):340-56.

473.   Kim YJ, Siegler EL, Siriwon N, Wang P. Therapeutic strategies for targeting cancer stem cells. J Cancer Metasta Treat 2016;2:233-42.

474.   Understanding and targeting cancer stem cells: therapeutic implications and challenges. Acta Pharmacologica Sinica. 2013;34(6):732.

475.   Facucho-oliveira JM, St john JC. The relationship between pluripotency and mitochondrial DNA proliferation during early embryo development and embryonic stem cell differentiation. Stem Cell Rev. 2009;5(2):140-58.

476.   Wanet A, Arnould T, Najimi M, Renard P. Connecting Mitochondria, Metabolism, and Stem Cell Fate. Stem Cells Dev. 2015;24(17):1957-71.

477.   Harris H. The analysis of malignancy by cell fusion: the position in 1988. Cancer Res. 1988;48(12):3302-6.

478.   Szent-györgyi A. The living state and cancer. Proc Natl Acad Sci USA. 1977;74(7):2844-7.

479.   Soto AM, Sonnenschein C. The somatic mutation theory of cancer: growing problems with the paradigm?. Bioessays. 2004;26(10):1097-107.

480.   Abdouh M, Zhou S, Arena V, et al. Transfer of malignant trait to immortalized human cells following exposure to human cancer serum. J Exp Clin Cancer Res. 2014;33:86.

481.   Gerschenson M, Graves K, Carson SD, Wells RS, Pierce GB. Regulation of melanoma by the embryonic skin. Proc Natl Acad Sci USA. 1986;83(19):7307-10.

482.   Postovit LM, Margaryan NV, Seftor EA, Hendrix MJ. Role of nodal signaling and the microenvironment underlying melanoma plasticity. Pigment Cell Melanoma Res. 2008;21(3):348-57.

483. Zhou S, Abdouh M, Arena V, Arena M, Arena GO. Reprogramming Malignant Cancer Cells toward a Benign Phenotype following Exposure to Human Embryonic Stem Cell Microenvironment. PLoS ONE. 2017;12(1):e0169899.

484. Abbott DE, Postovit LM, Seftor EA, Margaryan NV, Seftor RE, Hendrix MJ. Exploiting the convergence of embryonic and tumorigenic signaling pathways to develop new therapeutic targets. Stem Cell Rev. 2007;3(1):68-78.

485. D'angelo RC, Wicha MS. Stem cells in normal development and cancer. Prog Mol Biol Transl Sci. 2010;95:113-58.

486. Verney EL, Pierce GB, Dixon FJ. The biology of testicular cancer. III. Heterotransplanted choriocarcinomas. Cancer Res. 1959;19(6, Part 1):633-7.

487. Postovit LM, Seftor EA, Seftor RE, Hendrix MJ. Targeting Nodal in malignant melanoma cells. Expert Opin Ther Targets. 2007;11(4):497-505.

488. Hendrix MJ, Seftor EA, Kirschmann DA, Quaranta V, Seftor RE. Remodeling of the microenvironment by aggressive melanoma tumor cells. Ann N Y Acad Sci. 2003;995:151-61.

489. Hendrix MJ, Seftor EA, Seftor RE, Kasemeier-kulesa J, Kulesa PM, Postovit LM. Reprogramming metastatic tumour cells with embryonic microenvironments. Nat Rev Cancer. 2007;7(4):246-55.

490. Díez-torre A, Andrade R, Eguizábal C, et al. Reprogramming of melanoma cells by embryonic microenvironments. Int J Dev Biol. 2009;53(8-10):1563-8.

491. Lee LM, Seftor EA, Bonde G, Cornell RA, Hendrix MJ. The fate of human malignant melanoma cells transplanted into zebrafish embryos: assessment of migration and cell division in the absence of tumor formation. Dev Dyn. 2005;233(4):1560-70.

492. Seftor EA, Brown KM, Chin L, et al. Epigenetic transdifferentiation of normal melanocytes by a metastatic melanoma microenvironment. Cancer Res. 2005;65(22):10164-9.

493. Postovit LM, Seftor EA, Seftor RE, Hendrix MJ. Influence of the microenvironment on melanoma cell fate determination and phenotype. Cancer Res. 2006;66(16):7833-6.

494. Veselá A, Wilhelm J. The role of carbon dioxide in free radical reactions of the organism. Physiol Res. 2002;51(4):335-9.

495. Squadrito GL, Pryor WA. Oxidative chemistry of nitric oxide: the roles of superoxide, peroxynitrite, and carbon dioxide. Free Radic Biol Med. 1998;25(4-5):392-403.

496. Kogan AKh, Grachev SV, Eliseeva SV, Bolevich S. [Ability of carbon dioxide to inhibit generation of superoxide anion radical in cells and its biomedical role]. Vopr Med Khim. 1996;42(3):193-202.

497. Kogan AKh, Manuĭlov BM, Grachev SV, Bolevich S, Tsypin AB, Daniliak IG. [CO2--a natural inhibitor of active oxygen form generation by phagocytes]. Biull Eksp Biol Med. 1994;118(10):395-8.

498. Kogan AKh, Grachev SV, Eliseeva SV, Bolevich S. [Carbon dioxide--a universal inhibitor of the generation of active oxygen forms by cells (deciphering one enigma of evolution)]. Izv Akad Nauk Ser Biol. 1997;(2):204-17.

499. Boljevic S, Kogan AH, Gracev SV, Jelisejeva SV, Daniljak IG. [Carbon dioxide inhibits the generation of active forms of oxygen in human and animal cells and the significance of the phenomenon in biology and medicine]. Vojnosanit Pregl. 1996;53(4):261-74.

500. Baev VI, Vasil'eva IV, L'vov SN, Shugaleĭ IV. [The unknown physiological role of carbon dioxide]. Fiziol Zh Im I M Sechenova. 1995;81(2):47-52.

501. Kogan AKh, Bolevich S, Daniliak IG. [Comparative study of the effect of carbon dioxide on the generation of active forms of oxygen by leukocytes in health and in bronchial asthma]. Patol Fiziol Eksp Ter. 1995;(3):34-40.

502. Bolevich S, Kogan AH, Zivkovic V, et al. Protective role of carbon dioxide (CO2) in generation of reactive oxygen species. Mol Cell Biochem. 2016;411(1-2):317-30.

503. Sandulache VC, Parekh A, Li-korotky HS, Dohar JE, Hebda PA. Prostaglandin E2 differentially modulates human fetal and adult dermal fibroblast migration and contraction: implication for wound healing. Wound Repair Regen. 2006;14(5):633-43.

504. Vaughan RA, Garcia-smith R, Trujillo KA, Bisoffi M. Tumor necrosis factor alpha increases aerobic glycolysis and reduces oxidative metabolism in prostate epithelial cells. Prostate. 2013;73(14):1538-46.

505. Liechty KW, Adzick NS, Crombleholme TM. Diminished interleukin 6 (IL-6) production during scarless human fetal wound repair. Cytokine. 2000;12(6):671-6.

506. Liechty KW, Crombleholme TM, Cass DL, Martin B, Adzick NS. Diminished interleukin-8 (IL-8) production in the fetal wound healing response. J Surg Res. 1998;77(1):80-4.

507. Adzick NS, Lorenz HP. Cells, matrix, growth factors, and the surgeon. The biology of scarless fetal wound repair. Ann Surg. 1994;220(1):10-8.

508. Wilgus TA, Bergdall VK, Tober KL, et al. The impact of cyclooxygenase-2 mediated inflammation on scarless fetal wound healing. Am J Pathol. 2004;165(3):753-61.

509. Guido C, Whitaker-menezes D, Capparelli C, et al. Metabolic reprogramming of cancer-associated fibroblasts by TGF-β drives tumor growth: connecting TGF-β signaling with "Warburg-like" cancer metabolism and L-lactate production. Cell Cycle. 2012;11(16):3019-35.

510. Cho JS, Han IH, Lee HR, Lee HM. Prostaglandin E2 Induces IL-6 and IL-8 Production by the EP Receptors/Akt/NF-κB Pathways in Nasal Polyp-Derived Fibroblasts. Allergy Asthma Immunol Res. 2014;6(5):449-57.

511. Hinson RM, Williams JA, Shacter E. Elevated interleukin 6 is induced by prostaglandin E2 in a murine model of inflammation: possible role of cyclooxygenase-2. Proc Natl Acad Sci USA. 1996;93(10):4885-90.

512. Caristi S, Piraino G, Cucinotta M, Valenti A, Loddo S, Teti D. Prostaglandin E2 induces interleukin-8 gene transcription by activating C/EBP homologous protein in human T lymphocytes. J Biol Chem. 2005;280(15):14433-42.

513. Yu Y, Chadee K. Prostaglandin E2 stimulates IL-8 gene expression in human colonic epithelial cells by a posttranscriptional mechanism. J Immunol. 1998;161(7):3746-52.

514. Ramirez-yañez GO, Hamlet S, Jonarta A, Seymour GJ, Symons AL. Prostaglandin E2 enhances transforming growth factor-beta 1 and TGF-beta receptors synthesis: an in vivo and in vitro study. Prostaglandins Leukot Essent Fatty Acids. 2006;74(3):183-92.

515. Ricciotti E, Fitzgerald GA. Prostaglandins and inflammation. Arterioscler Thromb Vasc Biol. 2011;31(5):986-1000.

516. Guyenet SJ, Carlson SE. Increase in adipose tissue linoleic acid of US adults in the last half century. Adv Nutr. 2015;6(6):660-4.

517. Nourooz-zadeh J, Pereira P. Age-related accumulation of free polyunsaturated fatty acids in human retina. Ophthalmic Res. 1999;31(4):273-9.

518. Lee J, Yu BP, Herlihy JT. Modulation of cardiac mitochondrial membrane fluidity by age and calorie intake. Free Radic Biol Med. 1999;26(3-4):260-5.

519. Smídová L, Base J, Mourek J, Cechová I. Proportion of individual fatty acids in the non-esterified (free) fatty acid (FFA) fraction in the serum of laboratory rats of different ages. Physiol Bohemoslov. 1990;39(2):125-34.

520. Schäfer L, Overvad K, Thorling EB, Velander G. Adipose tissue levels of fatty acids and tocopherol in young and old women. Ann Nutr Metab. 1989;33(6):315-22.

521. Laganiere S, Yu BP. Modulation of membrane phospholipid fatty acid composition by age and food restriction. Gerontology. 1993;39(1):7-18.

522. Qi K, Hall M, Deckelbaum RJ. Long-chain polyunsaturated fatty acid accretion in brain. Curr Opin Clin Nutr Metab Care. 2002;5(2):133-8.

523. Guerra A, Demmelmair H, Toschke AM, Koletzko B. Three-year tracking of fatty acid composition of plasma phospholipids in healthy children. Ann Nutr Metab. 2007;51(5):433-8.

524. Crowe FL, Skeaff CM, Green TJ, Gray AR. Serum n-3 long-chain PUFA differ by sex and age in a population-based survey of New Zealand adolescents and adults. Br J Nutr. 2008;99(1):168-74.

525. Laganiere S, Yu BP. Anti-lipoperoxidation action of food restriction. Biochem Biophys Res Commun. 1987;145(3):1185-91.

526. Walker CG, Browning LM, Mander AP, et al. Age and sex differences in the incorporation of EPA and DHA into plasma fractions, cells and adipose tissue in humans. Br J Nutr. 2014;111(4):679-89.

527. Paradies G, Ruggiero FM, Petrosillo G, Quagliariello E. Age-dependent decline in the cytochrome c oxidase activity in rat heart mitochondria: role of cardiolipin. FEBS Lett. 1997;406(1-2):136-8.

528. Paradies G, Petrosillo G, Gadaleta MN, Ruggiero FM. The effect of aging and acetyl-L-carnitine on the pyruvate transport and oxidation in rat heart mitochondria. FEBS Lett. 1999;454(3):207-9.

529. Orrenius S, Zhivotovsky B. Cardiolipin oxidation sets cytochrome c free. Nat Chem Biol. 2005;1(4):188-9.

530. Iverson SL, Orrenius S. The cardiolipin-cytochrome c interaction and the mitochondrial regulation of apoptosis. Arch Biochem Biophys. 2004;423(1):37-46.

531. Paradies G, Paradies V, De benedictis V, Ruggiero FM, Petrosillo G. Functional role of cardiolipin in mitochondrial bioenergetics. Biochim Biophys Acta. 2014;1837(4):408-17.

532. Hanske J, Toffey JR, Morenz AM, Bonilla AJ, Schiavoni KH, Pletneva EV. Conformational properties of cardiolipin-bound cytochrome c. Proc Natl Acad Sci USA. 2012;109(1):125-30.

533. Lee HJ, Mayette J, Rapoport SI, Bazinet RP. Selective remodeling of cardiolipin fatty acids in the aged rat heart. Lipids Health Dis. 2006;5:2.

534. Bronnikov GE, Kulagina TP, Aripovsky AV. Dietary supplementation of old rats with hydrogenated peanut oil restores activities of mitochondrial respiratory complexes in skeletal muscles. Biochemistry Mosc. 2010;75(12):1491-7.

535. Ehrlich P. Ueber den jetzigen stand der karzinomforschung. Ned Tijdschr Geneeskd. 1909;5:73–290.

536. Kim R, Emi M, Tanabe K. Cancer immunoediting from immune surveillance to immune escape. Immunology. 2007;121(1):1-14.

537. Shankaran V, Ikeda H, Bruce AT, et al. IFNgamma and lymphocytes prevent primary tumour development and shape tumour immunogenicity. Nature. 2001;410(6832):1107-11.

538. Girardi M, Oppenheim DE, Steele CR, et al. Regulation of cutaneous malignancy by gammadelta T cells. Science. 2001;294(5542):605-9.

539. Dunn GP, Bruce AT, Sheehan KC, et al. A critical function for type I interferons in cancer immunoediting. Nat Immunol. 2005;6(7):722-9.

540. Kaplan DH, Shankaran V, Dighe AS, et al. Demonstration of an interferon gamma-dependent tumor surveillance system in immunocompetent mice. Proc Natl Acad Sci USA. 1998;95(13):7556-61.

541. Street SE, Trapani JA, Macgregor D, Smyth MJ. Suppression of lymphoma and epithelial malignancies effected by interferon gamma. J Exp Med. 2002;196(1):129-34.

542. Smyth MJ, Thia KY, Street SE, Macgregor D, Godfrey DI, Trapani JA. Perforin-mediated cytotoxicity is critical for surveillance of spontaneous lymphoma. J Exp Med. 2000;192(5):755-60.

543. Hayward AR, Levy J, Facchetti F, et al. Cholangiopathy and tumors of the pancreas, liver, and biliary tree in boys with X-linked immunodeficiency with hyper-IgM. J Immunol. 1997;158(2):977-83.

544. Mueller BU, Pizzo PA. Cancer in children with primary or secondary immunodeficiencies. J Pediatr. 1995;126(1):1-10.

545. Van der meer JW, Weening RS, Schellekens PT, Van munster IP, Nagengast FM. Colorectal cancer in patients with X-linked agammaglobulinaemia. Lancet. 1993;341(8858):1439-40.

546. Gatti RA, Good RA. Occurrence of malignancy in immunodeficiency diseases. A literature review. Cancer. 1971;28(1):89-98.

547. Kinlen LJ, Webster AD, Bird AG, et al. Prospective study of cancer in patients with hypogammaglobulinaemia. Lancet. 1985;1(8423):263-6.

548. Salavoura K, Kolialexi A, Tsangaris G, Mavrou A. Development of cancer in patients with primary immunodeficiencies. Anticancer Res. 2008;28(2B):1263-9.

549. Schreiber RD, Old LJ, Smyth MJ. Cancer immunoediting: integrating immunity's roles in cancer suppression and promotion. Science. 2011;331(6024):1565-70.

550. Boshoff C, Whitby D, Talbot S, Weiss RA. Etiology of AIDS-related Kaposi's sarcoma and lymphoma. Oral Dis. 1997;3 Suppl 1:S129-32.

551. Mueller N. Overview of the epidemiology of malignancy in immune deficiency. J Acquir Immune Defic Syndr. 1999;21 Suppl 1:S5-10.

552. George J. Friou, M.D., "Relationship of Malignancy, Autoimmunity, and Immunological Disease," Annals of the New York Academy of Sciences, March 18, 1974, 44-45, 48.

553. Goldstein MR, Mascitelli L. Surgery and cancer promotion: are we trading beauty for cancer?. QJM. 2011;104(9):811-5.

554. Sakai Y, Takayanagi K, Ohno M, Inose R, Fujiwara H. A trial of improvement of immunity in cancer patients by laughter therapy. Jpn Hosp. 2013;(32):53-9.

555. Hayashi K, Kawachi I, Ohira T, Kondo K, Shirai K, Kondo N. Laughter is the Best Medicine? A Cross-Sectional Study of Cardiovascular Disease Among Older Japanese Adults. J Epidemiol. 2016;26(10):546-552.

556. Fairey AS, Courneya KS, Field CJ, Mackey JR. Physical exercise and immune system function in cancer survivors: a comprehensive review and future directions. Cancer. 2002;94(2):539-51.

557. Gleeson M. Immune function in sport and exercise. J Appl Physiol. 2007;103(2):693-9.

558. Friedenreich CM, Cust AE. Physical activity and breast cancer risk: impact of timing, type and dose of activity and population subgroup effects. Br J Sports Med. 2008;42(8):636-47.

559. Giovannucci E, Ascherio A, Rimm EB, Colditz GA, Stampfer MJ, Willett WC. Physical activity, obesity, and risk for colon cancer and adenoma in men. Ann Intern Med. 1995;122(5):327-34.

560. Giovannucci E, Colditz GA, Stampfer MJ, Willett WC. Physical activity, obesity, and risk of colorectal adenoma in women (United States). Cancer Causes Control. 1996;7(2):253-63.

561. Thune I, Furberg AS. Physical activity and cancer risk: dose-response and cancer, all sites and site-specific. Med Sci Sports Exerc. 2001;33(6 Suppl):S530-50.

562. Bang O. The lactate content of blood during and after muscular exercise in man. Scand. Arch. Physiol. 1936;74:51–82.

563. Owles WH. Alterations in the lactic acid content of the blood as a result of light exercise, and associated changes in the co(2)-combining power of the blood and in the alveolar co(2) pressure. J Physiol (Lond). 1930;69(2):214-37.

564. Ghosh AK. Anaerobic threshold: its concept and role in endurance sport. Malays J Med Sci. 2004;11(1):24-36.

565. Meyer T, Faude O, Scharhag J, Urhausen A, Kindermann W. Is lactic acidosis a cause of exercise induced hyperventilation at the respiratory compensation point?. Br J Sports Med. 2004;38(5):622-5.

566. Nieman DC. Is infection risk linked to exercise workload?. Med Sci Sports Exerc. 2000;32(7 Suppl):S406-11.

567. Nieman DC. Immunonutrition support for athletes. Nutr Rev. 2008;66(6):310-20.

568. Gleeson M. Immune system adaptation in elite athletes. Curr Opin Clin Nutr Metab Care. 2006;9(6):659-65.

569. Jeurissen A, Bossuyt X, Ceuppens JL, Hespel P. [The effects of physical exercise on the immune system]. Ned Tijdschr Geneeskd. 2003;147(28):1347-51.

570. Mackinnon LT. Chronic exercise training effects on immune function. Med Sci Sports Exerc. 2000;32(7 Suppl):S369-76.

571. Shaikh SR, Edidin M. Immunosuppressive effects of polyunsaturated fatty acids on antigen presentation by human leukocyte antigen class I molecules. J Lipid Res. 2007;48(1):127-38.

572. Hughes DA, Pinder AC. n-3 polyunsaturated fatty acids inhibit the antigen-presenting function of human monocytes. Am J Clin Nutr. 2000;71(1 Suppl):357S-60S.

573. Geyeregger R, Zeyda M, Zlabinger GJ, Waldhäusl W, Stulnig TM. Polyunsaturated fatty acids interfere with formation of the immunological synapse. J Leukoc Biol. 2005;77(5):680-8.

574. Shaikh SR, Edidin M. Polyunsaturated fatty acids, membrane organization, T cells, and antigen presentation. Am J Clin Nutr. 2006;84(6):1277-89.

575. Van der heide JJ, Bilo HJ, Donker JM, Wilmink JM, Tegzess AM. Effect of dietary fish oil on renal function and rejection in cyclosporine-treated recipients of renal transplants. N Engl J Med. 1993;329(11):769-73.

576. Izgüt-uysal VN, Tan R, Bülbül M, Derin N. Effect of stress-induced lipid peroxidation on functions of rat peritoneal macrophages. Cell Biol Int. 2004;28(7):517-21.

577. Mascioli EA, Bistrian BR, Babayan VK, Blackburn GL. Medium chain triglycerides and structured lipids as unique nonglucose energy sources in hyperalimentation. Lipids. 1987;22(6):421-3.

578. Bennett WM, Carpenter CB, Shapiro ME, et al. Delayed omega-3 fatty acid supplements in renal transplantation. A double-blind, placebo-controlled study. Transplantation. 1995;59(3):352-6.

579. Mertin J. Letter: Unsaturated fatty acids and renal transplantation. Lancet. 1974;2(7882):717.

580. Mchugh MI, Wilkinson R, Elliott RW, et al. Immunosuppression with polyunsaturated fatty acids in renal transplantation. Transplantation. 1977;24(4):263-7.

581. Guimarães AR, Sitnik RH, Curi CM, Curi R. Polyunsaturated and saturated fatty acids-rich diets and immune tissues. 2. Maximal activities of key enzymes of glutaminolysis, glycolysis, pentose-phosphate-pathway and Krebs cycle in thymus, spleen and mesenteric lymph nodes. Biochem Int. 1990;22(6):1015-23.

582. C. J. Meade and J. Martin, Adv. Lipid Res., 127, 1978.

583. Popovici D, Mihai N, Urbanavicius V. Abnormalities of oxidative phosphorylation due to excess of deficiency of thyroid hormones. Endocrinologie. 1980;18(3):143-7.

584. Martinez B, Del hoyo P, Martin MA, Arenas J, Perez-castillo A, Santos A. Thyroid hormone regulates oxidative phosphorylation in the cerebral cortex and striatum of neonatal rats. J Neurochem. 2001;78(5):1054-63.

585. Harper ME, Seifert EL. Thyroid hormone effects on mitochondrial energetics. Thyroid. 2008;18(2):145-56.

586. Lanni A, Moreno M, Goglia F. Mitochondrial Actions of Thyroid Hormone. Compr Physiol. 2016;6(4):1591-1607.

587. Yehuda-shnaidman E, Kalderon B, Bar-tana J. Thyroid hormone, thyromimetics, and metabolic efficiency. Endocr Rev. 2014;35(1):35-58.

588. Verhoeven AJ, Kamer P, Groen AK, Tager JM. Effects of thyroid hormone on mitochondrial oxidative phosphorylation. Biochem J. 1985;226(1):183-92.

589. Singhal H, Greene ME, Tarulli G, et al. Genomic agonism and phenotypic antagonism between estrogen and progesterone receptors in breast cancer. Sci Adv. 2016;2(6):e1501924.

590. Behera MA, Dai Q, Garde R, Saner C, Jungheim E, Price TM. Progesterone stimulates mitochondrial activity with subsequent inhibition of apoptosis in MCF-10A benign breast epithelial cells. Am J Physiol Endocrinol Metab. 2009;297(5):E1089-96.

591. Kalra PS, Kalra SP. Progesterone stimulates testosterone secretion in male rats. Neuroendocrinology. 1980;30(3):183-6.

592. Schweizer MT, Antonarakis ES, Wang H, et al. Effect of bipolar androgen therapy for asymptomatic men with castration-resistant prostate cancer: results from a pilot clinical study. Sci Transl Med. 2015;7(269):269ra2.

593. Vallée M, Vitiello S, Bellocchio L, et al. Pregnenolone can protect the brain from cannabis intoxication. Science. 2014;343(6166):94-8.

594. Patel MA, Katyare SS. Dehydroepiandrosterone (DHEA) treatment stimulates oxidative energy metabolism in the cerebral mitochondria from developing rats. Int J Dev Neurosci. 2006;24(5):327-34.

595. Patel MA, Modi HR, Katyare SS. Stimulation of oxidative energy metabolism in liver mitochondria from old and young rats by treatment with dehydroepiandrosterone (DHEA). A comparative study. Age (Dordr). 2007;29(1):41-9.

596. Patel MA, Katyare SS. Treatment with dehydroepiandrosterone (DHEA) stimulates oxidative energy metabolism in the liver mitochondria from developing rats. Mol Cell Biochem. 2006;293(1-2):193-201.

597. Patel MA, Katyare SS. Treatment with dehydroepiandrosterone (DHEA) stimulates oxidative energy metabolism in the cerebral mitochondria. A comparative study of effects in old and young adult rats. Neurosci Lett. 2006;402(1-2):131-6.

598. Cleary MP. Effect of dehydroepiandrosterone treatment on liver metabolism in rats. Int J Biochem. 1990;22(3):205-10.

599. Muthusamy T, Murugesan P, Srinivasan C, Balasubramanian K. Sex steroids influence glucose oxidation through modulation of insulin receptor expression and IRS-1 serine phosphorylation in target tissues of adult male rat. Mol Cell Biochem. 2011;352(1-2):35-45.

600. Toro-urrego N, Garcia-segura LM, Echeverria V, Barreto GE. Testosterone Protects Mitochondrial Function and Regulates Neuroglobin Expression in Astrocytic Cells Exposed to Glucose Deprivation. Front Aging Neurosci. 2016;8:152.

601. Wang F, Yang J, Sun J, et al. Testosterone replacement attenuates mitochondrial damage in a rat model of myocardial infarction. J Endocrinol. 2015;225(2):101-11.

602. Parthasarathy C, Renuka VN, Balasubramanian K. Sex steroids enhance insulin receptors and glucose oxidation in Chang liver cells. Clin Chim Acta. 2009;399(1-2):49-53.

603. Tinker, B. (2015). Cholesterol in food not a concern, report says. CNN. [Online]. Available: http://www.cnn.com/2015/02/19/health/dietary-guidelines.[March 1, 2017].

604. Singh-manoux A, Gimeno D, Kivimaki M, Brunner E, Marmot MG. Low HDL cholesterol is a risk factor for deficit and decline in memory in midlife: the Whitehall II study. Arterioscler Thromb Vasc Biol. 2008;28(8):1556-62.

605. Huang X, Auinger P, Eberly S, et al. Serum cholesterol and the progression of Parkinson's disease: results from DATATOP. PLoS ONE. 2011;6(8):e22854.

606. Engelberg H. Low serum cholesterol and suicide. Lancet. 1992;339(8795):727-9.

607. Boscarino JA, Erlich PM, Hoffman SN. Low serum cholesterol and external-cause mortality: potential implications for research and surveillance. J Psychiatr Res. 2009;43(9):848-54.

608. Hawthon K, Cowen P, Owens D, Bond A, Elliott M. Low serum cholesterol and suicide. Br J Psychiatry. 1993;162:818-25.

609. Horwich TB, Hamilton MA, Maclellan WR, Fonarow GC. Low serum total cholesterol is associated with marked increase in mortality in advanced heart failure. J Card Fail. 2002;8(4):216-24.

610. Bae JM, Yang YJ, Li ZM, Ahn YO. Low cholesterol is associated with mortality from cardiovascular diseases: a dynamic cohort study in Korean adults. J Korean Med Sci. 2012;27(1):58-63.

611. Froom P, Kristal-boneh E, Melamed S, Harari G, Benbassat J, Ribak J. Serum total cholesterol and cardiovascular mortality in Israeli males: the CORDIS Study. Cardiovascular Occupational Risk Factor Determination in Israeli Industry. Isr Med Assoc J. 2000;2(9):668-71.

612. Ravnskov U, Diamond DM, Hama R, et al. Lack of an association or an inverse association between low-density-lipoprotein cholesterol and mortality in the elderly: a systematic review. BMJ Open. 2016;6(6):e010401.

613. Knekt P, Reunanen A, Aromaa A, Heliövaara M, Hakulinen T, Hakama M. Serum cholesterol and risk of cancer in a cohort of 39,000 men and women. J Clin Epidemiol. 1988;41(6):519-30.

614. Nago N, Ishikawa S, Goto T, Kayaba K. Low cholesterol is associated with mortality from stroke, heart disease, and cancer: the Jichi Medical School Cohort Study. J Epidemiol. 2011;21(1):67-74.

615. Behar S, Graff E, Reicher-reiss H, et al. Low total cholesterol is associated with high total mortality in patients with coronary heart disease. The Bezafibrate Infarction Prevention (BIP) Study Group. Eur Heart J. 1997;18(1):52-9.

616. Eichholzer M, Stähelin HB, Gutzwiller F, Lüdin E, Bernasconi F. Association of low plasma cholesterol with mortality for cancer at various sites in men: 17-y follow-up of the prospective Basel study. Am J Clin Nutr. 2000;71(2):569-74.

617. Illingworth DR, Harris WS, Connor WE. Inhibition of low density lipoprotein synthesis by dietary omega-3 fatty acids in humans. Arteriosclerosis. 1984;4(3):270-5.

618. Connor WE, Defrancesco CA, Connor SL. N-3 fatty acids from fish oil. Effects on plasma lipoproteins and hypertriglyceridemic patients. Ann N Y Acad Sci. 1993;683:16-34.

619. Karanth S, Tran VM, Kuberan B, Schlegel A. Polyunsaturated fatty acyl-coenzyme As are inhibitors of cholesterol biosynthesis in zebrafish and mice. Dis Model Mech. 2013;6(6):1365-77.

620. Spady DK. Regulatory effects of individual n-6 and n-3 polyunsaturated fatty acids on LDL transport in the rat. J Lipid Res. 1993;34(8):1337-46.

621. Illingworth DR, Harris WS, Connor WE. Inhibition of low density lipoprotein synthesis by dietary omega-3 fatty acids in humans. Arteriosclerosis. 1984;4(3):270-5.

622. O'brien T, Katz K, Hodge D, Nguyen TT, Kottke BA, Hay ID. The effect of the treatment of hypothyroidism and hyperthyroidism on plasma lipids and apolipoproteins AI, AII and E. Clin Endocrinol (Oxf). 1997;46(1):17-20.

623.   Canaris GJ, Manowitz NR, Mayor G, Ridgway EC. The Colorado thyroid disease prevalence study. Arch Intern Med. 2000;160(4):526-34.

624.   Turner KB, Steiner A. A LONG TERM STUDY OF THE VARIATION OF SERUM CHOLESTEROL IN MAN. J Clin Invest. 1939;18(1):45-9.

625.   Feld S, Dickey RA. An Association Between Varying Degrees of Hypothyroidism and Hypercholesterolemia in Women: The Thyroid-Cholesterol Connection. Prev Cardiol. 2001;4(4):179-182.

626.   Oribe H. [Clinical studies on lipid metabolism in hyperthyroidism and hypothyroidism--evaluation of serum apolipoprotein levels before and after treatment]. Nihon Naibunpi Gakkai Zasshi. 1989;65(8):781-93.

627.   Muls E, Blaton V, Rosseneu M, Lesaffre E, Lamberigts G, De moor P. Serum lipids and apolipoproteins A-I, A-II, and B in hyperthyroidism before and after treatment. J Clin Endocrinol Metab. 1982;55(3):459-64.

628.   Kung AW, Pang RW, Lauder I, Lam KS, Janus ED. Changes in serum lipoprotein(a) and lipids during treatment of hyperthyroidism. Clin Chem. 1995;41(2):226-31.

629.   Diekman MJ, Anghelescu N, Endert E, Bakker O, Wiersinga WM. Changes in plasma low-density lipoprotein (LDL)- and high-density lipoprotein cholesterol in hypo- and hyperthyroid patients are related to changes in free thyroxine, not to polymorphisms in LDL receptor or cholesterol ester transfer protein genes. J Clin Endocrinol Metab. 2000;85(5):1857-62.

630.   Meier C, Staub JJ, Roth CB, et al. TSH-controlled L-thyroxine therapy reduces cholesterol levels and clinical symptoms in subclinical hypothyroidism: a double blind, placebo-controlled trial (Basel Thyroid Study). J Clin Endocrinol Metab. 2001;86(10):4860-6.

631.   Iqbal A, Jorde R, Figenschau Y. Serum lipid levels in relation to serum thyroid-stimulating hormone and the effect of thyroxine treatment on serum lipid levels in subjects with subclinical hypothyroidism: the Tromsø Study. J Intern Med. 2006;260(1):53-61.

632.   Kung AW, Pang RW, Janus ED. Elevated serum lipoprotein(a) in subclinical hypothyroidism. Clin Endocrinol (Oxf). 1995;43(4):445-9.

633.   Mikhail GS, Alshammari SM, Alenezi MY, Mansour M, Khalil NA. Increased atherogenic low-density lipoprotein cholesterol in untreated subclinical hypothyroidism. Endocr Pract. 2008;14(5):570-5.

634.   Danese MD, Ladenson PW, Meinert CL, Powe NR. Clinical review 115: effect of thyroxine therapy on serum lipoproteins in patients with mild thyroid failure: a quantitative review of the literature. J Clin Endocrinol Metab. 2000;85(9):2993-3001.

635.   Shin DJ, Osborne TF. Thyroid hormone regulation and cholesterol metabolism are connected through Sterol Regulatory Element-Binding Protein-2 (SREBP-2). J Biol Chem. 2003;278(36):34114-8.

636.   Thompson GR, Soutar AK, Spengel FA, Jadhav A, Gavigan SJ, Myant NB. Defects of receptor-mediated low density lipoprotein catabolism in homozygous familial hypercholesterolemia and hypothyroidism in vivo. Proc Natl Acad Sci USA. 1981;78(4):2591-5.

637.   Pugsley LI. The effect of thyrotropic hormone upon serum cholesterol. Biochem J. 1935;29(3):513-6.

638.   Jung CH, Sung KC, Shin HS, et al. Thyroid dysfunction and their relation to cardiovascular risk factors such as lipid profile, hsCRP, and waist hip ratio in Korea. Korean J Intern Med. 2003;18(3):146-53.

639.   Luboshitzky R, Aviv A, Herer P, Lavie L. Risk factors for cardiovascular disease in women with subclinical hypothyroidism. Thyroid. 2002;12(5):421-5.

CANCER CURED

640. Pesić M, Antić S, Kocić R, Radojković D, Radenković S. [Cardiovascular risk factors in patients with subclinical hypothyroidism]. Vojnosanit Pregl. 2007;64(11):749-52.

641. Walsh JP, Bremner AP, Bulsara MK, et al. Thyroid dysfunction and serum lipids: a community-based study. Clin Endocrinol (Oxf). 2005;63(6):670-5.

642. Serter R, Demirbas B, Korukluoglu B, Culha C, Cakal E, Aral Y. The effect of L-thyroxine replacement therapy on lipid based cardiovascular risk in subclinical hypothyroidism. J Endocrinol Invest. 2004;27(10):897-903.

643. Milionis HJ, Tambaki AP, Kanioglou CN, Elisaf MS, Tselepis AD, Tsatsoulis A. Thyroid substitution therapy induces high-density lipoprotein-associated platelet-activating factor-acetylhydrolase in patients with subclinical hypothyroidism: a potential antiatherogenic effect. Thyroid. 2005;15(5):455-60.

644. Arinzon Z, Zuta A, Peisakh A, Feldman J, Berner Y. Evaluation response and effectiveness of thyroid hormone replacement treatment on lipid profile and function in elderly patients with subclinical hypothyroidism. Arch Gerontol Geriatr. 2007;44(1):13-9.

645. Miura S, Iitaka M, Yoshimura H, et al. Disturbed lipid metabolism in patients with subclinical hypothyroidism: effect of L-thyroxine therapy. Intern Med. 1994;33(7):413-7.

646. Dzugan SA, Arnold smith R. Hypercholesterolemia treatment: a new hypothesis or just an accident?. Med Hypotheses. 2002;59(6):751-6.

647. Althaus BU, Staub JJ, Ryff-de lèche A, Oberhänsli A, Stähelin HB. LDL/HDL-changes in subclinical hypothyroidism: possible risk factors for coronary heart disease. Clin Endocrinol (Oxf). 1988;28(2):157-63.

648. Thorell B, Svärdsudd K. Myocardial infarction risk factors and well-being among 50-year-old women before and after the menopause. The population study "50-year-old people in Kungsör". Scand J Prim Health Care. 1993;11(2):141-6.

649. Altınterim B. Anti-Thyroid Effects of PUFAs (polyunsaturated fats) and Herbs. 2012.

650. The Conscious Life. Fat Composition of Olive Oil. [Online]. Available: https://theconsciouslife.com/foods/olive-oil-04053.htm.[March 1, 2017].

651. Fukusen N, Kido H, Katunuma N. Inhibition of chymase activity by phosphoglycerides. Arch Biochem Biophys. 1985;237(1):118-23.

652. Tabachnick M, Korcek L. Effect of long-chain fatty acids on the binding of thyroxine and triiodothyronine to human thyroxine-binding globulin. Biochim Biophys Acta. 1986;881(2):292-6.

653. Chopra IJ, Huang TS, Beredo A, Solomon DH, Chua teco GN, Mead JF. Evidence for an inhibitor of extrathyroidal conversion of thyroxine to 3,5,3'-triiodothyronine in sera of patients with nonthyroidal illnesses. J Clin Endocrinol Metab. 1985;60(4):666-72.

654. Wiersinga WM, Chopra IJ, Teco GN. Inhibition of nuclear T3 binding by fatty acids. Metab Clin Exp. 1988;37(10):996-1002.

655. Rafael J, Patzelt J, Schäfer H, Elmadfa I. The effect of essential fatty acid deficiency on basal respiration and function of liver mitochondria in rats. J Nutr. 1984;114(2):255-62.

656. Wesson LG, Burr GO. The metabolic rate and respiratory quotients of rats on a fat-deficient diet. J. Biol. Chem. 1931;91:525-539.

657. Burr GO, Beber AJ. Metabolism studies with rats suffering from fat deficiency: six figures. J Nutr. 1937;14:553-566.

658. Goubern M, Yazbeck J, Senault C, Portet R. Non-shivering thermogenesis and brown adipose tissue activity in essential fatty acid deficient rats. Arch Int Physiol Biochim. 1990;98(4):193-9.

659. Rafael J, Patzelt J, Elmadfa I. Effect of dietary linoleic acid and essential fatty acid deficiency on resting metabolism, nonshivering thermogenesis and brown adipose tissue in the rat. J Nutr. 1988;118(5):627-32.

660. Yazbeck J, Goubern M, Senault C, Chapey MF, Portet R. The effects of essential fatty acid deficiency on brown adipose tissue activity in rats maintained at thermal neutrality. Comp Biochem Physiol A Comp Physiol. 1989;94(2):273-6.

661. O'reilly I, Murphy MP. Studies on the rapid stimulation of mitochondrial respiration by thyroid hormones. Acta Endocrinol. 1992;127(6):542-6.

662. Lombardi A, Moreno M, De lange P, Iossa S, Busiello RA, Goglia F. Regulation of skeletal muscle mitochondrial activity by thyroid hormones: focus on the "old" triiodothyronine and the "emerging" 3,5-diiodothyronine. Front Physiol. 2015;6:237.

663. Weitzel JM, Iwen KA, Seitz HJ. Regulation of mitochondrial biogenesis by thyroid hormone. Exp Physiol. 2003;88(1):121-8.

664. Wrutniak-cabello C, Casas F, Cabello G. Thyroid hormone action in mitochondria. J Mol Endocrinol. 2001;26(1):67-77.

665. Verhoeven AJ, Kamer P, Groen AK, Tager JM. Effects of thyroid hormone on mitochondrial oxidative phosphorylation. Biochem J. 1985;226(1):183-92.

666. Hoch FL, Lipmann F. THE UNCOUPLING OF RESPIRATION AND PHOSPHORYLATION BY THYROID HORMONES. Proc Natl Acad Sci USA. 1954;40(10):909-21.

667. Wooten WL, Cascarano J. The effect of thyroid hormone on mitochondrial biogenesis and cellular hyperplasia. J Bioenerg Biomembr. 1980;12(1-2):1-12.

668. Lesmana R, Sinha RA, Singh BK, Zhou J, Obha K, Wu Y, Yau WWY, Bay BH, Yen PM. Thyroid hormone stimulation of autophagy is essential for mitochondrial biogenesis activity in skeletal muscle. Endocrinology. 2015;157(1).

669. Weitzel JM, Iwen KA. Coordination of mitochondrial biogenesis by thyroid hormone. Mol Cell Endocrinol. 2011;342(1-2):1-7.

670. Marín-garcía J. Thyroid hormone and myocardial mitochondrial biogenesis. Vascul Pharmacol. 2010;52(3-4):120-30.

671. Cioffi F, Senese R, Lanni A, Goglia F. Thyroid hormones and mitochondria: with a brief look at derivatives and analogues. Mol Cell Endocrinol. 2013;379(1-2):51-61.

672. Nelson BD. Thyroid hormone regulation of mitochondrial function. Comments on the mechanism of signal transduction. Biochim Biophys Acta. 1990;1018(2-3):275-7.

673. Pottinger TG, Carrick TR, Hughes SE, Balm PH. Testosterone, 11-ketotestosterone, and estradiol-17 beta modify baseline and stress-induced interrenal and corticotropic activity in trout. Gen Comp Endocrinol. 1996;104(3):284-95.

674. Katoh K, Asari M, Ishiwata H, Sasaki Y, Obara Y. Saturated fatty acids suppress adrenocorticotropic hormone (ACTH) release from rat anterior pituitary cells in vitro. Comp Biochem Physiol, Part A Mol Integr Physiol. 2004;137(2):357-64.

675. Oh YT, Kim J, Kang I, Youn JH. Regulation of hypothalamic-pituitary-adrenal axis by circulating free fatty acids in male Wistar rats: role of individual free fatty acids. Endocrinology. 2014;155(3):923-31.

676. Jankord R, Ganjam VK, Turk JR, Hamilton MT, Laughlin MH. Exercise training alters effect of high-fat feeding on the ACTH stress response in pigs. Appl Physiol Nutr Metab. 2008;33(3):461-9.

677. Van schalkwijk DB, Pasman WJ, Hendriks HF, et al. Dietary medium chain fatty acid supplementation leads to reduced VLDL lipolysis and uptake rates in comparison to linoleic acid supplementation. PLoS ONE. 2014;9(7):e100376.

678. Goodfriend TL, Ball DL, Raff H, Bruder ED, Gardner HW, Spiteller G. Oxidized products of linoleic acid stimulate adrenal steroidogenesis. Endocr Res. 2002;28(4):325-30.

679. Bruder ED, Ball DL, Goodfriend TL, Raff H. An oxidized metabolite of linoleic acid stimulates corticosterone production by rat adrenal cells. Am J Physiol Regul Integr Comp Physiol. 2003;284(6):R1631-5.

680. Abou-samra AB, Catt KJ, Aguilera G. Role of arachidonic acid in the regulation of adrenocorticotropin release from rat anterior pituitary cell cultures. Endocrinology. 1986;119(4):1427-31.

681. Montero D, Terova G, Rimoldi S, et al. Modulation of adrenocorticotrophin hormone (ACTH)-induced expression of stress-related genes by PUFA in inter-renal cells from European sea bass (Dicentrarchus labrax). J Nutr Sci. 2015;4:e16.

682. Ganga R, Bell JG, Montero D, et al. Adrenocorticotrophic hormone-stimulated cortisol release by the head kidney inter-renal tissue from sea bream (Sparus aurata) fed with linseed oil and soyabean oil. Br J Nutr. 2011;105(2):238-47.

683. Ganga R, Tort L, Acerete L, Montero D, Izquierdo MS. Modulation of ACTH-induced cortisol release by polyunsaturated fatty acids in interrenal cells from gilthead seabream, Sparus aurata. J Endocrinol. 2006;190(1):39-45.

684. Won JG, Orth DN. Role of lipoxygenase metabolites of arachidonic acid in the regulation of adrenocorticotropin secretion by perifused rat anterior pituitary cells. Endocrinology. 1994;135(4):1496-503.

685. Reed MJ, Beranek PA, Cheng RW, James VH. Free fatty acids: a possible regulator of the available oestradiol fractions in plasma. J Steroid Biochem. 1986;24(2):657-9.

686. Bruning PF, Bonfrer JM. Possible relevance of steroid availability and breast cancer. Ann N Y Acad Sci. 1988;538:257-64.

687. Benassayag C, Rigourd V, Mignot TM, et al. Does high polyunsaturated free fatty acid level at the feto-maternal interface alter steroid hormone message during pregnancy?. Prostaglandins Leukot Essent Fatty Acids. 1999;60(5-6):393-9.

688. Reed MJ, Dunkley SA, Singh A, Thomas BS, Haines AP, Cruickshank JK. The role of free fatty acids in regulating the tissue availability and synthesis of sex steroids. Prostaglandins Leukot Essent Fatty Acids. 1993;48(1):111-6.

689. Vaiopoulos AG, Athanasoula KCh, Papavassiliou AG. NF-κB in colorectal cancer. J Mol Med. 2013;91(9):1029-37.

690. Denton RM, Ashcroft SJ. A tribute to the life and work of Philip Randle. Diabetologia. 2007;50(7):1359-61.

691. Randle PJ. Regulatory interactions between lipids and carbohydrates: the glucose fatty acid cycle after 35 years. Diabetes Metab Rev. 1998;14(4):263-83.

692. Hosios AM, Hecht VC, Johnson M, Rathmell JC, Manalis SR, Vander Heiden MG. Amino acids rather than glucose accounts for the majority of cell mass in rapidly proliferating mammalian cells. Molecular Cancer Research. 2016;14(1):A36.

693. Rajagopalan KN, Egnatchik RA, Calvaruso MA, et al. Metabolic plasticity maintains proliferation in pyruvate dehydrogenase deficient cells. Cancer Metab. 2015;3:7.

694. Seyfried TN. Is mitochondrial glutamine fermentation a missing link in the metabolic theory of cancer? 2012. Pp. 133-144.

695. Gu Y, Chen T, Fu S, et al. Perioperative dynamics and significance of amino acid profiles in patients with cancer. J Transl Med. 2015;13:35.

696. Dereziński P, Klupczynska A, Sawicki W, Pałka JA, Kokot ZJ. Amino Acid Profiles of Serum and Urine in Search for Prostate Cancer Biomarkers: a Pilot Study. Int J Med Sci. 2017;14(1):1-12.

697. Andersen DK. Diabetes and cancer: placing the association in perspective. Curr Opin Endocrinol Diabetes Obes. 2013;20(2):81-6.

698. Cui Y, Andersen DK. Diabetes and pancreatic cancer. Endocr Relat Cancer. 2012;19(5):F9-F26.

699. Salvatore T, Marfella R, Rizzo MR, Sasso FC. Pancreatic cancer and diabetes: A two-way relationship in the perspective of diabetologist. Int J Surg. 2015;21 Suppl 1:S72-7.

700. Muniraj T, Chari ST. Diabetes and pancreatic cancer. Minerva Gastroenterol Dietol. 2012;58(4):331-45.

701. Sciacca L, Vigneri R, Tumminia A, et al. Clinical and molecular mechanisms favoring cancer initiation and progression in diabetic patients. Nutr Metab Cardiovasc Dis. 2013;23(9):808-15.

702. Toriola AT, Stolzenberg-solomon R, Dalidowitz L, Linehan D, Colditz G. Diabetes and pancreatic cancer survival: a prospective cohort-based study. Br J Cancer. 2014;111(1):181-5.

703. Rosta A. [Diabetes and cancer risk: oncologic considerations]. Orv Hetil. 2011;152(29):1144-55.

704. Buysschaert M, Sadikot S. Diabetes and cancer: a 2013 synopsis. Diabetes Metab Syndr. 2013;7(4):247-50.

705. Mcdermott WV. Metabolism and toxicity of ammonia. N Engl J Med. 1957;257(22):1076-81.

706. Leke R, Bak LK, Anker M, et al. Detoxification of ammonia in mouse cortical GABAergic cell cultures increases neuronal oxidative metabolism and reveals an emerging role for release of glucose-derived alanine. Neurotox Res. 2011;19(3):496-510.

707. Kala G, Hertz L. Ammonia effects on pyruvate/lactate production in astrocytes--interaction with glutamate. Neurochem Int. 2005;47(1-2):4-12.

708. Muntz JA, Hurwitz J. Effect of potassium and ammonium ions upon glycolysis catalyzed by an extract of rat brain. Arch Biochem Biophys. 1951;32(1):124-36.

709. Pascual G, Avgustinova A, Mejetta S, Martin M, Castellanos A, Attolini SO, Berenguer A, Prats N, Toll A, Hueto JA, Bescos C, Di Croce L, Benitah SA. Targeting metastasis-intitating cells through the fatty acid receptor CD36. Nature. 2017;541:41-45.

710. Slebe F, Rojo F, Vinaixa M, et al. FoxA and LIPG endothelial lipase control the uptake of extracellular lipids for breast cancer growth. Nat Commun. 2016;7:11199.

711. Cohen LA. Fat and endocrine-responsive cancer in animals. Prev Med. 1987;16(4):468-74.

712. Rao CV, Hirose Y, Indranie C, Reddy BS. Modulation of experimental colon tumorigenesis by types and amounts of dietary fatty acids. Cancer Res. 2001;61(5):1927-33.

713. Zusman I, Gurevich P, Madar Z, et al. Tumor-promoting and tumor-protective effects of high-fat diets on chemically induced mammary cancer in rats. Anticancer Res. 1997;17(1A):349-56.

714. Carroll KK. Neutral fats and cancer. Cancer Res. 1981;41(9 Pt 2):3695-9.

715. Chan PC, Ferguson KA, Dao TL. Effects of different dietary fats on mammary carcinogenesis. Cancer Res. 1983;43(3):1079-83.

716. Dayton S, Hashimoto S, Wollman J. Effect of high-oleic and high-linoleic safflower oils on mammary tumors induced in rats by 7,12-dimethylbenz(alpha)anthracene. J Nutr. 1977;107(8):1353-60.

717. Carroll KK, Hopkins GJ. Dietary polyunsaturated fat versus saturated fat in relation to mammary carcinogenesis. Lipids. 1979;14(2):155-8.

718. Karmali RA, Donner A, Gobel S, Shimamura T. Effect of n-3 and n-6 fatty acids on 7,12 dimethylbenz (a) anthracene-induced mammary tumorigenesis. Anticancer Res. 1989;9(4):1161-7.

CANCER CURED

719.   Aylsworth CF, Jone C, Trosko JE, Meites J, Welsch CW. Promotion of 7,12-dimethylbenz[a]anthracene-induced mammary tumorigenesis by high dietary fat in the rat: possible role of intercellular communication. J Natl Cancer Inst. 1984;72(3):637-45.

720.   Cohen LA, Thompson DO, Maeura Y, Choi K, Blank ME, Rose DP. Dietary fat and mammary cancer. I. Promoting effects of different dietary fats on N-nitrosomethylurea-induced rat mammary tumorigenesis. J Natl Cancer Inst. 1986;77(1):33-42.

721.   Kuno T, Hirose Y, Yamada Y, et al. Promoting effects of high-fat corn oil and high-fat mixed lipid diets on 7,12-dimethylbenz[a]anthracene-induced mammary tumorigenesis in F344 rats. Oncol Rep. 2003;10(3):699-703.

722.   Cohen LA, Thompson DO, Choi K, Karmali RA, Rose DP. Dietary fat and mammary cancer. II. Modulation of serum and tumor lipid composition and tumor prostaglandins by different dietary fats: association with tumor incidence patterns. J Natl Cancer Inst. 1986;77(1):43-51.

723.   Hopkins GJ, Kennedy TG, Carroll KK. Polyunsaturated fatty acids as promoters of mammary carcinogenesis induced in Sprague-Dawley rats by 7,12-dimethylbenz[a]anthracene. J Natl Cancer Inst. 1981;66(3):517-22.

724.   Carroll KK. Dietary fat in relation to mammary carcinogenesis. Int Symp Princess Takamatsu Cancer Res Fund. 1985;16:255-63.

725.   Welsch CW. Dietary fat, calories, and mammary gland tumorigenesis. Adv Exp Med Biol. 1992;322:203-22.

726.   Oyaizu N, Morii S, Saito K, Katsuda Y, Matsumoto J. Mechanism of growth enhancement of 7,12-dimethylbenz[a]-anthracene-induced mammary tumors in rats given high polyunsaturated fat diet. Jpn J Cancer Res. 1985;76(8):676-83.

727.   Selenskas SL, Ip MM, Ip C. Similarity between trans fat and saturated fat in the modification of rat mammary carcinogenesis. Cancer Res. 1984;44(4):1321-6.

728.   Cohen LA, Choi K, Weisburger JH, Rose DP. Effect of varying proportions of dietary fat on the development of N-nitrosomethylurea-induced rat mammary tumors. Anticancer Res. 1986;6(2):215-8.

729.   Griffini P, Fehres O, Klieverik L, et al. Dietary omega-3 polyunsaturated fatty acids promote colon carcinoma metastasis in rat liver. Cancer Res. 1998;58(15):3312-9.

730.   Twining, C. W., Brenna, J. T., Hairston, N. G. and Flecker, A. S. (2016), Highly unsaturated fatty acids in nature: what we know and what we need to learn. Oikos, 125: 749–760.

731.   Mehta RS, Gunnett CA, Harris SR, Bunce OR, Hartle DK. High fish oil diet increases oxidative stress potential in mammary gland of spontaneously hypertensive rats. Clin Exp Pharmacol Physiol. 1994;21(11):881-9.

732.   Sauer LA, Dauchy RT. Blood nutrient concentrations and tumor growth in vivo in rats: relationships during the onset of an acute fast. Cancer Res. 1987;47(4):1065-8.

733.   Kline BE, Miller JA. The carcinogenicity of p-dimethylaminoazobenzene in diets containing the fatty acids of hydrogenated coconut oil or of corn oil. Cancer Res. 1946;6:1-4.

734.   Roebuck BD, Longnecker DS, Baumgartner KJ, Thron CD. Carcinogen-induced lesions in the rat pancreas: effects of varying levels of essential fatty acid. Cancer Res. 1985;45(11 Pt 1):5252-6.

735.   Carroll KK. Summation: which fat/how much fat--animals. Prev Med. 1987;16(4):510-5.

736.   Hopkins GJ, Carroll KK. Relationship between amount and type of dietary fat in promotion of mammary carcinogenesis induced by 7,12-dimethylbenz[a]anthracene. J Natl Cancer Inst. 1979;62(4):1009-12.

737.   Ip C, Carter CA, Ip MM. Requirement of essential fatty acid for mammary tumorigenesis in the rat. Cancer Res. 1985;45(5):1997-2001.

738. Singer MM, Wright F, Stanley LK, Roe BB, Hamilton WK. Oxygen toxicity in man. A prospective study in patients after open-heart surgery. N Engl J Med. 1970;283(27):1473-8.

739. Baeyens DA, Hoffert JR, Fromm PO. A comparative study of oxygen toxicity in the retina, brain and liver of the teleost, amphibian and mammal. Comp Biochem Physiol A Comp Physiol. 1973;45(4):925-32.

740. Brown JR, Dubois RN. Cyclooxygenase as a target in lung cancer. Clin Cancer Res. 2004;10(12 Pt 2):4266s-4269s.

741. Riedl K, Krysan K, Põld M, et al. Multifaceted roles of cyclooxygenase-2 in lung cancer. Drug Resist Updat. 2004;7(3):169-84.

742. Harris RE. Cyclooxygenase-2 (cox-2) and the inflammogenesis of cancer. Subcell Biochem. 2007;42:93-126.

743. Sandler AB, Dubinett SM. COX-2 inhibition and lung cancer. Semin Oncol. 2004;31(2 Suppl 7):45-52.

744. Spano JP, Chouahnia K, Morère JF. [Cyclooxygenase 2 inhibitors and lung carcinoma]. Bull Cancer. 2004;91 Spec No:S109-12.

745. Zelenay S, Reis e sousa C. Reducing prostaglandin E2 production to raise cancer immunogenicity. Oncoimmunology. 2016;5(5):e1123370.

746. Fujita H, Koshida K, Keller ET, et al. Cyclooxygenase-2 promotes prostate cancer progression. Prostate. 2002;53(3):232-40.

747. Carroll KK, Braden LM. Dietary fat and mammary carcinogenesis. Nutr Cancer. 1984;6(4):254-9.

748. Jiang J, Dingledine R. Prostaglandin receptor EP2 in the crosshairs of anti-inflammation, anti-cancer, and neuroprotection. Trends Pharmacol Sci. 2013;34(7):413-23.

749. Wang MT, Honn KV, Nie D. Cyclooxygenases, prostanoids, and tumor progression. Cancer Metastasis Rev. 2007;26(3-4):525-34.

750. Castellone MD, Teramoto H, Williams BO, Druey KM, Gutkind JS. Prostaglandin E2 promotes colon cancer cell growth through a Gs-axin-beta-catenin signaling axis. Science. 2005;310(5753):1504-10.

751. Wu WK, Sung JJ, Lee CW, Yu J, Cho CH. Cyclooxygenase-2 in tumorigenesis of gastrointestinal cancers: an update on the molecular mechanisms. Cancer Lett. 2010;295(1):7-16.

752. Castellone MD, Teramoto H, Gutkind JS. Cyclooxygenase-2 and colorectal cancer chemoprevention: the beta-catenin connection. Cancer Res. 2006;66(23):11085-8.

753. Wang D, Dubois RN. Eicosanoids and cancer. Nat Rev Cancer. 2010;10(3):181-93.

754. Hiraga T, Myoui A, Choi ME, Yoshikawa H, Yoneda T. Stimulation of cyclooxygenase-2 expression by bone-derived transforming growth factor-beta enhances bone metastases in breast cancer. Cancer Res. 2006;66(4):2067-73.

755. Singh B, Berry JA, Shoher A, Ayers GD, Wei C, Lucci A. COX-2 involvement in breast cancer metastasis to bone. Oncogene. 2007;26(26):3789-96.

756. Singh B, Berry JA, Shoher A, Lucci A. COX-2 induces IL-11 production in human breast cancer cells. J Surg Res. 2006;131(2):267-75.

757. Fosslien E. Review: molecular pathology of cyclooxygenase-2 in cancer-induced angiogenesis. Ann Clin Lab Sci. 2001;31(4):325-48.

758. Gately S, Kerbel R. Therapeutic potential of selective cyclooxygenase-2 inhibitors in the management of tumor angiogenesis. Prog Exp Tumor Res. 2003;37:179-92.

759. Wolfe RR, Martini WZ, Irtun O, Hawkins HK, Barrow RE. Dietary fat composition alters pulmonary function in pigs. Nutrition. 2002;18(7-8):647-53.

760. Kramer JK, Farnworth ER, Thompson BK, Corner AH, Trenholm HL. Reduction of myocardial necrosis in male albino rats by manipulation of dietary fatty acid levels. Lipids. 1982;17(5):372-82.

761. Davidson MB, Carroll KK. Inhibitory effect of a fat-free diet on mammary carcinogenesis in rats. Nutr Cancer. 1982;3(4):207-15.

762. Buckingham KW. Effect of dietary polyunsaturated/saturated fatty acid ratio and dietary vitamin E on lipid peroxidation in the rat. J Nutr. 1985;115(11):1425-35.

763. Jenkinson AM, Collins AR, Duthie SJ, Wahle KW, Duthie GG. The effect of increased intakes of polyunsaturated fatty acids and vitamin E on DNA damage in human lymphocytes. FASEB J. 1999;13(15):2138-42.

764. Debry G. Polyunsaturated fatty acids and vitamin E : their importance in human nutrition. Ann Nutr Aliment. 1980;34(2):337-50.

765. Dubois RN, Abramson SB, Crofford L, et al. Cyclooxygenase in biology and disease. FASEB J. 1998;12(12):1063-73.

766. Chan TA. Prostaglandins and the colon cancer connection. Trends Mol Med. 2006;12(6):240-4.

767. Buchanan FG, Dubois RN. Connecting COX-2 and Wnt in cancer. Cancer Cell. 2006;9(1):6-8.

768. Roelofs HM, Te morsche RH, Van heumen BW, Nagengast FM, Peters WH. Over-expression of COX-2 mRNA in colorectal cancer. BMC Gastroenterol. 2014;14:1.

769. Bodey B, Siegel SE, Kaiser HE. Cyclooxygenase-2 (COX-2) overexpression in childhood brain tumors. In Vivo. 2006;20(4):519-25.

770. Petkova DK, Clelland C, Ronan J, et al. Overexpression of cyclooxygenase-2 in non-small cell lung cancer. Respir Med. 2004;98(2):164-72.

771. Turini ME, Dubois RN. Cyclooxygenase-2: a therapeutic target. Annu Rev Med. 2002;53:35-57.

772. Dempke W, Rie C, Grothey A, Schmoll HJ. Cyclooxygenase-2: a novel target for cancer chemotherapy?. J Cancer Res Clin Oncol. 2001;127(7):411-7.

773. Harris RE. Cyclooxygenase-2 (cox-2) blockade in the chemoprevention of cancers of the colon, breast, prostate, and lung. Inflammopharmacology. 2009;17(2):55-67.

774. Williams CS, Mann M, Dubois RN. The role of cyclooxygenases in inflammation, cancer, and development. Oncogene. 1999;18(55):7908-16.

775. Spinella F, Rosanò L, Di castro V, Nicotra MR, Natali PG, Bagnato A. Inhibition of cyclooxygenase-1 and -2 expression by targeting the endothelin a receptor in human ovarian carcinoma cells. Clin Cancer Res. 2004;10(14):4670-9.

776. Gridelli C, Maione P, Airoma G, Rossi A. Selective cyclooxygenase-2 inhibitors and non-small cell lung cancer. Curr Med Chem. 2002;9(21):1851-8.

777. Sawaoka H, Tsuji S, Tsujii M, et al. Cyclooxygenase inhibitors suppress angiogenesis and reduce tumor growth in vivo. Lab Invest. 1999;79(12):1469-77.

778. Tsuji S, Tsujii M, Kawano S, Hori M. Cyclooxygenase-2 upregulation as a perigenetic change in carcinogenesis. J Exp Clin Cancer Res. 2001;20(1):117-29.

779. Liu XH, Kirschenbaum A, Yao S, Lee R, Holland JF, Levine AC. Inhibition of cyclooxygenase-2 suppresses angiogenesis and the growth of prostate cancer in vivo. J Urol. 2000;164(3 Pt 1):820-5.

780. Yoshida S, Amano H, Hayashi I, et al. COX-2/VEGF-dependent facilitation of tumor-associated angiogenesis and tumor growth in vivo. Lab Invest. 2003;83(10):1385-94.

781. Chu J, Lloyd FL, Trifan OC, Knapp B, Rizzo MT. Potential involvement of the cyclooxygenase-2 pathway in the regulation of tumor-associated angiogenesis and growth in pancreatic cancer. Mol Cancer Ther. 2003;2(1):1-7.

782. Rozic JG, Chakraborty C, Lala PK. Cyclooxygenase inhibitors retard murine mammary tumor progression by reducing tumor cell migration, invasiveness and angiogenesis. Int J Cancer. 2001;93(4):497-506.

783. Goldyne ME. Prostaglandins and the modulation of immunological responses. Int J Dermatol. 1977;16(9):701-12.

784. Muthuswamy R, Okada NJ, Jenkins FJ, et al. Epinephrine promotes COX-2-dependent immune suppression in myeloid cells and cancer tissues. Brain Behav Immun. 2017;62:78-86.

785. Goodwin JS, Ceuppens J. Regulation of the immune response by prostaglandins. J Clin Immunol. 1983;3(4):295-315.

786. Langhendries JP, Maton P, François-adant A, Chantrain C, Bury F, Philippet P. [Prostaglandins and the immune response at the intestinal submucosal level. A potential site for interference with the repeated use of paracetamol and ibuprofen at a young age?]. Arch Pediatr. 2015;22(3):311-9.

787. Remes lenicov F, Varese A, Merlotti A, Geffner J, Ceballos A. Prostaglandins in semen compromise the immune response against sexually transmitted pathogens. Med Hypotheses. 2014;83(2):208-10.

788. Barone J, Hebert JR. Dietary fat and natural killer cell activity. Med Hypotheses. 1988;25(4):223-6.

789. Robertson GL, Kermode WJ. Salicylic acid in fresh and canned fruit and vegetables. J. Sci. Food. Ag. 1981;32(8):833-836.

790. Spencer, B. (2016). How liquid aspirin could help fight brain cancer. DailyMail. [Online]. Available: http://www.dailymail.co.uk/sciencetech/article-3663188/How-liquid-aspirin-help-fight-brain-cancer-Special-version-drug-ten-times-effective-killing-cancer-cells-chemotherapy.html.[March 2, 2017].

791. US Preventive Services Task Force. (2016). Aspirin Use to Prevent Cardiovascular Disease and Colorectal Cancer: Preventive Medication. [Online]. Available: https://www.uspreventiveservicestaskforce.org/Page/Document/UpdateSummaryFinal/aspirin-to-prevent-cardiovascular-disease-and-cancer.[March 1, 2017].

792. Uyttebrouck, O. (2016). Death rates for most cancers in decline. Albuquerque Journal. [Online]. Available: https://www.abqjournal.com/754139/death-rates-for-most-cancers-in-decline.html.[March 1, 2017].

793. Agus DB, Gaudette É, Goldman DP, Messali A. The Long-Term Benefits of Increased Aspirin Use by At-Risk Americans Aged 50 and Older. PLoS ONE. 2016;11(11):e0166103.

794. Emilsson L, Holme Ø, Bretthauer M, et al. Systematic review with meta-analysis: the comparative effectiveness of aspirin vs. screening for colorectal cancer prevention. Aliment Pharmacol Ther. 2017;45(2):193-204.

795. Schönhöfer PS, Sohn J, Peters HD, Dinnendahl V. Effects of sodium salicylate and acetylsalicylic acid on the lipolytic system of fat cells. Biochem Pharmacol. 1973;22(5):629-37.

796. Hundal RS, Petersen KF, Mayerson AB, et al. Mechanism by which high-dose aspirin improves glucose metabolism in type 2 diabetes. J Clin Invest. 2002;109(10):1321-6.

797. Meester WD, Schut GE, Hamp JA, Sekhar NC. Effect of aspirin on epinephrine-induced lipolysis and platelet aggregation in rats. Res Commun Chem Pathol Pharmacol. 1972;4(2):405-11.

798. Nixon M, Wake DJ, Livingstone DE, et al. Salicylate downregulates 11β-HSD1 expression in adipose tissue in obese mice and in humans, mediating insulin sensitization. Diabetes. 2012;61(4):790-6.

799. De cristóbal J, Cárdenas A, Lizasoain I, et al. Inhibition of glutamate release via recovery of ATP levels accounts for a neuroprotective effect of aspirin in rat cortical neurons exposed to oxygen-glucose deprivation. Stroke. 2002;33(1):261-7.

800. Singh AK, Zajdel J, Mirrasekhian E, et al. Prostaglandin-mediated inhibition of serotonin signaling controls the affective component of inflammatory pain. J Clin Invest. 2017.

801. Cotlier E. Senile cataracts: evidence for acceleration by diabetes and deceleration by salicylate. Can J Ophthalmol. 1981;16(3):113-8.

802. Cotlier E. Aspirin effect on cataract formation in patients with rheumatoid arthritis alone or combined with diabetes. Int Ophthalmol. 1981;3(3):173-7.

803. Gomes I. Aspirin: a neuroprotective agent at high doses?. Natl Med J India. 1998;11(1):14-7.

804. Asanuma M, Nishibayashi-asanuma S, Miyazaki I, Kohno M, Ogawa N. Neuroprotective effects of non-steroidal anti-inflammatory drugs by direct scavenging of nitric oxide radicals. J Neurochem. 2001;76(6):1895-904.

805. Choi HW, Tian M, Manohar M, et al. Human GAPDH Is a Target of Aspirin's Primary Metabolite Salicylic Acid and Its Derivatives. PLoS ONE. 2015;10(11):e0143447.

806. Smith JW, Al-khamees O, Costall B, Naylor RJ, Smythe JW. Chronic aspirin ingestion improves spatial learning in adult and aged rats. Pharmacol Biochem Behav. 2002;71(1-2):233-8.

807. Guan XT, Shao F, Xie X, Chen L, Wang W. Effects of aspirin on immobile behavior and endocrine and immune changes in the forced swimming test: comparison to fluoxetine and imipramine. Pharmacol Biochem Behav. 2014;124:361-6.

808. Schwarz KB, Arey BJ, Tolman K, Mahanty S. Iron chelation as a possible mechanism for aspirin-induced malondialdehyde production by mouse liver microsomes and mitochondria. J Clin Invest. 1988;81(1):165-70.

809. Verheij M, Stewart FA, Oussoren Y, Weening JJ, Dewit L. Amelioration of radiation nephropathy by acetylsalicylic acid. Int J Radiat Biol. 1995;67(5):587-96.

810. Wang HF, Li XD, Chen YM, Yuan LB, Foye WO. Radiation-protective and platelet aggregation inhibitory effects of five traditional Chinese drugs and acetylsalicylic acid following high-dose gamma-irradiation. J Ethnopharmacol. 1991;34(2-3):215-9.

811. Sjaarda LA, Radin RG, Silver RM, Mitchell E, Mumford SL, Wilcox B, Galai N, Perkins NJ, Wactawski-Wende J, Stanford JB, Schisterman EF. Preconception low-dose aspirin restores diminished pregnancy and live birth rates in women with low grade inflammation: a secondary analysis of a randomized trial. J Clin. Endocrinol. Metab. Jc.2016-2917.

812. Wada I, Hsu CC, Williams G, Macnamee MC, Brinsden PR. The benefits of low-dose aspirin therapy in women with impaired uterine perfusion during assisted conception. Hum Reprod. 1994;9(10):1954-7.

813. Wan QL, Zheng SQ, Wu GS, Luo HR. Aspirin extends the lifespan of Caenorhabditis elegans via AMPK and DAF-16/FOXO in dietary restriction pathway. Exp Gerontol. 2013;48(5):499-506.

814. Ayyadevara S, Bharill P, Dandapat A, et al. Aspirin inhibits oxidant stress, reduces age-associated functional declines, and extends lifespan of Caenorhabditis elegans. Antioxid Redox Signal. 2013;18(5):481-90.

815. Strong R, Miller RA, Astle CM, et al. Nordihydroguaiaretic acid and aspirin increase lifespan of genetically heterogeneous male mice. Aging Cell. 2008;7(5):641-50.

816. Lutchman, Vicky; Medkour, Younes; Samson, Eugenie; Arlia-Ciommo, Anthony; Dakik, Pamela; Cortes, Berly; Feldman, Rachel; Mohtashami, Sadaf; McAuley, Mélissa; Chancharoen, Marisa; Rukundo, Belise; Simard, Éric; Titorenko, Vladimir I. Discovery of plant extracts that greatly delay yeast chronological aging and have different effects on longevity-defining cellular processes. Oncotarget. 7(13):16542.

817. Arango HA, Icely S, Roberts WS, Cavanagh D, Becker JL. Aspirin effects on endometrial cancer cell growth. Obstet Gynecol. 2001;97(3):423-7.

818. Redlak MJ, Power JJ, Miller TA. Aspirin-induced apoptosis in human gastric cancer epithelial cells: relationship with protein kinase C signaling. Dig Dis Sci. 2007;52(3):810-6.

819. Rioux N, Castonguay A. Prevention of NNK-induced lung tumorigenesis in A/J mice by acetylsalicylic acid and NS-398. Cancer Res. 1998;58(23):5354-60.

820. Valdéz JC, Perdigón G. Piroxicam, indomethacin and aspirin action on a murine fibrosarcoma. Effects on tumour-associated and peritoneal macrophages. Clin Exp Immunol. 1991;86(2):315-21.

821. Maity G, De A, Das A, Banerjee S, Sarkar S, Banerjee SK. Aspirin blocks growth of breast tumor cells and tumor-initiating cells and induces reprogramming factors of mesenchymal to epithelial transition. Lab Invest. 2015;95(7):702-17.

822. Mitral, P. (2016). Aspirin lifeline for end-stage cancer. Times of India. [Online]. Available: http://timesofindia.indiatimes.com/city/kolkata/Aspirin-lifeline-for-end-stage-cancer/articleshow/53407589.cms.[March 1, 2017].

823. Mitrugno A, Sylman JL, Ngo AT, et al. Aspirin therapy reduces the ability of platelets to promote colon and pancreatic cancer cell proliferation: Implications for the oncoprotein c-MYC. Am J Physiol, Cell Physiol. 2017;312(2):C176-C189.

824. Saini T, Bagchi M, Bagchi D, Jaeger S, Hosoyama S, Stohs SJ. Protective ability of acetylsalicylic acid (aspirin) to scavenge radiation induced free radicals in J774A.1 macrophage cells. Res Commun Mol Pathol Pharmacol. 1998;101(3):259-68.

825. Shi X, Ding M, Dong Z, et al. Antioxidant properties of aspirin: characterization of the ability of aspirin to inhibit silica-induced lipid peroxidation, DNA damage, NF-kappaB activation, and TNF-alpha production. Mol Cell Biochem. 1999;199(1-2):93-102.

826. Beckmann I, Ben-efraim S, Vervoort M, Wallenburg HC. Release of tumor necrosis factor-alpha and prostanoids in whole blood cultures after in vivo exposure to low-dose aspirin. Mediators Inflamm. 2001;10(2):81-8.

827. Shackelford R, Alford PB, Xue Y, Thai SF, Adams DO, Pizzo S. Aspirin Inhibits Tumor Necrosis Factor-α Gene Expression in Murine Tissue Macrophages. Molecular Pharmacology. 1997;52(3):421.

828. Vervoordeldonk MJ, Pineda torra IM, Aarsman AJ, Van den bosch H. Aspirin inhibits expression of the interleukin-1beta-inducible group II phospholipase A2. FEBS Lett. 1996;397(1):108-12.

829. Marshall H. Aspirin inhibits IL-4 production. Trends Immunol. 2001;22(5):242.

830. Cianferoni A, Schroeder JT, Kim J, et al. Selective inhibition of interleukin-4 gene expression in human T cells by aspirin. Blood. 2001;97(6):1742-9.

831. Hovens MM, Snoep JD, Groeneveld Y, Frölich M, Tamsma JT, Huisman MV. Effects of aspirin on serum C-reactive protein and interleukin-6 levels in patients with type 2 diabetes without cardiovascular disease: a randomized placebo-controlled crossover trial. Diabetes Obes Metab. 2008;10(8):668-74.

832. Kim SR, Bae MK, Kim JY, Wee HJ, Yoo MA, Bae SK. Aspirin induces apoptosis through the blockade of IL-6-STAT3 signaling pathway in human glioblastoma A172 cells. Biochem Biophys Res Commun. 2009;387(2):342-7.

833. Ogston NC, Karastergiou K, Hosseinzadeh-attar MJ, et al. Low-dose acetylsalicylic acid inhibits the secretion of interleukin-6 from white adipose tissue. Int J Obes (Lond). 2008;32(12):1807-15.

834. Goldstein SL, Leung JC, Silverstein DM. Pro- and anti-inflammatory cytokines in chronic pediatric dialysis patients: effect of aspirin. Clin J Am Soc Nephrol. 2006;1(5):979-86.

835. Wu D, Sheu JS, Liu HC, et al. Increase of toll-like receptor 4 but decrease of interleukin-8 mRNA expression among ischemic stroke patients under aspirin treatment. Clin Biochem. 2012;45(16-17):1316-9.

836. Yang YY, Hu CJ, Chang SM, Tai TY, Leu SJ. Aspirin inhibits monocyte chemoattractant protein-1 and interleukin-8 expression in TNF-alpha stimulated human umbilical vein endothelial cells. Atherosclerosis. 2004;174(2):207-13.

837. Perez-g M, Melo M, Keegan AD, Zamorano J. Aspirin and salicylates inhibit the IL-4- and IL-13-induced activation of STAT6. J Immunol. 2002;168(3):1428-34.

838. Bhatt S, Pundarikakshudu K, Patel P, et al. Beneficial effect of aspirin against interferon-α-2b-induced depressive behavior in Sprague Dawley rats. Clin Exp Pharmacol Physiol. 2016;43(12):1208-1215.

839. Di luigi L, Rossi C, Sgrò P, et al. Do non-steroidal anti-inflammatory drugs influence the steroid hormone milieu in male athletes?. Int J Sports Med. 2007;28(10):809-14.

840. Schönhöfer PS, Sohn J, Peters HD, Dinnendahl V. Effects of sodium salicylate and acetylsalicylic acid on the lipolytic system of fat cells. Biochem Pharmacol. 1973;22(5):629-37.

841. Maharaj H, Maharaj DS, Saravanan KS, Mohanakumar KP, Daya S. Aspirin curtails the acetaminophen-induced rise in brain norepinephrine levels. Metab Brain Dis. 2004;19(1-2):71-7.

842. Hundal RS, Petersen KF, Mayerson AB, et al. Mechanism by which high-dose aspirin improves glucose metabolism in type 2 diabetes. J Clin Invest. 2002;109(10):1321-6.

843. Meester WD, Schut GE, Hamp JA, Sekhar NC. Effect of aspirin on epinephrine-induced lipolysis and platelet aggregation in rats. Res Commun Chem Pathol Pharmacol. 1972;4(2):405-11.

844. Yang H, Pellegrini L, Napolitano A, et al. Aspirin delays mesothelioma growth by inhibiting HMGB1-mediated tumor progression. Cell Death Dis. 2015;6:e1786.

845. Choi HW, Tian M, Song F, et al. Aspirin's Active Metabolite Salicylic Acid Targets High Mobility Group Box 1 to Modulate Inflammatory Responses. Mol Med. 2015;21:526-35.

846. Nadar S, Blann AD, Lip GY. Effects of aspirin on intra-platelet vascular endothelial growth factor, angiopoietin-1, and p-selectin levels in hypertensive patients. Am J Hypertens. 2006;19(9):970-7.

847. Zandomeneghi R, Serra L, Pavesi C, Baumgartl U, Poppi C, Montanari P. Effect of aspirin and indomethacin on epidermal growth factor secretion in duodenal tissue fragments cultivated in vitro. Digestion. 1992;51(1):37-41.

848. Chiow KH, Tan Y, Chua RY, et al. SNX3-dependent regulation of epidermal growth factor receptor (EGFR) trafficking and degradation by aspirin in epidermoid carcinoma (A-431) cells. Cell Mol Life Sci. 2012;69(9):1505-21.

849. Amin AR, Vyas P, Attur M, et al. The mode of action of aspirin-like drugs: effect on inducible nitric oxide synthase. Proc Natl Acad Sci USA. 1995;92(17):7926-30.

850. Carvalho-filho MA, Ropelle ER, Pauli RJ, et al. Aspirin attenuates insulin resistance in muscle of diet-induced obese rats by inhibiting inducible nitric oxide synthase production and S-nitrosylation of IRbeta/IRS-1 and Akt. Diabetologia. 2009;52(11):2425-34.

851. Chen B, Zhao J, Zhang S, Wu W, Qi R. Aspirin inhibits the production of reactive oxygen species by downregulating Nox4 and inducible nitric oxide synthase in human endothelial cells exposed to oxidized low-density lipoprotein. J Cardiovasc Pharmacol. 2012;59(5):405-12.

852. Carnovale DE, Fukuda A, Underhill DC, Laffan JJ, Breuel KF. Aspirin dose dependently inhibits the interleukin-1 beta-stimulated increase in inducible nitric oxide synthase, nitric oxide, and prostaglandin E(2) production in rat ovarian dispersates cultured in vitro. Fertil Steril. 2001;75(4):778-84.

853. De cristóbal J, Cárdenas A, Lizasoain I, et al. Inhibition of glutamate release via recovery of ATP levels accounts for a neuroprotective effect of aspirin in rat cortical neurons exposed to oxygen-glucose deprivation. Stroke. 2002;33(1):261-7.

854. Ashoori MR, Bathaie SZ, Heidarzadeh H. Long-term, high-dose aspirin therapy increases the specific activity of complex III of mitochondrial respiratory chain in the kidney of diabetic rats. Phys. Pharm. 2015; 158-166.

855. Cheshire RM, Park MV. The inhibition of lactate dehydrogenase by salicylate. Int. J. Bio. 1977; 8(9):637-643.

856. Harris RE, Robertson FM, Abou-issa HM, Farrar WB, Brueggemeier R. Genetic induction and upregulation of cyclooxygenase (COX) and aromatase (CYP19): an extension of the dietary fat hypothesis of breast cancer. Med Hypotheses. 1999;52(4):291-2.

857. Terry MB, Gammon MD, Zhang FF, et al. Association of frequency and duration of aspirin use and hormone receptor status with breast cancer risk. JAMA. 2004;291(20):2433-40.

858. Gates MA, Tworoger SS, Eliassen AH, Missmer SA, Hankinson SE. Analgesic use and sex steroid hormone concentrations in postmenopausal women. Cancer Epidemiol Biomarkers Prev. 2010;19(4):1033-41.

859. Shen L, Shen J, Pu J, He B. Aspirin attenuates pulmonary arterial hypertension in rats by reducing plasma 5-hydroxytryptamine levels. Cell Biochem Biophys. 2011;61(1):23-31.

860. Daya S, Anoopkumar-dukie S. Acetaminophen inhibits liver trytophan-2,3-dioxygenase activity with a concomitant rise in brain serotonin levels and a reduction in urinary 5-hydroxyindole acetic acid. Life Sci. 2000;67(3):235-40.

861. Starke RM, Chalouhi N, Ding D, Hasan DM. Potential role of aspirin in the prevention of aneurysmal subarachnoid hemorrhage. Cerebrovasc Dis. 2015;39(5-6):332-42.

862. Wehbeh A, Tamim HM, Abu daya H, et al. Aspirin Has a Protective Effect Against Adverse Outcomes in Patients with Nonvariceal Upper Gastrointestinal Bleeding. Dig Dis Sci. 2015;60(7):2077-87.

863. Elwood PC, Morgan G, Galante J, et al. Systematic Review and Meta-Analysis of Randomised Trials to Ascertain Fatal Gastrointestinal Bleeding Events Attributable to Preventive Low-Dose Aspirin: No Evidence of Increased Risk. PLoS ONE. 2016;11(11):e0166166.

864. Peat, R. Aspirin, brain and cancer. [Online]. Available: http://raypeat.com/articles/aging/aspirin-brain-cancer.shtml. [March 1, 2017].

865. Somasundaram S, Sigthorsson G, Simpson RJ, et al. Uncoupling of intestinal mitochondrial oxidative phosphorylation and inhibition of cyclooxygenase are required for the development of NSAID-enteropathy in the rat. Aliment Pharmacol Ther. 2000;14(5):639-50.

866. Brzozowski T, Konturek PC, Konturek SJ, Stachura J. Gastric adaptation to aspirin and stress enhances gastric mucosal resistance against the damage by strong irritants. Scand J Gastroenterol. 1996;31(2):118-25.

867. Brzozowski T, Konturek PC, Konturek SJ, Ernst H, Stachura J, Hahn EG. Gastric adaptation to injury by repeated doses of aspirin strengthens mucosal defence against subsequent exposure to various strong irritants in rats. Gut. 1995;37(6):749-57.

868. Coleman WB, Wennerberg AE, Smith GJ, Grisham JW. Regulation of the differentiation of diploid and some aneuploid rat liver epithelial (stemlike) cells by the hepatic microenvironment. Am J Pathol. 1993;142(5):1373-82.

869. Yoshimura K. Biphasic activation of nuclear factor-kappa B in chondrocyte death induced by interleukin-1beta: The expression of inducible nitric oxide synthase and phagocyte-type NADPH oxidase through immediate and monocarboxylate transporter-1-mediated late-phase activation of nuclear factor-kappa B. 2016; 58(2):39-44.

870. Ando M, Uehara I, Kogure K, et al. Interleukin 6 enhances glycolysis through expression of the glycolytic enzymes hexokinase 2 and 6-phosphofructo-2-kinase/fructose-2,6-bisphosphatase-3. J Nippon Med Sch. 2010;77(2):97-105.

871. Kawauchi K, Araki K, Tobiume K, Tanaka N. p53 regulates glucose metabolism through an IKK-NF-kappaB pathway and inhibits cell transformation. Nat Cell Biol. 2008;10(5):611-8.

872. Vaughan OR, Davies KL, Ward JW, De blasio MJ, Fowden AL. A physiological increase in maternal cortisol alters uteroplacental metabolism in the pregnant ewe. J Physiol (Lond). 2016;594(21):6407-6418.

873. Blecher M. EFFECTS OF CORTISOL ON THE METABOLISM OF GLUCOSE BY LYMPHOID TISSUE. J Biol Chem. 1964;239:1299-300.

874. Laurent D, Petersen KF, Russell RR, Cline GW, Shulman GI. Effect of epinephrine on muscle glycogenolysis and insulin-stimulated muscle glycogen synthesis in humans. Am J Physiol. 1998;274(1 Pt 1):E130-8.

875. Shi, S., Xu, J., Zhang, B., Ji, S., Xu, W., Liu, J., ... Yu, X. (2016). VEGF promotes glycolysis in pancreatic cancer via HIF1α up-regulation. Current Molecular Medicine, 16(4), 394-403.

876. Sumi S, Ichihara K, Kono N, Nonaka K, Tarui S. Insulin and epidermal growth factor stimulate glycolysis in quiescent 3T3 fibroblasts with no changes in key glycolytic enzyme activities. Endocrinol Jpn. 1984;31(2):117-25.

877. Caneba CA, Yang L, Baddour J, Curtis R, Win J, Hartig S, Marini J, Nagrath D. Nitric oxide is a positive regulator of the Warburg effect in ovarian cancer cells. Cell Death & Disease. 2014;5(6):e1302.

878. Thomas M, Monet JD, Brami M, et al. Comparative effects of 17 beta-estradiol, progestin R5020, tamoxifen and RU38486 on lactate dehydrogenase activity in MCF-7 human breast cancer cells. J Steroid Biochem. 1989;32(2):271-7.

879. Iwai M, Jungermann K. Leukotrienes increase glucose and lactate output and decrease flow in perfused rat liver. Biochem Biophys Res Commun. 1988;151(1):283-90.

880. Koren-schwartzer N, Chen-zion M, Ben-porat H, Beitner R. Serotonin-induced decrease in brain ATP, stimulation of brain anaerobic glycolysis and elevation of plasma hemoglobin; the protective action of calmodulin antagonists. Gen Pharmacol. 1994;25(6):1257-62.

881. Novak M, Hall CL, Blackburn BJ. A nuclear magnetic resonance study of the glucose metabolism of Hymenolepis diminuta exposed to histamine and serotonin in vitro. Int J Parasitol. 1991;21(5):589-96.

882. Braggion-santos MF, Volpe GJ, Pazin-filho A, Maciel BC, Marin-neto JA, Schmidt A. Sudden cardiac death in Brazil: a community-based autopsy series (2006-2010). Arq Bras Cardiol. 2015;104(2):120-7.

883. Barclay AW, Brand-miller J. The Australian paradox: a substantial decline in sugars intake over the same timeframe that overweight and obesity have increased. Nutrients. 2011;3(4):491-504.

884. Anderson KE, Rosner W, Khan MS, et al. Diet-hormone interactions: protein/carbohydrate ratio alters reciprocally the plasma levels of testosterone and cortisol and their respective binding globulins in man. Life Sci. 1987;40(18):1761-8.

885. Lane AR, Duke JW, Hackney AC. Influence of dietary carbohydrate intake on the free testosterone: cortisol ratio responses to short-term intensive exercise training. Eur J Appl Physiol. 2010;108(6):1125-31.

886. Henderson, Y. Carbon Dioxide. [Online]. Available: http://www.learnbuteyko.org/information-about-learnbuteykoorg/carbon-dioxide-by-yandell-henderson. [March 1, 2017].

887. Girardis M, Busani S, Damiani E, et al. Effect of Conservative vs Conventional Oxygen Therapy on Mortality Among Patients in an Intensive Care Unit: The Oxygen-ICU Randomized Clinical Trial. JAMA. 2016;316(15):1583-1589.

888. Yip K, Alonzi R. Carbogen gas and radiotherapy outcomes in prostate cancer. Ther Adv Urol. 2013;5(1):25-34.

889. Ferguson ND. Oxygen in the ICU: Too Much of a Good Thing?. JAMA. 2016;316(15):1553-1554.

890. Kavanagh B. Normocapnia vs hypercapnia. Minerva Anestesiol. 2002;68(5):346-50.

891. Austin MA, Wills KE, Blizzard L, Walters EH, Wood-baker R. Effect of high flow oxygen on mortality in chronic obstructive pulmonary disease patients in prehospital setting: randomised controlled trial. BMJ. 2010;341:c5462.

892. Liu Y, Rosenthal RE, Haywood Y, Miljkovic-lolic M, Vanderhoek JY, Fiskum G. Normoxic ventilation after cardiac arrest reduces oxidation of brain lipids and improves neurological outcome. Stroke. 1998;29(8):1679-86.

893. Lundy JS. Carbon dioxide as an aid in general anesthesia. JAMA. 1925;85(25):1953-1955.

894. Henderson Y. Resuscitation: from carbon monoxide asphyxia, from ether or alcohol intoxication, and from respiratory failure due to other causes; with some remarks also on the use of oxygen in pneumonia, and inhalational therapy in general. JAMA. 1924;83(10):758-764.

895. Fisher JA, Iscoe S, Fedorko L, Duffin J. Rapid elimination of CO through the lungs: coming full circle 100 years on. Exp Physiol. 2011;96(12):1262-9.

896. Henderson, Y., and Haggard, H.W., J. Pharmacol. And Exp. Therap., 16, 11 (1920).

897. Henderson, Y., and Haggard, H.W., J.Am. Med. Assn.,79, 1137 (1922).

898. Henderson, Y., Haggard, H.W., Coryllos, P.N., Birnbaum, G.L., and Radloff, E.M., Arch. Int. Med., 45, 72 (1930).

899. Henderson Y. Reasons for the use of carbon dioxide with oxygen in the treatment of pneumonia. N Engl. J. Med. 1932; 206:151-155.

900. Fosslien E. Cancer morphogenesis: role of mitochondrial failure. Ann Clin Lab Sci. 2008;38(4):307-29.

901. Briva A, Lecuona E, Sznajder JI. [Permissive and non-permissive hypercapnia: mechanisms of action and consequences of high carbon dioxide levels]. Arch Bronconeumol. 2010;46(7):378-82.

902. Curley G, Laffey JG, Kavanagh BP. Bench-to-bedside review: carbon dioxide. Crit Care. 2010;14(2):220.

903. O'croinin D, Ni chonghaile M, Higgins B, Laffey JG. Bench-to-bedside review: Permissive hypercapnia. Crit Care. 2005;9(1):51-9.

904. Ismaiel NM, Henzler D. Effects of hypercapnia and hypercapnic acidosis on attenuation of ventilator-associated lung injury. Minerva Anestesiol. 2011;77(7):723-33.

905. Rogovik A, Goldman R. Permissive hypercapnia. Emerg Med Clin North Am. 2008;26(4):941-52, viii-ix.

906. Bautista AF, Akca O. Hypercapnia: is it protective in lung injury?. Med Gas Res. 2013;3(1):23.

907. Laffey JG, Kavanagh BP. Carbon dioxide and the critically ill--too little of a good thing?. Lancet. 1999;354(9186):1283-6.

908. Gao W, Liu DD, Li D, Cui GX. Effect of Therapeutic Hypercapnia on Inflammatory Responses to One-lung Ventilation in Lobectomy Patients. Anesthesiology. 2015;122(6):1235-52.

909. Nardelli LM, Rzezinski A, Silva JD, et al. Effects of acute hypercapnia with and without acidosis on lung inflammation and apoptosis in experimental acute lung injury. Respir Physiol Neurobiol. 2015;205:1-6.

910. Ni chonghaile M, Higgins B, Laffey JG. Permissive hypercapnia: role in protective lung ventilatory strategies. Curr Opin Crit Care. 2005;11(1):56-62.

911. Contreras M, Masterson C, Laffey JG. Permissive hypercapnia: what to remember. Curr Opin Anaesthesiol. 2015;28(1):26-37.

912. De smet HR, Bersten AD, Barr HA, Doyle IR. Hypercapnic acidosis modulates inflammation, lung mechanics, and edema in the isolated perfused lung. J Crit Care. 2007;22(4):305-13.

913. Bannenberg GL, Giammarresi C, Gustafsson LE. Inhaled carbon dioxide inhibits lower airway nitric oxide formation in the guinea pig. Acta Physiol Scand. 1997;160(4):401-5.

914. Brogan TV, Hedges RG, Mckinney S, Robertson HT, Hlastala MP, Swenson ER. Pulmonary NO synthase inhibition and inspired CO_2: effects on V'/Q' and pulmonary blood flow distribution. Eur Respir J. 2000;16(2):288-95.

915. Adding LC, Agvald P, Persson MG, Gustafsson LE. Regulation of pulmonary nitric oxide by carbon dioxide is intrinsic to the lung. Acta Physiol Scand. 1999;167(2):167-74.

916. Nichol AD, O'cronin DF, Naughton F, Hopkins N, Boylan J, Mcloughlin P. Hypercapnic acidosis reduces oxidative reactions in endotoxin-induced lung injury. Anesthesiology. 2010;113(1):116-25.

917. Maurer M, Riesen W, Muser J, Hulter HN, Krapf R. Neutralization of Western diet inhibits bone resorption independently of K intake and reduces cortisol secretion in humans. Am J Physiol Renal Physiol. 2003;284(1):F32-40.

918. Rojas vega S, Strüder HK, Wahrmann BV, Bloch W, Hollmann W. Bicarbonate reduces serum prolactin increase induced by exercise to exhaustion. Med Sci Sports Exerc. 2006;38(4):675-80.

919. Strüder HK, Hollmann W, Donike M, Platen P, Weber K. Effect of O2 availability on neuroendocrine variables at rest and during exercise: O2 breathing increases plasma prolactin. Eur J Appl Physiol Occup Physiol. 1996;74(5):443-9.

920. Nielsen FU, Daugaard P, Bentzen L, et al. Effect of changing tumor oxygenation on glycolytic metabolism in a murine C3H mammary carcinoma assessed by in vivo nuclear magnetic resonance spectroscopy. Cancer Res. 2001;61(13):5318-25.

921. Sabatini S, Kurtzman NA. Bicarbonate therapy in severe metabolic acidosis. J Am Soc Nephrol. 2009;20(4):692-5.

922. Malov luS, Kulikov AN. [Bicarbonate deficiency and duodenal peptic ulcer]. Ter Arkh. 1998;70(2):28-32.

923. Pepelko WE. The effect of cortisol upon lipolysis during cypercapnia and after beta-andrenergic blockade. Anat & Phys Pharmac. 1971. Available: http://oai.dtic.mil/oai/oai?verb=getRecord&metadataPrefix=html&identifier=AD0731124. [February 15, 2017].

924. Haylor J, Toner JM, Jackson PR, Ramsay LE, Lote CJ. Is the urinary excretion of prostaglandin E in man dependent on urine pH?. Clin Sci. 1985;68(4):475-7.

925. Strider JW, Masterson CG, Durham PL. Treatment of mast cells with carbon dioxide suppresses degranulation via a novel mechanism involving repression of increased intracellular calcium levels. Allergy. 2011;66(3):341-50.

926. Onishi Y, Kawamoto T, Ueha T, et al. Transcutaneous application of carbon dioxide (CO_2) induces mitochondrial apoptosis in human malignant fibrous histiocytoma in vivo. PLoS ONE. 2012;7(11):e49189.

927. Pagourelias ED, Zorou PG, Tsaligopoulos M, Athyros VG, Karagiannis A, Efthimiadis GK. Carbon dioxide balneotherapy and cardiovascular disease. Int J Biometeorol. 2011;55(5):657-63.

928. Hartmann BR, Bassenge E, Pittler M. Effect of carbon dioxide-enriched water and fresh water on the cutaneous microcirculation and oxygen tension in the skin of the foot. Angiology. 1997;48(4):337-43.

929. Hartmann B, Drews B, Burnus C, Bassenge E. [Increase in skin blood circulation and transcutaneous oxygen partial pressure of the top of the foot in lower leg immersion in water containing carbon dioxide in patients with arterial occlusive disease. Results of a controlled study compared with fresh water]. VASA. 1991;20(4):382-7.

930. Hartmann B, Drews B, Bassenge E. [CO2-induced acral blood flow and the oxygen partial pressure in arterial occlusive disease]. Dtsch Med Wochenschr. 1991;116(43):1617-21.

931. Hartmann BR, Bassenge E, Hartmann M. Effects of serial percutaneous application of carbon dioxide in intermittent claudication: results of a controlled trial. Angiology. 1997;48(11):957-63.

932. Resch KL, Just U. [Possibilities and limits of CO2 balneotherapy]. Wien Med Wochenschr. 1994;144(3):45-50.

933. Sato M, Kanikowska D, Iwase S, et al. Effects of immersion in water containing high concentrations of CO2 (CO2-water) at thermoneutral on thermoregulation and heart rate variability in humans. Int J Biometeorol. 2009;53(1):25-30.

934. Schmidt KL. Carbon dioxide bath (carbon dioxide spring). Center for Clinical Research in Rheumatology, Physical Medicine and Balneotherapy, Germany. Available: http://www.mesotherapyworldwide.com/images/pdf/Carbon_Dioxide_Bath.pdf. [April 1, 2017].

935. Strec V, Dukát A, Aksamitová K, Adolf P, Stalmaseková B. [Response to a series of carbon dioxide baths]. Vnitr Lek. 1992;38(2):148-54.

936. Hartmann B, Pohl U, Wohltmann D, Holtz J, Bassenge E. [The effect of carbon dioxide baths on blood pressure of borderline hypertensive patients]. Z Kardiol. 1989;78(8):526-31.

937. Akamine T, Taguchi N. Effects of an artificially carbonated bath on athletic warm-up. J Hum Ergol (Tokyo). 1998;27(1-2):22-9.

938. Miao P, Sheng S, Sun X, Liu J, Huang G. Lactate dehydrogenase A in cancer: a promising target for diagnosis and therapy. IUBMB Life. 2013;65(11):904-10.

939. Mcswain SD, Hamel DS, Smith PB, et al. End-tidal and arterial carbon dioxide measurements correlate across all levels of physiologic dead space. Respir Care. 2010;55(3):288-93.

940. Tolner EA, Hochman DW, Hassinen P, et al. Five percent CO_2 is a potent, fast-acting inhalation anticonvulsant. Epilepsia. 2011;52(1):104-14.

941. Lee HJ, Park CY, Lee JH, et al. Therapeutic effects of carbogen inhalation and lipo-prostaglandin E1 in sudden hearing loss. Yonsei Med J. 2012;53(5):999-1004.

942. Griffiths JR, Taylor NJ, Howe FA, et al. The response of human tumors to carbogen breathing, monitored by Gradient-Recalled Echo Magnetic Resonance Imaging. Int J Radiat Oncol Biol Phys. 1997;39(3):697-701.

943. Taylor NJ, Baddeley H, Goodchild KA, et al. BOLD MRI of human tumor oxygenation during carbogen breathing. J Magn Reson Imaging. 2001;14(2):156-63.

944. Baddeley H, Brodrick PM, Taylor NJ, et al. Gas exchange parameters in radiotherapy patients during breathing of 2%, 3.5% and 5% carbogen gas mixtures. Br J Radiol. 2000;73(874):1100-4.

945. Mcsheehy PM, Port RE, Rodrigues LM, et al. Investigations in vivo of the effects of carbogen breathing on 5-fluorouracil pharmacokinetics and physiology of solid rodent tumours. Cancer Chemother Pharmacol. 2005;55(2):117-28.

946. Teicher BA, Schwartz GN, Dupuis NP, et al. Oxygenation of human tumor xenografts in nude mice by a perfluorochemical emulsion and carbogen breathing. Artif Cells Blood Substit Immobil Biotechnol. 1994;22(4):1369-75.

947. Alonzi R, Padhani AR, Maxwell RJ, et al. Carbogen breathing increases prostate cancer oxygenation: a translational MRI study in murine xenografts and humans. Br J Cancer. 2009;100(4):644-8.

948. Khan N, Li H, Hou H, et al. Tissue pO2 of orthotopic 9L and C6 gliomas and tumor-specific response to radiotherapy and hyperoxygenation. Int J Radiat Oncol Biol Phys. 2009;73(3):878-85.

949. Khan N, Mupparaju S, Hekmatyar SK, et al. Effect of hyperoxygenation on tissue pO2 and its effect on radiotherapeutic efficacy of orthotopic F98 gliomas. Int J Radiat Oncol Biol Phys. 2010;78(4):1193-200.

950. Powell ME, Collingridge DR, Saunders MI, Hoskin PJ, Hill SA, Chaplin DJ. Improvement in human tumour oxygenation with carbogen of varying carbon dioxide concentrations. Radiother Oncol. 1999;50(2):167-71.

951. Hou H, Krishnamurthy nemani V, Du G, et al. Monitoring oxygen levels in orthotopic human glioma xenograft following carbogen inhalation and chemotherapy by implantable resonator-based oximetry. Int J Cancer. 2015;136(7):1688-96.

952. Aquino-parsons C, Green A, Minchinton AI. Oxygen tension in primary gynaecological tumours: the influence of carbon dioxide concentration. Radiother Oncol. 2000;57(1):45-51.

953. Core Writing Team, Pachauri, R.K. and Reisinger, A. 2007. Climate Change 2007: Synthesis Report. IPCC, Geneva, Switzerland. pp 104.

954. Valentino FL, Leuenberger M, Uglietti C and Staburm P. Measurements and trend analysis of O2, CO2 and from high altitude research station Junfgraujoch, Switzerlnd – a comparison with the observations from the remote site Puy de Dôme, France. Science of the Total Environment 2008, 203-10.

955. Sirignano C, Neubert REM, Jeijer HAJ and Rödenbeck C. Atmospheric oxygen and carbon dioxide observations from two European coastal stations 2000-2005: continental influence trend changes and APO climatology. Atmos Chem Phy Discuss 2008, 8, 20113-54.

956. Tohjima Y, Muai H, Machida T, Nojiri Y. Gas-chromatographic measurements of the atmospheric oxygen/nitrogen ratio at haterumna island and Cape Ochi-ishi, Japan. Geophys Res Lett 2003, 30, 1653.

957. Earth System Research Laboratory. 2017. Trends in Atmospheric Carbon Dioxide. [Online]. Available: https://www.esrl.noaa.gov/gmd/ccgg/trends/global.html.[March 1, 2017].

958. Kelly, M. (2016). Ice cores reveal a slow decline in atmospheric oxygen over the last 800,000 years. Princeton University [Online]. Available: https://blogs.princeton.edu/research/2016/09/23/ice-cores-reveal-a-slow-decline-in-atmospheric-oxygen-over-the-last-800000-years-science/.[March 1, 2017].

959. Schmidtko S, Stramma L, Visbeck M. Decline in global oceanic oxygen content during the past five decades. Nature. 2015;542:335-339.

960. Kulish OP. [Effect high-altitude conditions on the antitumor activity of cyclophosphane and its action on lymphoid tissue cells]. Eksp Onkol. 1985;7(3):60-3.

961. Kulish OP, Galkina KA. [Effect of high-altitude hypoxia on the effectiveness of chemotherapy in tumors]. Biull Eksp Biol Med. 1983;95(2):33-5.

962. Yu L, Hales CA. Long-term exposure to hypoxia inhibits tumor progression of lung cancer in rats and mice. BMC Cancer. 2011;11:331.

963. Basciano L, Nemos C, Foliguet B, et al. Long term culture of mesenchymal stem cells in hypoxia promotes a genetic program maintaining their undifferentiated and multipotent status. BMC Cell Biol. 2011;12:12.

964. Benedict, F.G., and Higgins, H.L.: Am. J. Physiol. 30:217, 1912.

965. Higgins, H.L.,; Peabody, F.W., and Fitz, R.: J. M. Research. 29:263, 1916.

966. Hawley, E.E.; Johnson, C.W., and Murlin, J.R.: J. Nutrition. 6:523, 1933.

CONCLUSION

The cancer establishment maintains that cancer is a genetic disease, but the metabolic nature of cancer was established almost 100 years ago by Dr. Otto Warburg. Since then the genetic theory of cancer has been disproven repeatedly and Warburg's metabolic theory confirmed repeatedly, yet the cancer industry continues to ignore the truth. To this day, the public remains 'officially' uninformed that cancer is a metabolic disease which is both preventable and reversible.

Dr. Otto Warburg observed that cancer cells were nothing but normal cells with malfunctioning mitochondria – not a biological terrorist-type cell that's on a killing spree. This observation has been validated numerous times since Warburg, perhaps most notably by the elite Russian Scientist Konstantin Buteyko. Buteyko's conclusion after a lifetime of work in search of the root cause of disease was that all people with suboptimal health, including cancer, have one thing in common: A deficiency of carbon dioxide in the body. This situation arises because in cells with malfunctioning mitochondria, lactate is rendered as a byproduct of metabolism instead of carbon dioxide.

PARADIGM SHIFT: A BIOLOGICAL UNDERSTANDING OF CANCER

The development of cancer is characterized by a shift inside the body from high levels of carbon dioxide and low levels of lactate to low levels of carbon dioxide and high levels of lactate. This altered environment is the result of cells progressively losing their ability to utilize oxygen and glucose efficiently. When cells utilize oxygen and glucose efficiently, they render the healing carbon dioxide that is required for health. When cells lose their ability to utilize oxygen and glucose efficiently, they render lactate, which perpetuates the cancer metabolism.

It should be known by all that the most accurate ways to diagnose cancer are either to test for lactate levels in the blood (or other body fluids) or for carbon dioxide in the exhaled breath. Many doctors have realized this in recent years and are beginning to put it into practice.

If elevated lactate or a deficiency of carbon dioxide is found in the body, it means that a significant number of cells are inefficiently producing energy. Instead of deriving energy from the complete oxidation of glucose within the mitochondria of cells, cancer cells derive their energy from the fermentation of glucose, and then once the body is out of glucose, from the use of amino acids and fatty acids. This 'cancer metabolism' tends to be self-promoting, and brings about the excessive and prolonged production of the cancer-promoting hormones and inflammatory substances that have been identified within the bodies of cancer patients, particularly within the tumor microenvironment.

Most of the cancer-causing substances within the tumor microenvironment of cancer patients exist initially as a means to help the body heal the damaged, 'cancerous' tissue. But due to the presence of unsaturated free fatty acids and the toxic metabolites rendered from their oxididation, the presence of these cancer-causing substances becomes prolonged and the body loses its capacity to 'switch off' the stress metabolism and complete the healing process.

If a cancer patient is not thrashed with so-called treatments involving knives, poison injections and deadly high-dose ionizing radiation they often heal cancer on their own, which is testament to the remarkable healing capacity of the human body. And when healing foods and medicines like oranges, coconut oil, sodium bicarbonate, red light and aspirin are employed to enhance immunity, protect the body from oxidative damage and inhibit the self-perpetuating cycle of stress, the tumor microenvironment and overall environment of the body can be quickly altered and a reduction of cancer symptoms or a complete resolution of the disease can occur.

MOVING FORWARD

In book 1 of this series it was established using evidence from existing scientific publications that cancer treatments are doing far more harm than good. This has been known for decades, and many doctors and scientists have done everything they can to warn the public, but to this day their warnings remain mostly unknown. I hope this series of books plays a substantial part in making this universally understood. In this exciting age of information, where communication between people anywhere in the world is instant and books can be easily self-published, the opportunity to create real, lasting change in the world has never been greater.

This shift in our understanding of cancer begins with understanding what the disease truly is and isn't, which has been the goal of this book. It is with this understanding that a more rational approach to the prevention and treatment of cancer can begin.

It can now be said with certainty that cancer is not a disease of genetic origin, but one of damaged metabolism. And, rather than a disease involving mutant 'terrorist' cells whose goal is to murder the host, cancer cells are simply normal cells that are damaged from not getting everything they need to function properly.

A complete evidence-based understanding of all the nutritional and lifestyle factors that can shift the metabolism to and away from cancer is the final objective of this book series. An evidence-based protocol for alternative cancer treatment is all that stands between us and a world without cancer.

If you've made it this far in the series, it's clear that you are willing to 'carry your own cross' and take responsibility for your thoughts and for your existence. The path of seeking truth, of caring about the world around you and wanting to make a difference can be a difficult path to walk, but those willing to do so will be rewarded with health and the knowledge and power to change the world.

In the final book of this series, an evidence-based anti-cancer nutritional, exercise and medicinal protocol will be presented so that all the most effective healing strategies can be combined in a bulk approach to safely and effectively prevent and heal cancer.

ABOUT THE AUTHOR

MARK SLOAN has written over 300 articles and is the author of *The Cancer Industry, Cancer: The Metabolic Disease Unravelled* and the 6x international #1 bestseller *Red Light Therapy: Miracle Medicine.* Mark lives in Ontario, Canada and his goal is to build his home from scratch, entirely off grid and live a self-sufficient, resilient and responsible life as God had intended. Mark is passionate about learning and his ultimate goal in life is to reduce the suffering in this world and to make a better place for every human being alive and for future generations.

PLEASE REVIEW THIS!

I hope you enjoyed this book and that it has given you the confidence you need to make your own health decisions. Above all, I hope it gives you hope for a brighter future.

If this book helped or entertained you in any way, all I ask in return is that you take a moment to write an honest, sincere review of this book on Amazon. It will only take a few minutes, and it will help me out more than you can imagine.

Made in the USA
Monee, IL
20 May 2024

58711164R00193